DISEASES OF FEMALES.

THE

HOMŒOPATHIC TREATMENT

OF THE

Diseases of Females,

AND

INFANTS AT THE BREAST.

BY

DR. G. H. G. JAHR.

TRANSLATED FROM THE FRENCH BY

CHARLES J. HEMPEL, M. D.

Fellow, and Corresponding Member of the Homœopathic College of Pennsylvania, Honorary Member of the London Hahnemannian Society, etc., etc., etc.

NEW YORK:
PUBLISHED BY WM. RADDE, 300 BROADWAY.

PHILADELPHIA:
RADEMACHER & SHEEK, 239 ARCH STREET.
1856.

KING & BAIRD, PRS., SANSOM ST. PHILAD'A.

EDITOR'S PREFACE.

THIS work has enjoyed such a distinguished reception in Europe by all classes of Homœopathic practitioners, that we felt confident a translation of the work into the English language would be hailed with satisfaction by our American Homœopathic brethren. The work being very complete in the original, we have not deemed it necessary to encumber it with notes of our own. We have confined ourselves to supplying a few omissions concerning doses, principally for the benefit of lay practitioners and professional beginners: we have no doubt that all intelligent friends of our art will derive pleasure and profit from a perusal of this work to whose pages all who are in need of the instruction afforded by them, may refer with perfect safety and reliance in every curable case of female disease.

CHARLES J. HEMPEL.

Philadelphia, August, 1856.

PREFACE.

THIS new work is composed after the same plan and according to the same principles as our Treatise on Nervous Diseases. We have especially endeavored to place in the hands of our readers a complete Materia Medica of the affections of the uterine system, such as the limits of our Homœopathic Manual did not allow us to offer. We have attempted to join it to the article on dysmenorrhœa in general, (§§ 5 to 10); and here the reader will likewise find a complete repertory of the symptoms exhibited by the female organs of generation and their functions, so that practitioners will find placed at their disposal, all the elements which the actual condition of our science offers for the successful treatment and the rapid cure of the numerous diseases to which woman is so frequently subject, and the treatment of which, with the means offered by the Old School, has always remained problematical.

A perusal of the Table of Contents, will show the reader that our plan embraces a complete list of all the diseases to which women are subject, both during the period of nursing, and at any other time, and we have even added some remarks concerning the cases required by new-born or nursing infants, whose lives are so intimately connected with that of the mother. Among these affections, and especially among the organic lesions peculiar to females, there are some, it is true, for which Homœopathy has done little or nothing, and for which we have consequently been unable to indicate any positive treatment based upon clinical experience; but being persuaded that all these diseases are no less accessible to internal treatment than many others which were formerly, before they had been successfully treated with Homœopathic remedies, supposed equally incapable of being removed by internal medicines, we have not omitted a single case without at least indicating the remedies which seemed to us to deserve in preference to others, the attention of the profession in regard to its treatment.

The usefulness of the pathological, symptomatological and diagnostic notes, with which we have accompanied each article of our Treatise on Nervous Affections, having been generally appreciated, we have enriched the present work with similar notes, and we have availed ourselves for this purpose not only of what the principal French authors, such as Velpeau, Desormeaux, Lisfranc, Chailly, Nouvre, Fabre, etc., have published on this subject, but likewise of what the most celebrated and recent authors in Germany have contributed to the study of these affections. However, since it is not the object of our work to present a nosographical treatise of these maladies, but only to furnish therapeutical indications, we have often been obliged, without however omitting any thing of the substance, to content ourselves with furnishing a general statement of the well established facts contained in the works which we have consulted.

Among the observations which have been addressed to us concerning some of our previous publications, we find complaints from various quarters that the dose of the medicine to be prescribed, has not been indicated. In the present work, we have furnished here and there a few indications in reference to this matter, but rather with a view of preventing the employment of too large doses, than for the purpose of furnishing general rules which are to be followed blindly. It is impossible to indicate the dose in every single case; one must not have the least idea of the practice of medicine in order to imagine that every affection, notwithstanding its greater or less degree of intensity, has its particular doses which cure all the varieties and forms thereof, no matter how or under what circumstances. Nothing varies more than the doses, and it is more particularly in the administration of the medicines that the practitioner ought to be the sole judge of what is required to be done. He who does not feel competent to assume this responsibility, had better never meddle with the practice of medicine, for there is no treatise extant on this subject, that will give him all the light he desires. On the other hand, it must be conceded that works like the present, sometimes fall into the hands of new converts, who have as yet little knowledge of homœopathic medication, or of the principles of our art in general, and who nevertheless feel anxious to use the remedies which are here recommended for various diseases. We advise all such beginners to read elementary works where the principles of Homœopathy are taught, such as S. Hahnemann's Organon, or our own Elements of Homœopathy. In these works they will find every thing that they require to know concerning doses, and they will likewise obtain a knowledge of the general rules, which they may afterwards apply to all particular cases.

G. H. G. JAHR.

Paris, September, 1855.

TABLE OF CONTENTS.

ARTICLE VII.

ARTICLE VIII.

ARTICLE IX.

ARTICLE X.

ARTICLE XI.

ARTICLE XII.

ARTICLE XIII.

SECOND SECTION.

ARTICLE I.

ARTICLE II.

ARTICLE III.

ARTICLE XIV.

ARTICLE II.

ARTICLE III.

HOMŒOPATHIC TREATMENT

OF

DISEASES OF FEMALES.

FIRST SECTION.

FUNCTIONAL LESIONS AND NERVOUS AFFECTIONS OF THE UTERINE SYSTEM.

SECTION 1.

WE have divided this work in three sections: the first contains *functional and nervous derangements peculiar to females;* the second, *organic lesions* of the uterus and the other sexual organs: the third, affections of females from the period of conception, to the end of the nursing period. (1) In this first section, we intend to treat successively; 1st, of dysmenorrhœa or retarded and painful menstruation; 2d, of menstrual colic; 3d, of the various menstrual irregularities; 4th, of amenorrhœa or menstrual suppression; 5th, of anæmia of young girls at the age of pubescence; 6th, of the derangements peculiar to the climacteric period; 7th, of irregularities of the menstrual blood; 8th, of metrorrhagia; 9th, of leucorrhœa; 10th, of hysteralgia; 11th, of nymphomania; 12th, of chlorosis.

(1) For the study and the treatment of the diseases of children, we refer our readers to F. Hartmann's treatise, entitled, "Homœopathic Treatment of the Diseases of Children," translated by Charles J. Hempel, M. D., for sale by W. Radde, 322 Broadway, New York, and Rademacher & Sheek, 239 Arch street, Philadelphia.

Having treated of hysteria elsewhere in a detailed manner, we shall content ourselves with referring the reader to that work. (1)

ARTICLE I.

DYSMENORRHŒA IN GENERAL.

SECTION 2.

General Characteristics.—By dysmenorrhœa, we not only understand *painful menstruation* accompanied by more or less extensive derangements of the nervous system, but also any abnormal secretion of blood, both as regards quantity and quality. Dysmenorrhœa being distinguished from amenorrhœa and menorrhagia only by a greater or less degree of intensity, it will be readily perceived that all that can be said of the causes, the essential and accessory symptoms, the characteristic signs and the treatment as amenorrhœa and menorrhagia, likewise applies to a certain extent to the various forms of dysmenorrhœa. This is the reason why we will give here all the details applicable to all possible menstrual disorders; this will permit us to use more brevity in describing the other forms, and simply to add that which is peculiar to each variety. We may distinguish dysmenorrhœa into three distinct forms, namely: 1st, *excessive or profuse menstruation*, known by the term *menorrhagia;* 2d, *scanty menstruation*, known under the name of *menoschesia;* 3d, *painful menstruation*, or dysmenorrhœa, properly speaking. It is, however, of very rare occurrence in practice, to find the various forms of dysmenorrhœa as perfectly distinct as they are here drawn on paper; difficult menstruation is almost always an accompaniment of menorrhagia and menoschesia; and, on the other hand, when the catamenia are painful, they are generally either too profuse or insufficient. Moreover, inasmuch as *menorrhagia* has almost always the same symptoms and

(1) Homœopathic Treatment of Nervous and Mental Diseases; translated by Charles J. Hempel, M. D., and for sale by W. Radde, 322 Broadway, New York, and Rademacher & Sheek, 239 Arch street, Philadelphia.

results from the same causes as *metrorrhagia;* and inasmuch as *menoschesia* is, in these respects, nearly related to *amenorrhœa*, we prefer arraying the remarks we may have to offer concerning these irregularities, under the heads of *metrorrhagia* and *amenorrhœa*, and we shall confine ourselves here to *dysmenorrhœa*, properly speaking, whether characterised by a too profuse or too scanty discharge of the menstrual fluid. In most cases the menstrual secretion is difficult, and painful menstruation is too scanty; sometimes the blood is discharged only in drops, in small quantity, and with remarkable slowness; but even if the quantity is sufficient, the flow is always preceded by more or less acute pains, especially by nervous colic, which is known by the name of menstrual colic. These colics are often accompanied by various nervous and other accessory symptoms, such as lassitude in the extremities, shiverings, pains in the lumbar regions, headache, vertigo, nose-bleed, oppression, labored breathing, cough, hæmoptysis, gastralgia, nausea, vomiting, weeping, hysteria, chlorosis. If the discharge of blood is too scanty, the head feels heavy; the face is alternately red and pale; there is rising of heat to the face; violent but transitory palpitation of the heart; quick, full and vibratory pulse; vicarious hæmorrhages from the nose, bladder, bronchial tubes, or from ulcers and other cutaneous lesions; sense of weight at the epigastric region; uterine colicky pains; labor-pains in the small of the back, and sub-acute irritation of the uterus. If the blood flows too profusely, the nervous and accessory symptoms which exist previous to the appearance of the menses, generally cease in proportion as the menstrual discharge increases; in such cases, the flow may continue pretty profusely for several days without causing a loss of strength or the least appearance of illness in the looks of the patient.

Section 3.

Causes, course and *diagnostic signs.*—Among the predisposing causes of dysmenorrhœa, authors generally mention onanism, venereal infection, amorous excesses, or else the contrary of these, strict abstemiousness; but in many cases it is undoubtedly induced by a nervous constitution, an impoverished state of the blood, a sickly condition of the system, or general debility resulting from some former sickness. Sometimes it sets in in consequence of some sudden emotion, fright, fear, chagrin, wrath, &c.; other causes are, an improper mode of life, deficient exercise, insalubrity of the air, and the like. As regards the *proximate cause*, it is almost always difficult to determine it; in some cases the irregularity has been attributed to chronic inflammations of the uterus, or to scirrhous and tuberculous degenerations of this organ; but in most cases, there is nothing unusual in the patient's constitution to which the disease could positively be traced. As regards the course and termination of this disease, scanty dysmenorrhœa generally ends in complete suppression of the menses, with all the consequences incidental to such a condition; profuse dysmenorrhœa frequently degenerates in metrorrhagia; and if the menses are succeeded by leucorrhœa, they frequently change to this latter secretion entirely. In difficult menstruation, if the tension and swelling of the uterus are of long duration, chronic inflammation or schirrus of the uterus may supervene. In some cases scanty menses are accompanied by vicarious discharges of blood, such as nose-bleed, bloody expectorations from the chest, vomiting of blood, piles, hæmaturia, hæmorrhage from the eyes and mouth, discharge of blood from sores, ulcers, or bloody sweat; also, in particular localities only. As regards the *diagnostic signs*, scanty dysmenorrhœa might sometimes be confounded with superficial metritis, which affection sometimes accompanies dysmenorrhœa, either as the cause or effect of the disease; but all doubt as to the precise character of the disease is easily removed by a knowledge of the origin and causes of the existing symptoms. The uterine cramps which precede miscarriage, are sometimes confounded with difficult menstruation; but the discharge of the water which would soon supervene in a case of miscarriage, would indicate the precise nature of the flow. Hæmorrhoidal colic can scarcely be mistaken for menstrual colic, since the former affection is never accompanied by the nervous symptoms that are always present in the latter; the absence of all morbid signs in the uterine region would of course preclude the possibility of establishing a wrong diagnosis.

Section 4.

Treatment; what is to be done during the flow.—Nothing is more difficult than the treatment of menstrual disorders, unless the patient is willing to assist the physician by observing a careful diet and avoiding every thing that might tend to keep up the irregularity. Frequent walking, muscular exercise, all sorts of amusements, absence of all violent and especially unpleasant emotions, such as chagrin, vexations, etc., are indispensable requisites to a restoration of the menstrual functions to their normal standard. As regards therapeutic means, we have a sufficient number in homœopathy, each of which, if used in season, may be able to effect a perfect cure. We have to observe, however, that in habitual dysmenorrhœa, which generally results from constitutional causes, the accidental treatment has to be distinguished from the constitutional. The former aims at quieting for the time time being the distressing symptoms inherent in difficult menstruation; whereas the latter, or the radical treatment, endeavors to prevent the return of these symptoms, and to restore the regularity of the menstrual discharges. In this paragraph we will first point out the principal means of the immediate or accidental treatment, and in the subsequent paragraphs, we will furnish a complete list of the remedies that have a tendency to regulate the menstrual secretions; at the close of the article we will furnish an expose of the leading symptoms by which the respective remedies are indicated. The most useful medicines which may have to be used for accidents that may occur during the menstrual flow, are, in general, *Belladonna*, *Bryonia*, *Calcarea*, *Chamomilla*,

Cocculus, Coffea, Graphites, Ignatia, Nux vomica; among these remedies the most efficacious are,

a. For MENSTRUAL COLIC: *Belladonna, Chamomilla, Coffea, Nux vomica, Veratrum.* (Compare Sections 11—14.)

b. For UTERINE CRAMPS: 1. *Coffea, Pulsatila, Secale.* 2. *Cocculus, Cuprum, Ignatia.* 3. *Chamomilla, Veratrum.*

c. For TOO EARLY MENSES: 1. *Calcarea, Chamomilla, Ipecacuanha, Nux vomica.* 2. *Ignatia, Platina.* (Compare Section 16.)

d. For LATE MENSES: 1. *Cuprum, Kali, Pulsatilla, Sulphur.* 2. *Lachesis, Phosphorus.* (Compare Section 19.)

e. TOO LONG: 1. *Cuprum, Nux vomica, Platina.* 2. *China, Ignatia.* 3. *Aconite, Sulphur.* (Compare Section 18.)

f. TOO PROFUSE: 1. *Belladonna, Calcarea, Ipecacuanha, Nux vomica.* 2. *Chamomilla, Ignatia, Sulphur.* (Compare Section 17.)

g. TOO SCANTY: 1. *Kali, Pulsatilla, Sulphur.* 2. *Cocculus, Lachesia.* 3. *Aconite, Cuprum,* 4. *Bryonia, Chamomilla, Nux vomica, Veratrum.* (Compare Section 20.)

h. TOO SHORT: 1. *Pulsatilla, Sulphur.* 2. *Phosphorus.* 3. *Lachesis.* 4. *Platina.* 5. *Bryonia, Kali, Nux vomica.* (Compare Section 21.)

For the details concerning the selection of these remedies, we refer the reader to the following paragraphs:

SECTION 5.

Radical treatment; principal remedies.—After having indicated, in the preceding paragraph, the principal remedies for most important symptoms which sometimes supervene in the course of an irregular menstrual flow, we will now furnish a list of all the remedies which correspond to menstrual irregularities, and likewise give all possible indications for their rational use, both in the treatment of the accidental symptoms as well as the germs of the disease. The principal remedies for menstrual irregularities in general are: 1. *Calcarea, Graphites, Kali, Kreosotum, Lachesis. Lycopodium,*

Magnesia carb., *Natrum mur.*, *Nux vom.*, *Phosphorus*, *Platina*, *Pulsatilla*, *Sepia*, *Sulphur.* The following remedies will be found particularly efficacious:

CALCAREA, for the following symptoms: *Premature menses*, three or four days too soon, or *too copious. Previous to the catamenia:* lascivious dreams, headache, swelling and sensitiveness of the breasts, leucorrhœa, nervous prostration, and tendency to start; nocturnal shivering, and pains in the bowels. *During the catamenia:* rush of blood to the head, with heat in the head; pressure at the vertex; nocturnal agglutination of the lids, with lachrymation in the day-time, heaviness of the head, and dizziness; tearing and boring headache, worse during a change in the weather, and after a sudden and keen emotion; excoriation; pain in the throat and at the uvula, when swallowing; *toothache*, boring in the decayed teeth; inclination to vomit, and ineffectual desire to go to stool; vomiting and nausea; crampy pains in the small of the back, with griping pains; asthmatic oppression; drawing, with pressure and shooting pains in the abdomen, with restlessness even unto fainting; contractive pinching in the abdomen when the secretion of blood is interrupted; involuntary discharge of urine during emotion. *After the catamenia:* drawing and shooting in the teeth, day and night, worse by inclining the head to the right or left, and preventing sleep. *Mucous leucorrhœa, resembling milk*, also with itching of the parts; itching of the parts, with shootings, heat, excoriation, pain, and smarting; inflammation, redness and swelling of the vulva; eruption on the parts; dampness and smarting between the parts and the thighs; pressure in the vulva; shooting in the os tincæ; sensation of pleasure in the parts. *Symptoms of chlorosis.—Polypi in the uterus.*

GRAPHITES.—The menses return tardily, and are too scanty, do not last long enough, with discharge of a thick and black blood; uterine cramps, cutting pains, pressive headache, nausea, pains in the chest, bronchial or nasal catarrh; great weakness, rheumatic pains in the extremities, œdematous swelling of the feet and legs, *herpetic eruptions*, toothache, with rheumatic pain in the cheek, heaviness in the abdomen, dulness of the head, heaviness in the arms and legs, pains in the sides, pressure and heat in the bowels, fatiguing cough. *Previous to the menses:* itching in the parts; cutting pains at the commencement of the menses. *During the menses: violent headache*, especially in the evening, with eructations and nausea; nausea in the morning, with weakness and trembling in the day-time; pain in the epigastrium, as if everything would be torn; bearing-down pains in the abdomen, with pain in the back and sides, eructations, pricking pain in the teeth, and soreness of the parts and between the thighs; hoarseness, coryza, with fever; dry cough, with profuse perspiration; swelling of the feet and catarrhal affection of the cheek; painfulness of the varices; obscuration of sight, with deadness of the hands and formication in the anus and lips: pains in the extremities; discharge of blood from the anus; cramps in the abdomen; colic; pains in the chest; weakness; the ulcers get worse. *After the menses:* shiverings, cutting, griping pains, diarrhœa; *leucorrhœa*, especially before or after the menses, resembling water or white mucus, with weakness in the back and loins, or with tension of the bowels; leucorrhœa, day and night: *bearing-down on the parts*, especially when standing; smarting in the vagina; prickings and vesicles at the labia; itching at the vulva, especially before the menses, with pimples; *soreness of the parts and between the thighs*, with pimples, blotches, and ulcers; swelling and hardness of one of the ovaries.

KALI CARBONICUM.—The menses are either *too scanty* and *too late*, or else *too copious*, *too early*, and *last too long*, with weariness, desire to sleep, colic, and toothache; the menstrual blood is acrid, fetid, and excoriating. *Before the menses:* in the morning, on waking, pleasurable sensation, as during an embrace; a good deal of heat, with frequent thirst, and restless sleep; frequent shivering, with trembling of the limbs, crampy sensation in the abdomen, sour eructations, rheumatic swelling of the cheek, with prickings, and swelling of the gums. *During the menses:* headache in the morning, with heaviness of the head; nausea after eating, with sense of fulness and vomiting; colic, with foul taste in the mouth; rumbling, lassitude, and drowsiness; wind in the bowels, with foul taste in the mouth, and bitter, bilious eructations; griping colic, with pressure on the parts, as if everything would be pressed out; constipation; painful sensation of weight in the loins; *nasal catarrh*, with colic, toothache, pains in the back, stitches in the ears, restless sleep, and anxious dreams; violent startings in the whole body; dozing at night, with anxious reveries, and dizziness on waking. *After the menses:* nocturnal gastralgia, with sense of coldness in the back and stomach; yellowish, mucous leucorrhœa, with itching and smarting at the parts; erythematous soreness, itching and titillation of the parts, with smarting and gnawing pimples; tearing on the parts extending up to the chest; pricking in the labia majora; stitches through the vulva; pricking or excoriation; pain in the vagina during an embrace; aversion to an embrace, or excessive sexual irritation.

KREASOTUM.—The menses are *too early*, *too copious*, and *last too long*, with discharge of dark-colored and coagulated blood, or with violent colic, and discharge of clear and watery blood. *Before the menses:* hard bearing; regurgitation of a whitish and tasteless froth, or watery vomiting; considerable distention of the abdomen; colic, with cramp, pains at the navel; followed by whitish leucorrhœa; restless and nervous excitement. *During the menses:* buzzing in the head, with pressure from within outwards, worse by stooping; hard hearing; flatulence that smells like rotten eggs; retention of stool and wind, with discharge of coagulated blood after the discharge of flatulence; frequent shivering; stitch in the side of the chest, with cutting pains above the navel; profuse sweat on the back and chest; report in the abdomen, followed by diarrhœa. *After the menses:* violent abdominal cramps, especially in the groin; pressure on the parts, as if the menses would reappear; contractive pains in the vagina, followed by leucorrhœa; discharge of a fetid, acrid, bloody serum, with gnawing, tickling and itching of the parts; frequent and violent distress after too copious and long-lasting catamenia; whitish or acrid leucorrhœa, with itching and gnawing at the parts; serous leucorrhœa, having a foul smell; discharge of bloody mucus from the vagina; leucorrhœa, with debility; cramp-pains in the external parts; stitches passing from the abdomen through the vagina, like electric shocks; frequent itching in the vagina, with smarting, heat, excoriating pain on urinating, *swelling, heat and hardness of the labia;* frequent prolapsus of the womb; ulcerative pain at the neck of the uterus, during an embrace; and indurations at the neck; sexual desire more active in the matin; burning in the parts, during an embrace; after an embrace, the menses appear, with profuse discharge of a dark blood, and followed by a grayish leucorrhœa, with swelling, burning pain, and gnawing itching of the parts.

LACHESIS.—The menses are *too scanty, too short and late*, with hæmorrhoidal pains, nose-bleed, bloody stool, constipation, with burning pain and pressure in the bowels, toothache, leucorrhœa, and many other sufferings, *especially at the critical age*, or after the fruitless exhibition of *Sepia. Before the menses:* headache with vertigo, nose-bleed; gastralgia with pressure, spasms in the chest and eructations; nervous distress; leucorrhœa; urine with mucous sediment; colic with sense of malaise. *During the menses:* Tearing in the abdomen; beating in the head; violent pains at times in the loins, at others in the bowels, or lameness in the hips; pushing pain from the loins to the private parts; violent cramps in the bowels, as if cut with knives; viscous and acrid blood. *Leucorrhœa*, especially previous to the menses, profuse, smarting, mucous, staining the linen greenish and stiffening it, with scanty and short menses. Pain in the parts as if swollen, with inability to bear contact, and obliging her to keep her thighs apart: cramps that seem to extend up to the chest; *swelling of the parts and cramps in the uterus*, with sexual excitement, thrill, tickling from the thighs to the genital organs, and circular contraction from the uterus to the right side of the abdomen and chest, with heat, uneasiness, tickling under the skin from the anus to the sides and between the shoulder-blades. Is often indispensable in dysmenorrhœa *at the critical period*, especially when *Belladonna* or *Sepia* have proved inefficient.

LYCOPODIUM.—The menses are too short or too late, or else too profuse and too early, reappearing every six or eight days; the menses become suppressed by the least fright. *Before the menses:* distention of the abdomen; heaviness in the limbs; cold feet; *shivering*, sometimes violent and long-lasting, with general malaise; fever after midnight, with restlessness and shivering followed by heat in the face; *great sadness, melancholy*, peevish and timorous mood; weeping and nonsense, as if she would lose her reason; dilatation of the pupils. *During the menses:* violent itching in the vulva, not allowing her any rest, with swelling of the parts; contractive pain in the temples, as if the forehead would fly in pieces; dull headache; acidity in the mouth, with coated tongue; nausea; pain in the sides, in the morning on rising, hindering motion; swelling of the feet; lassitude; fainting turn at church, while standing, with loss of sight and hearing, heat in the head, pale face, has to sit down, dizziness followed by tightness of the head. *After the menses:* stitches in the head. *Leucorrhœa*, coming off by fits and starts, milky or serous (at full-moon); the leucorrhœa is preceded by cutting colic in the hypogastrium. Pricking in the parts; violent burning in the vagina during and after an embrace; *bearing-down in the groin as if the menses would appear; obstinate dryness of the vagina;* itching, burning and gnawing at the vulva; pressure from within outwards, above the pubis, when stooping; stitches in the labia when lying down; wind passes out of the vagina.

MAGNESIA CARBONICA.—The menses are *too early*, with toothache, pain in the sides, or bearing-down pain in the groin; the blood is profuse, thick and black; *profuse* and *long* catamenia, with colic; retarded catamenia, with coagula and preceded by sore throat; the menstrual discharge is more copious at night than in the day-time; the discharge is more copious when walking or standing. The menstrual blood is dark, black, thick, sticky. *Before the menses:* canine hunger and stomachache; nausea and frequent eructations; *pain in the side*, with laming and aching pains, bearing-down and contraction; colic with pressure on the parts. *At the commencement of the menses:* coryza with stoppage of the nose. *During the menses:* diarrhœic stools, with trembling of the limbs; peevish mood; *headache with heaviness of the head* and a good deal of heat; bruised pain at the vertex; tearing in the head and nape of the neck; pulling in the forehead as far as the occiput, with heaviness of the head; agglutination of the eyelids, in the morning; the eyes are dull, dry and burning; burning rhagades at the lobe of the ear; pale face; insipid taste in the mouth, with anorexia; ptyalism; nausea and desire to vomit; violent colic; cutting pain at the navel, eased by emitting wind; violent pressure in the hypogastrium, interrupting sleep, night and morning; frequent sneezing; *drawing pain* in the sides, eased by stooping and worse when stretching one's-self; luxation pain in the right shoulder; pain in the knees, when walking, as if broken; painful sensitiveness of the feet, even in bed; itching at the neck and shoulders; *lassitude*, sometimes with sweat or drowsiness; frequent waking in the night; chilliness and shivering; shivering at night, on waking or when uncovering one's-self. *After the menses:* pain in the sides as if broken, towards evening; leucorrhœa. Watery, acrid, or else slimy and whitish leucorrhœa, with pinching round the navel or preceded by crampy-colic. Frequent itching at the parts.

Natrum muriaticum.—1. The menses are *too scanty, late and short*, with tightness of the head and determination of blood to the head, or pain in the bowels as if raw; *tendency of the menses to become suppressed*, especially in young girls at the age of pubescence; 2, the menses are *too early*, with scanty discharge and headache when coughing, sneezing or stooping as if the forehead would split; this remedy seems especially to agree when the menses are too early, with scanty or profuse discharge; 3, *the menses are more copious*, the blood being black and flowing day and night, sometimes with shivering and frequent yawning; 4, the menses last *too long*. *Before the menses:* attacks of anxiety, *melancholy* irascible mood; headache; qualmishness, with sweetish taste rising to the throat, and bloody saliva. *During the menses:* sadness, anxiety and fainting, with cold cheeks and internal heat; headache; heat in the face, in the evening; lancinating and tearing toothache in the open air; heaviness in the abdomen; crampy colic in the hypogastrium; burning and cutting in the groin, when urinating and during a meal, in a sitting posture; hard stool; violent fever at night, with burning thirst and complete loss of sleep. *After the menses:* tightness and heaviness of the head as from rush of blood; aversion to sexual intercourse, with dryness and soreness of the vagina during an embrace. Profuse, thick, whitish and transparent leucorrhœa, or else acrid, itching, smarting, greenish, with contraction in the abdomen or pressure on the parts, yellowish face, mucous diarrhœa with headache and colic. Bearing-down pressure towards the parts, as if prolapses would come on; *itching at the vulva;* pimples at the pubes; falling off of the hair. Aversion to sexual intercourse; after it, irritable and irascible mood.

Nux Vomica.—The menses are *too early* and last *too long*, preceded by drawing pain in the posterior cervical muscles. *During the menses*, nausea with fainting, especially in the morning; lassitude, with goose-flesh and rheumatic pains in extremities; debility, after every stool, also in the afternoon; with headache and chattering of teeth, followed by internal heat and dryness of the lips; *restlessness*, *irritable* and *quarrelsome mood;* congestion with vertigo and pressive headache; headache as if the eyes would start out of their sockets, with weakness and fever; headache, as if the brain were ulcerated, worse when lying; formication in the fauces, in the evening, in bed; nausea with shivering and lassitude; pressure in the side of the abdomen, from within, outwards; distention of the abdomen, as if it would burst; *crampy colic*, with shivering, lassitude and nausea; *uterine cramps*, with pressure in the hypogastrium, as far as the thighs; *constipation*, with ineffectual urging to stool; frequent and ineffectual urging to urinate; *pain in the sides as if lamed and bruised;* hæmorrhoidal pains; tearing and rheumatic pains in the arms and thighs. Fetid leucorrhœa, tinging the linen yellow. Frequent, digging, contractive and clawing uterine cramps, with more copious discharge of coagula; pressure with pushing towards the parts, especially in the morning in bed, or during a walk in the open air, with contraction in the hypogastrium; *congestion of blood towards the uterus;* irritation of the uterus, with heaviness, burning heat, stitches and pressure; *prolapsus of the womb;* hardness and swelling of the os tincæ; *swelling of the vagina*, like prolapsus, with burning and inability to bear contact; burning in the parts, with sexual exaltation; itching and gnawing eruption at the vulva.

PHOSPHORUS.—1. The menses are *too early*, *too copious* and *last too long*, with colic and pain in the sides; discharge of blood between the menstrual periods. 2. The menses are *too scanty*, preceded by leucorrhœa, or accompanied by colic, with cutting pains, as if caused by knives, weeping mood and vomiting of bile mixed with mucus and food. 3. The menses are *retarded*, but in this case *too copious*, with debility, rings around the eyes, loss of flesh and anxiety. Leucorrhœa in the place of the menses. *Before the menses:* bleeding of the ulcers; *leucorrhœa*, with weeping mood and frequent desire to urinate; catarrhal affection of the cheek and *swelling of the gums*. *During the menses:* lameness of the limbs; weakness and weariness, with pain in the back, palpitation, anxiety, pain in the stomach and violent nausea, obliging her to lie down; pricking, itching over the whole body; frequent shiverings, with coldness of the hands and feet; *fever in the afternoon*, with chattering of the teeth, followed by heat and headache; tightness of the head, with prostration and drowsiness; *lancinating headache* in the forehead, with desire to remain in bed; vertigo, when walking; violent toothache, commencing during a meal; violent nausea, obliging her to lie down; nausea when raising herself in bed, with sour vomiting, oppression, cold sweat on the forehead and vertigo when walking; contractive gastralgia and pinching in the stomach; *violent colic; pains as if cut with knives*, with pain in the back and vomiting; *fermentation in the abdomen;* violent pains in the back, as if lamed and bruised, with jerking in the body, anxiety, pains in the stomach, great weakness and nausea; *blood spitting, palpitation of the heart;* crampy contraction of the limbs. *After the menses:* weakness, with rings around the eyes, and anxiety; swelling of the gums or cheek. Milky, mucous or *acrid, smarting, corrosive* and *blistering leucorrhœa;* reddish leucorrhœa. *Stitches through the pelvis*, from the vagina to the uterus; tearing pain in the parts, as if caused by an ulcer; stinging and burning blotches at the border of the labia. *Aversion to sexual intercourse.*

PLATINA.—The menses are *too early, too copious* and last *too long*, with discharge of a black and viscous blood, and preceded or followed by leucorrhœa. *Before the menses:* labor pains; cramps at the commencement of the menses. *During the menses:* paroxysms of anxiety, with restlessness and tears; sleeplessness at night; suspicious moods, headache, frequent attacks of vertigo; *cramp colic*, with pressure above the vulva; sensitiveness of the parts, with pressure downwards; pressure in the hypogastrium, with ill-humor; *colic;* pulling in the groin; *constipation* or hard stool; frequent urging to urinate; short breath. *After the menses:* weakness or leucorrhœa. Albuminous *leucorrhœa*, coming off sometimes after urinating, and at other times after rising from a chair. *Pains in the abdomen as if the menses would come on*, with pulling in the groin and hypogastrium, or with cutting pains and pulling in the head; *pressure on the parts*, through the groin, towards the sacrum, with urging to stool; *congestion of blood to the uterus;* painful sensitiveness and pressure at the pubes and in the parts, with internal chilliness and shiverings; in the evening, in bed, the painful pressure downwards ceases, but comes on again as soon as she gets up in the morning. *Hardness of the womb;* cramps and stitches in the hardened part of the womb. *Excessive sexual desire, like nymphomania; voluptuous titillation in the genitals* and lower abdomen, with anxious oppression, palpitation of the heart; pressure in the parts, general weariness and stitches in the forepart of the head. *Polypi of the uterus.*

PULSATILLA.—*Retarded menses*, especially among young girls at the age of pubescence, or among women at the critical period, with *cramp-colic, chilliness, desire to vomit*, and other distresses; the menses *flow only in the day-time;* the menstrual blood is *thick, viscous, black and coagulated*, or else pale and watery. *Before the menses*, goose flesh, with pale face, yawning and stretching; weeping mood, sadness, *melancholy* or anxiety; *vertigo*, with eructation; megrim; mucus on the stomach; *nausea* and desire to vomit; *sour or mucous vomiting;* gastralgia; *pains in the liver; spasmodic colic; pains in the bowels, with vomiting;* heaviness in the abdomen like a stone; pressure on the rectum as if she had to go to stool; frequent urging to urinate, or to go to stool; *leucorrhœa; pain in the sides. During the menses: shivering, with pale face;* nervousness; headache on one side; obscuration of sight, worse in a warm room; *gastralgia;* nocturnal nausea, with mucus on the stomach; cramp-colic, with heat; pressure in the abdomen and loins as from a stone, with ineffectual urging to stool, and tendency of the limbs to go to sleep, when sitting; stitches in the chest when breathing; stitch in the side when moving the arm or drawing breath, also when laughing, almost laming the arm; pain in the side, removed by drawing breath. *Milky, thick, mucous and whitish*, or else *watery, burning, acrid leucorrhœa*, with swelling of the vulva; leucorrhœa before or after the menses, with colic. *Tractive tension* in the hypogastrium, like labor-pains; contractive pains in the left side of the uterus, obliging her to bend double; pulling pressure in the lower part of the womb in the morning, with drowsiness; *uterine cramps* like labor-pains; incisive pains at the os tincæ; irritation on the chest: burning stitches in the vagina and labia.

Sepia.—The menses are *too early* and *too copious*, with stiffness of the limbs, leucorrhœa, cramp-colic and pressure above the parts, headache, toothache and melancholy. Menstrual irregularities at the critical age. *Before the menses:* goose flesh all over, the whole day; violent colic, with fainting; pressure in the abdomen, followed by soreness at the perinæum and swelling of the vulva; sensation as if the vulva were dilated; burning at the vulva; smarting leucorrhœa, with soreness of the vulva. *During the menses:* prostration in the morning; *lameness and soreness* in the extremities; has to lie down in consequence of great uneasiness in the body, with pulling in the limbs and abdomen, borborygmis, palpitation of the heart, and embarrassed perspiration; great weakness in the evening, with obscuration of sight; sleeplessness at night, on account of a tearing pain in the back, with shivering and heat, thirst and painful contraction in the chest; *melancholy mood* in the morning; violent frontal headache, with discharge of hard and fetid mucus from the nose; nose-bleed, for three days; toothache, with throbbing in the gums; pulling in the teeth, as far as the cheek which swells; *crampy colic*, with pressure downwards; tearing in the tibia. *Acrid*, *corrosive*, *yellowish*, *watery* and *milky* leucorrhœa, or else reddish-green, fetid, bloody or purulent, with stitches in the uterus, itching in the vagina or vulva, distention and weight of the abdomen; a good deal of pain when walking, pulling in the hypogastrium, or burning and soreness between the thighs. Pains or painful rigidity in the region of the uterus; *pressure downwards,* as if every thing would issue through the vulva, with oppression, cutting colic and jelly-like leucorrhœa; *prolapsus of the vagina or uterus;* hardness of the neck of the uterus; heat in the parts and on the outside; swelling and humid itching and eruption at the labia minora; *redness and excoriation* of the parts and between the thighs; itching of the parts and in the vagina; stitches in the vagina as far as the navel; contractive pain in the vagina.—*Tendency to miscarriage.*

SULPHUR.—Retarded menses, with a good deal of distress, oppression, constipation and distention of the abdomen; *premature menses*, either too profuse or too scanty, with colic and pains in the sides; menses too profuse, the blood smelling sour, it is thick, black, acrid and excoriates the parts; the menses last too long: the *menstrual blood is too pale. Before the menses:* restlessness and uneasiness; headache; stinging toothache in a bad tooth in the morning; pyrosis; cramp under the left hypochondrium; itching at the vulva; leucorrhœa; cough in the evening, in bed, obliging her to leave her bed, after which the cough ceases; fulness on the chest, obliging her to draw a long breath. *During the menses: epileptiform convulsions*, with violent pains in the lower part of the bowels, shiverings, coldness of the forehead and hands, and distortion of the mouth; drowsiness in the day-time; rush of blood to the head; frontal headache; nose-bleed; pressure at the pit of the stomach; violent cramp-colic in the hypogastrium, with cutting pains, pinching, contraction, shivering in the whole body, and pain in the sides; pain in the epigastrium as if all the bowels were drawn up by strings in a ball, so that she is neither able to walk nor to lie down; *violent pains* in the loins and bowels, eased by exercise and by a more profuse discharge of menstrual blood. *After the menses:* itching at the nose for several days; leucorrhœa, nose-bleed. *Acrid, smarting, excoriating leucorrhœa*, or burning and watery, yellowish or slimy, with cutting or pinching pains in the bowels. Feeling of weakness in the parts; pressure on the parts; congestion of blood to the uterus; itching at the vulva and in the vagina, with or without pimples; painless vesicles at the vulva; *burning* at the vulva and in the vagina, not permitting her to remain seated; inflammation of one of the labia, with burning when urinating; excoriated spots at the vulva and perinæum; violent itching of the clitoris; sense of soreness in the vagina during an embrace.—*Tendency to miscarriage.*

Section 6.

Remedies of the Second Class.—Beside the above-mentioned remedies, the following will likewise be found more or less indicated by the symptoms: *Alumina*, *Ammonium*, *Belladonna*, *Carbo vegetabilis*, *Causticum*, *Chamomilla*, *China*, *Cocculus*, *Conium*, *Iodium*, *Magnesia muriatica*, *Mercurius*, *Natrum*, *Nitri acidum*, *Sabina*, *Silicia*, *Sulphuris acidum*, *Zincum*, more particularly:

Alumina, for the following symptoms: The menses are *too scanty* and *too pale*, or else too soon and too short; retarded menses also too short, only a discharge of a little colored water; the menses are too early and too profuse, preceded by colic. *Before the menses:* restless sleep, full of dreams, waking with a headache, heat in the face, excitement in the circulation, palpitation of the heart; colic at stool, with pinching, pressure and labor-pains; profuse leucorrhœa, with trembling, weariness and sensation as if the bowels would fall through the vulva. *During the menses:* headache when the discharge stops; fluent coryza, with pain at the forehead and nose; distension of the abdomen, with profuse discharge; colic with lassitude; diarrhœa with colic; frequent urination, with acrid and excoriating urine; leucorrhœa. *After the menses:* prostration of body and mind, with lowness of spirits, and weariness after working or walking ever so little; leucorrhœa. *Leucorrhœa, acrid, profuse*, like flesh-water, or *transparent mucus*, stiffening the linen, or *yellowish*, with itching at the vulva, burning and soreness. Stitch at the vulva, up to the chest; throbbing in the left side of the vagina as if there were an abscess.

Ammonium.—The menses are *too early;* or too feeble and short; *profuse menses*, especially at night, when sitting or riding in a carriage, with loss of appetite, colic; retarded menses. The menstrual blood is black, coagulated, with cramp-colic, hard and difficult stool; acrid blood, with burning and soreness of the parts; pale blood. *Before the menses:* pale face, colic and pain in the sides. *During the menses:*

prostration of the body, especially the thighs, with yawning, pain in the sides, toothache and chilliness; pale face; *toothache;* violent coryza; *violent colic*, with pressure, tension and crackling between the shoulder blades; tearing in the abdomen; pressure downwards, with cutting colic, tearing in the back and parts, and desire to remain in bed. Watery discharge from the vagina. *Acrid*, profuse, corrosive leucorrhœa, or else watery and burning. *Swelling*, *itching and burning of the vulva;* soreness of the parts and anus, with much pain when urinating,

Belladonna.—The menses are *too profuse*, too early, or else retarded, and *too pale.* Discharge of blood between the menses. The menstrual blood is fetid, bright-red, coagulated. *Before the menses:* weariness, blur before the eyes, annorexia and colic. *During the menses:* tearing pains in the limbs, at times in the back, at others in the arms; *rush of blood to the head*, with throbbing pain, heat in the head, red and puffed face, especially among full-blooded young females; anguish about the heart, violent thirst; colic, with pressure, as if everything would pass through the vulva, with weight in the bowels, like a stone; *pains in the sides*, and cramp-pains in the back; nocturnal sweat on the chest, with frequent yawning, shiverings over the back, and colic; leucorrhœa, with colic: stitches in the inner privates; dryness of the vagina: prolapsus and hardness of the uterus.

Carbo vegetabilis.—The menses are *too soon* and *too copious*, or too feeble and pale; retarded menses, with acrid, corrosive, thick and strong-smelling blood. *Before the menses:* violent itching, tetter; itching eruption at the back of the neck and between the shoulder-blades; headache; drawing pain from the hypogastrium to the sides: colic from morning till evening; *leucorrhœa* and smarting at the vulva. *During the menses:* headache, with contraction of the eyes; toothache; vomiting; colic, especially when the blood ceases to flow, with pains in the back and lameness in all the bones; burning in the hands, and soles of the feet; whitish, mucous, thick, yellowish, or milky leucorrhœa, or greenish, profuse and excoriating; discharge of bloody mucus from the vagina; *itching at the vulva and anus;* heat and redness in the vulva; *burning*, *excoriation*, and *swelling of the parts;* aphthæ at the vulva; red, sore spots, resembling little ulcers, with itching and leucorrhœa.

Causticum.—Retarded menses; or else too early and profuse; the menses are *too feeble*, do not flow at night; the menstrual blood smells badly, and causes an itching of the parts. *Before the menses:* dark melancholy; pains in the sides and anxious dreams; drawing colic. *During the menses:* weariness and ill-humor; vertigo, especially when stooping; *yellow complexion;* colic, as if the bowels would be torn, with lameness in the loins, and discharge of coagulated blood; cutting pains, with tearing in the back and loins, especially during emotion; diarrhœa, with cutting pains; *pain in the back;* stitch under the left breast; *leucorrhœa* at night, or very profuse and smelling like the menses; leucorrhœa, preceded by cramp-pains, with much flatulence; burning in the parts; soreness of the parts and between the thighs; *aversion to an embrace.*

Chamomilla.—Menses *too copious* and *early*, with *dark and coagulated blood*, and followed by distress; retarded menses, with anasarca, swelling of the bowels, labor-pains, and bloating of the pit of the stomach, with hard, aching pains in the præcordia. *Before the menses:* cramp pains, with pulling in the thighs; peevishness, with quarrelsome and capricious mood at the commencement of the menses. *During the menses:* fainting, with thirst, cold limbs, pale and hollow face; nausea, eructations, and desire to vomit, with yellowish tongue and bitter mouth; *crampy colic*, and *acute pains in the sides; labor-pains;* squeezing and pressing in the uterus; greenish or watery diarrhœa; tearing in the veins of the legs. *After the menses:* violent colic, with sensitiveness of the abdomen to contact, as if the parts within were ulcerated; *yellowish*, *smarting*, or watery and acrid leucorrhœa; *pressure on the parts*, like labor-pains, with frequent urging to urinate; burning, smarting in the vagina.

China.—Menses *too profuse,* like metrorrhagia, with black coagula, uterine cramps, cutting colic, and frequent urging to urinate, fainting, and convulsions; retarded menses. *Before the menses:* painful pressure on the groin and anus, with leucorrhœa. *During the menses:* convulsions, with abdominal cramps, and spasm of the chest; rush of blood to the head, with throbbing of the carotids, puffed face, protruded and weeping eyes, twitching of the eyelids, and loss of consciousness; serous or *bloody* leucorrhœa, with discharge of a fetid or purulent substance, painful itching, and crampy contractions in the inner parts; *congestion of blood to the womb,* with sense of fulness and painful pressure on the parts, especially when walking.

Cocculus.—The menses are *too early,* with *crampy colic;* the menses are *too feeble,* only a few doses being discharged; *the blood is black and coagulated,* with leucorrhœa between the bloody discharges, or with fainting and pressive colic; instead of the menses, a serous leucorrhœa, mixed with blood and pus; *retarded menses, preceded by cramp-colic,* flatulence, paralytic weakness, spasms in the chest, convulsions, nausea, unto fainting. *During the menses: distention of the abdomen,* with contractive colic, and contractions in the rectum; hard pressure in the abdomen, as from acute stones, with pain, as from an internal sore, when touching the abdomen. *After the menses:* hæmorrhoidal distress; *uterine cramps* from the least menstrual irregularity.

Conium.—The menses are *too slow,* with drawing pains down to the sacrum, day and night; the menses are *too early, too feeble;* discharge of a brownish blood in the place of the menses. *Before the menses:* tired feeling in the limbs, restlessness, weeping mood, anxiety about every trifle; dry heat in the body, without thirst; anxious dreams; stitches in the hepatic region, especially at night, when lying and drawing breath; pains in the sides. *During the menses: crampy colic,* very painful; pressure on the parts, and pulling in the thighs; contractive pain in the hypogastrium, disappearing during a walk in the open air; *acrid, smarting, ex-*

coriating leucorrhœa; thick or whitish, milky, preceded or accompanied by colic, or followed by lassitude or hoarseness, with loose cough; *itching at the vulva and in the vagina; pressure downwards* in the womb; stitches in the parts, especially in the labia and vagina; incisive pain between the labia when urinating; large pimple at the pubes, painful to contact; *uterine cramps*, with digging, pinching, smarting, distention, and stitches up to the left side of the chest.

IODIUM.—*Retarded menses*, with vertigo and beating of the heart; *profuse menses*, like flooding, especially at stool, accompanied by cutting colic, with pain in the sides and back. *Before the menses;* a good deal of distress; mounting of heat to the head, with palpitation of the heart, tension about the neck, which swells. *During the menses;* distress, weakness, pains in the sides. *After the menses;* beating of the heart; obstinate, excoriating leucorrhœa; cramp colic like labor-pain, violent pressure in the hypogastrium, towards the parts, hardness of the uterus.

MAGNESIA MURIATICA.—*Menses too copious* and *too soon*, with black coagula; retarded menses, with pains in the sides, pressure on the groin, and frequent yawning. *Before the menses:* leucorrhœa, nervous excitement. *During the menses:* weariness unto fainting, with lameness of the limbs and wakefulness in the evening, in bed; frequent yawning; pains in the sides and thighs; profuse leucorrhœa, watery or thick, especially after stool and urinating; *leucorrhœa*, preceded by cramp-colic. Discharge of blood previous to the menses. *Uterine cramps*, with pains extending to the thighs, and followed by leucorrhœa; schirrous indurations at the uterus.

MERCURIUS.—*Profuse menses*, with colic; suppressed menses; discharge of blood between the menses. *Before the menses:* dry heat, excited circulation and rush of blood to the head; itching of the labia. *During the menses:* anxiety which leaves one no rest; scorbutic affection, with red tongue or covered with red spots, burning, salt taste, teeth on edge and pale gums. Mild and whitish leucorrhœa, or else smarting, purulent, gnawing, or greenish, burning, with nightly itching in the parts; discharge of mucous and purulent flocks from the vagina. *Itching pimples* and *nodes at the labia;* swelling of the labia, with heat, hardness, shining redness, sensitiveness to the least contact, burning, throbbing and stinging; inflammatory swelling of the vagina, with redness and excoriation; falling of the vagina.

NATRUM CARBONICUM.—Menses too late, like serum, and scanty; menses too soon, profuse, and too long, like flooding. *Before the menses:* hardness, with stiffness of the nape of the neck; cutting pains in the hypogastrium. *During the menses:* tearing and stitches here and there; chattering of the teeth in the evening; tearing and throbbing headache; nausea and loathing, with prostration; painful distention of the abdomen, with diarrhœa, which affords ease; pains in the sides; lameness and tearing in the right hip. Putrid or thick yellowish leucorrhœa, especially when urinating or afterwards; leucorrhœa preceded by cutting pain; discharge of mucus from the vagina, after coit. Tearing in the parts; movements in the womb as from a fetus; malformation of the os tincæ; soreness of the parts, and between the thighs; pressure on the parts as if everything would fall out.

NITRI ACIDUM.—Menses *too profuse, too soon*, or too late, with colic and headache; suppressed menses. *Before the menses:* lameness of the limbs; colic; headache; cramp-colic in the hypogastrium and pains in the sides, at the commencement of the menses. *During the menses:* weakness, so that she is unable to breathe, and has to lie down; burning of the eyes; headache; swelling of the gums; pressure in the hepatic region; distention of the bowels; *cramp-colic*, as if the hypogastrium would burst, with eructation and constant desire to move about; pressure on the abdomen and pains in the sides; violent labor-pains, with pressure in the hypogastrium as far as the vagina; *pressure downwards* in the hypogastrium, with pains in the sides and pulling in the thighs and legs; contraction in the abdomen towards the parts; *palpitation*, with anguish, heat, and trembling of the limbs. *After the menses:* leucorrhœa. Profuse, mucous, flesh-colored, greenish, brownish, fetid or foul leucorrhœa. *Itching and soreness* at the vulva; irritation and inflammation of the labia; *stitches in the vagina;* dry burning at the parts; swelling of one side of the vagina and labia, with burning itching.

SABINA.—Menses *too profuse* and *too early*, with coagula or discharge of bright red blood, *violent colic*, labor-pains, scanty and red urine, dysuria and stranguria, opening of the mouth of the womb, discharge of a mucous liquid from the vagina; flow of blood during motion; menses last *too long*. Suppressed menses, in their stead leucorrhœa. *Milky*, yellowish, sanious, foul leucorrhœa, or like pitch, or flesh-colored, or with itching of the parts. Tendency to miscarriage. Excited sexual desire. Drawing pains in the lumbar vertebræ, like labor-pains; contractive uterine cramps; *heavy pressure* in the hypogastrium, as if the menses would appear; violent stitches deep in the vagina.

SILICEA.—The menses are *too soon*, or *too profuse*, or too scanty; strong smell of the menstrual blood. *Before the menses;* headache above the eyes; obstinate constipation; *diarrhœa;* icy coldness in the whole body at the commencement of the flow. *During the menses;* melancholy and anxiety in the præcordial region, with thoughts of suicide; everything *looks pale;* burning and soreness at the vulva, with eruption on the inside of the thighs; *colic;* nocturnal pulling between the shoulder-blades, she has to bend backwards. *After the menses;* bloody and mucous discharge from the vagina. Smarting, acrid, corrosive, or serous and milky leucorrhœa; leucorrhœa preceded by pinching at the navel. *Itching at the vulva;* labor-pains in the vagina, nausea during coit.

SULPHURIS ACIDUM.—Retarded menses, with colic and pains in the sides; menses *too copious*, *too early*, and *too long*. *Before the menses;* nightmare-like choking. *During the menses;* thirst, stitches in the abdomen and vagina. *After the menses; sexual excitement*, or aversion to intercourse. Transparent, milky, acrid and burning, or gnawing leucorrhœa; bloody mucous from the vagina. Excessive sexual desire, with little enjoyment during coit; lascivious dreams, with emission; violent desire for an embrace on waking in the morning, as if in the clitoris.

ZINCUM.—Retarded menses; *profuse menses*, especially at night and when walking, with coagula. *Before the menses:* lassitude, especially in the hands and feet; chilliness; irascible and weeping mood; anxiety; headache in the evening, like a weight in the forehead, drawing the head back; opthalmia; sudden oppression in the stomach; *distention of the abdomen;* burning when urinating; itching and stinging of the parts, with sense of swelling; leucorrhœa; heaviness in the legs, and pulling about the knees. *After the menses:* discharge of bloody mucous from the vagina. *Mucous, thick* leucorrhœa, preceded by colic, yawning, or after stool. Sexual desire; desire for self-gratification; pressure on the parts and rectum; varices at the feet.

SECTION 7.

Remedies that are less frequently indicated.—If none of the abovementioned remedies should be indicated, we may sometimes find a suitable remedy among the following: 3. *Aconitum, Ambra, Ammonium muriaticum, Arsenicum, Baryta, Berberis, Borax, Bovista, Bryonia, Cantharis, Carbo animalis, Ferrum, Hepar, Hyoscyamus, Ignatia, Moschus, Nitrum, Petroleum, Rhus toxicodendron, Ruta, Sarsaparilla, Secale, Stannum, Staphysagria, Stramonium, Thuja, Veratrum.*

ACONITUM.—*Profuse menses*, especially among plethoric females, young girls, like flooding; *suppression* occasioned by fright, or retarded menses among lively girls of a sanguineous temperament and leading a sedentary life. *Furor* at the commencement of the menses. Profuse, yellowish and sticky leucorrhœa.

AGNUS.—Retarded menses, with drawing colic; leucorrhœa, sterility.

AMBRA.—*Menses too early:* discharge of blood between the menses. *During the menses:* varices at the left leg, bluish and painful on pressure. Thick leucorrhœa at night, with stinging in the vagina, discharge of bluish and whitish mucus. Burning in the parts, with discharge of a few drops of blood after walking or hard stool; sore pain and *violent itching* of the parts; swelling and soreness of the labia.

AMMONIUM MURIATICUM.—*Menses too early,* with colic, during which the flow is more profuse. *During the menses:* vomiting and diarrhœa; *pressure* and *contraction* in the back and abdomen; pain in the back; tearing in the feet. Albuminous, or bluish and slimy leucorrhœa, with pinching about the navel.

ARSENICUM.—Menses *too profuse* and *too early;* suppressed menses, with pain at the coccyx and in the shoulders. *During the menses:* distress, cutting colic, stitches from the pit of the stomach to the hypogastrium, eructations, sighs, weeping. *After the menses:* discharge of bloody mucus. Stitches from the hypogastrium to the vagina; sexual desire with involuntary emission. *Acrid, corrosive,* thick, yellowish leucorrhœa; or coming off in drops, with flatulence from the vagina.

BARYRA.—Menses too scanty and short, or too profuse and early. *Before the menses:* toothache, leucorrhœa. *During the menses:* colic with pinching and cutting; lameness in the loins. Bloody leucorrhœa, with anxious palpitation, fainting weakness. Tearing in the vulva, by fits and starts; aversion to coit.

BERBERIS.—Menses *too feeble, long, watery,* grayish or slimy. *Before the menses:* pains in the limbs. *During the menses:* prostration, peevish mood, loathing of life; fainting; shiverings; headache; painful distension of the abdomen; stitch in the left side as far as the vagina; pains in the kidneys; burning at the anus; smarting in the vagina; stitches in the chest; *violent pains in the sacrum and loins,* as if bruised; tension in the nape of the neck, shoulders and arms; pain in the hip-bones; pressure in the thighs and legs.

After the menses: weariness, stinging and tearing headache. Suppressed sexual desire, with stitches in the parts during coit; *the vagina is sensitive to contact;* smarting and burning, with excoriation pain in the vagina as far the labia; pricking in the perinæum.

BORAX.—Menses *too soon* and *too profuse*, like flooding. *Before the menses:* heaviness on the chest, morning and evening, buzzing in the ears. *During the menses:* lassitude, pulsative headache and buzzing in the ears; colic from the stomach to the sides low down, with desire to vomit; crampy pressure in the groin. *After the menses:* gastralgia, with heaviness from the right hypochondrium to the shoulder blade, cramp pain in the sides, leucorrhœa. White, albuminous, thick or corrosive leucorrhœa. Stitches in the womb; pricking at the clitoris, at night.

BOVISTA.—Menses *too scanty* or retarded, watery. *Before the menses:* diarrhœa. *During the menses:* lassitude, headache, toothache, colic, soreness at the groin. *After the menses:* leucorrhœa. *Thick, viscous, albuminous* leucorrhœa of a yellowish-green color, acrid, corrosive.

BRYONIA.—*Suppressed menses*, with nose-bleed; menses *too early*; *too profuse*, like blooding, with dark blood, headache, pains in the sides. *During the menses:* rheumatic pains in the limbs; frequent shivering; *congestion of the blood to the head*, with nose-bleed; burning gastralgia; pressure and, fulness at the epigastrium; *constipation;* leucorrhœa; congestion of the chest with hacking cough.

CANTHARIS.—The menses are *too early* and *too copious*, with black blood; retarded menses. *Before the menses:* burning at urinating; urine with white sediment. *After the menses:* discharge of bloody mucus. Burning in the vulva; violent itching in the vagina; pressure towards the parts; *swelling of the neck of the uterus*, with burning in the bladder, colic, continual vomiting and febrile heat. Inflammation of the ovaria.

CARBO ANIMALIS.—The menses are *too early*, with pains in the sides, groin, and with headache; delaying menses.

Before the menses: heat with anxiety; headache; weakness in the thighs. *During the menses:* weariness which incapacitates her from speaking, with yawning and stretching; distention of the abdomen; *pressure in the groin*, sides and thighs, with ineffectual attempts to raise wind, with shivering and yawning. Burning, smarting, or watery leucorrhœa, or staining the linen yellow.

COFFEA.—The menses are *too copious*, with excessive sexual desire, voluptuous itching, and profuse mucous secretion; extremely distressing *menstrual colic*, so painful that they drive her to despair.

FERRUM.—Menses *too late* and *scanty*, with watery and pale blood; menses *too profuse*, like flooding, with excited circulation, heat in the face, black coagula, and labor-pains in the abdomen and sides. *Before the menses:* stinging headache, with ringing in the ears; rumbling in the abdomen, with discharge of long pieces of mucus from the vagina. *During the menses:* violent cutting pains, with watery blood. Milky, smarting and corrosive leucorrhœa. Sensitiveness of the vagina during an embrace; falling of the vagina.

HEPAR.—Menses too late or too scanty; discharge of blood between the menses. *Before the menses:* contractive headache; distention of the abdomen. *During the menses:* itching of the vulva. Smarting leucorrhœa at the vulva. Soreness at the vulva and between the thighs.

HYOSCYAMUS.—Menses too late or too early, or *profuse-like flooding*, with bright-red blood, delirious talk, cramp-pains. *Before the menses:* hysteric convulsions; almost constant and loud laughter; labor-pains in the abdomen, with pulling in the back and sides; headache, with nausea and sweat, at the commencement of the menses. *During the menses:* nonsense; *convulsive trembling* of the hands and feet; *profuse urine* and sweat. Excited sexual desire; soreness and burning at the entrance of the vagina.

IGNATIA.—The menses are *too early* and *too copious;* coagulated menstrual blood; the menses are scanty and smell foul. *During ths menses:* uterine cramps; contractive colic, with headache; heaviness and heat in the head, photophobia, anguish, palpitation of the heart, and lassitude unto fainting. Uterine cramps, with cutting pains, or pressive and contractive pains, like labor-pains, with embarrassed breathing, or followed by leucorrhœa.

IPECACUANHA.—The menses are *too copious* and *too early, like flooding*, with bright-red coagula. Pressure towards the parts and anus.

KALI JODATUM.—The menses are too feeble, or cease entirely. *Before the menses:* frequent urging to urinate. *During the menses*: uterine cramps and painful colic, with violent squeezing pain down to the thighs; frequent yawning; restlessness; chilliness, with goose-flesh; uneasiness and heat in the head; eructations; rumbling; nausea; pressure at the stomach; desire to vomit; shuddering over the face and hands. Clear, watery, corrosive, smarting leucorrhœa.

MOSCHUS.—The menses are *too early* and *too copious.* Violent drawing pains at the commencement of the menses. *Pulling and pressure on the parts, like labor-pains. Violent sexual desires.*

NITRUM.—The menses are too early, too copious, too long, with black and coagulated blood. *During the menses:* thirst, water-brash, *colic*, with pain in the sides and thighs; burning in the right groin when bending forward while sitting; weariness and pain in the limbs, with staggering gait. Light-colored, white leucorrhœa, stiffening the linen, with lameness of the small of the back.

NUX MOSCHATA.—The menses are too late, preceded by pains in the small of the back, headache, weariness, pressure at the stomach, water-brash, pain in the liver, thick, dark blood. Menses too late, with pressure in the abdomen and pulling in the limbs.

PETROLEUM.—The menses are too *early* and *scanty;* the menses are too late, with acrid blood and itching. *During the menses:* weariness and lameness all over; heat in the palms of the hands and soles of the feet; ringing and buzzing in the ears; tearing in the thighs; the limbs are sensitive to contact, here and there. *Albuminous* leucorrhœa, with lascivious dreams. Aversion to coit; itching in the urethra, when urinating; soreness at the vulva and between the thighs; burning in the parts, with discharge of blood.

PHOSPHORI ACIDUM.—Suppressed menses. *During the menses:* hepatic pains. *After the menses:* yellowish leucorrhœa, with itching. Tympanitic distension of the womb.

PRUNUS SPINOSA.—The menses are too early and too copious, like flooding, with light-colored and watery blood, and pains in the sides; daily discharge of blood from the vagina, between the menses. Weakening leucorrhœa, staining the linen yellow and excoriating the parts. Painless throbbing in the parts; tickling in the region of the ovaries.

RHUS TOXICODENDRON.—The menses are *too copious* and *too early*, with acrid blood, causing an itching of the parts, or with coagula and labor-pains. Drawing labor-pains in the womb; stitches in the vagina; excoriation-pains in the parts.

RUTA.—Menses *too soon*, *too copious*, or to scanty and short, followed by leucorrhœa. Corrosive leucorrhœa, after the menses.

SARSAPARILLA.—Retarded menses, with frequent urging to urinate; menses too scanty, with acrid and burning blood. *Before the menses:* itching and humid eruption on the forehead; soreness in the right groin, and urging to urinate, at the commencement of the courses. *During the menses:* colic, with pinching in the abdomen; griping in the pit of the stomach, down to the sacrum. Watery leucorrhœa, especially when walking.

SECALE.—Menses *too profuse* and *too long*, like flooding, with violent cramps, tingling in the legs, and great weakness; black, liquid blood, which is discharged only during a walk. Leucorrhœa. Tendency to miscarriage. Swelling and wens at the neck of the uterus; distention of the uterus; chronic metritis.

STANNUM.—Menses too profuse. *Before the menses:* anguish, gloom; pain at the malar bones, as from a blow.

Transparent, mucous, yellowish leucorrhœa. Pressure in the hypogastrium, as if the menses would appear; uterine cramps; prolapsus of the vagina during hard stool.

STAPHYSAGRIA.—Suppression. Painful sensitiveness of the parts, especially when sitting; cramp-pain in the parts, and in the vagina; itching of the vulva; blotch on one of the labia majora, itching and sore when touched.

STRAMONIUM.—*Menses like flooding*, with coagula; the menstrual blood is watery; black blood between the menses. *During the menses:* the body smells of semen; loquacious mood; drawing in the abdomen, thighs and limbs. *After the menses:* sighs and moans; erysipelas of the left cheek.

TARTARUS.—*Profuse* and *premature menses:* watery blood. Viscous leucorrhœa, white, slimy. Nettle-rash at the vulva.

THUYA.—Menses scanty. Leucorrhœa. Mucous discharge from the urethra. Burning, itching and stinging in the parts, especially when walking; crampy pain down to the hypogastrium, especially on rising; pressure and contraction when sitting; *swelling of the labia*, with burning pain when walking and touching the parts; whitish ulcer at one of the labia, with excoriation, pain when touching it; wen at the neck of the uterus.

VERATRUM.—*Menses premature and profuse. Before the menses:* nose-bleed; pimples on the labia; vertigo in the day-time, with sweat at night. Diarrhœa, with nausea and shiverings at the commencement of the menses. *During the menses:* tearing headache, with desire to vomit; buzzing in the ears; pains in all the limbs, with much thirst. *After the menses:* Gritting the teeth and bluish color of the face.

SECTION 8.

Indications derived from the nature of the menses.—In conformity with what we have stated in Section 4, we now furnish a general list of all the remedies that have reference to menstrual irregularities, in order to place before the eyes of the practitioner every thing that may serve him as a guide in the selection of a remedial agent, in case the usual remedies should not avail.

MENSES TOO COPIOUS:—1. *Belladonna, Calcarea, Chamomilla, Ferrum, Ipecacuanha, Nux vomica, Platina, Sabina, Secale, Stramonium.*

2. *Arsenicum, Bryonia, Cantharides, Carbo vegetabilis, Coffea, Crocus, Hyoscyamus, Ignatia, Magnes australis, Mercurius, Natrum muriat., Nitric acid, Nux moschata, Phosphorus, Sepia, Sulphur, Sulphuric acid.*

3. *Chelidonium, Cina, Kreosote, Lycopodium, Moschus, Ruta, Sambucus, Silicea.*

4. *Aconitum, Agaricus, Ambra, Ammonium muriaticum, Antimonium, Borax, Bovista, Carbo animalis, Causticum, Cyclamen, Hepar, Iodium, Laurocerasus, Ledum, Magnesia muriat., Muriatic acid, Natrum, Nitrum, Phosphoric acid, Pulsatilla, Rhus, Selenium, Stannum, Veratrum.*

5. *Ammoniacum, Arnica, Baryta, Cannabis, Capsicum, Clematis, Cocculus, Colocynthis, Cuprum, Dulcamara, Magnesia carb., Mezereum, Opoponax, Plumbum, Rhododendron, Sabadilla, Spongia, Strontian, Zincum.*

MENSES TOO LONG:—1. *Aconitum, Chininum, Ignatia, Lycopodium, Natrum muriaticum, Nux vomica, Platina, Secale, Silicea, Sulphur.*

2. *Baryta, Bryonia, Calcarea, Cantharides, Coffea, Crocus, Cuprum, Ferrum, Kreosotum, Magnes australis, Mercurius, Phosphorus, Rhus, Sabina, Sepia.*

3. *Arsenicum, Asarum, Belladonna. Causticum, Chelidonium, Dulcamara, Kali, Laurocerasus, Stramonium.*

4. *Agaricus, Belladonna, Borax, Bovista, Cina, Hyoscyamas, Ledum, Magnesia carbonica, Natrum, Nitrum, Sabadilla, Stannum, Sulphuric acid, Zincum.*

MENSES PREMATURE:—1. *Ambra, Belladonna, Calcarea, Carbo vegetabilis, Chamomilla, Ignatia, Ipecacuanha, Natrum muriaticum, Nux vomica, Phosphorus, Rhus, Sabina.*

2. *Ammoniacum, Ammonium muriaticum, Asarum, Bovista, Cantharides, Cina, Cocculus, Colchicum, Crocus, Kali, Kreosotum, Laurocerasus, Magnes australis, Manganum, Platina, Secale, Sepia, Sulphuric acid.*

3. *Alumina, Arnica, Asarum, Belladonna, Borax, Bryonia, Carbo animalis, China, Colocynthis, Hepar, Iodium, Lachesis, Ledum, Magnesia muriatic, Muriatic acid, Natrum, Nitrum, Nitric acid, Nux moschata, Phosphoric acid, Plumbum, Pulsatilla, Ruta, Silicea, Spongia, Stannum, Sulphur.*

4. *Aconitum, Arsenicum, Baryta, Cannabis, Causticum, Clematis, Coffea, Conium, Digitalis, Dulcamara, Ferrum, Graphites, Helleborus, Hyoscyamus, Lycopodium, Magnesia carbonica, Mezereum, Natrum muriaticum, Petroleum, Pulsatilla, Rhododendron, Ruta, Spigelia, Staphysagria, Stramonium, Strontiana.*

MENSES RETARDED, DELAYING:—1. *Causticum, Cuprum, Dulcamara, Graphites, Kali, Lycopodium, Magnesia carbonica, Natrum muriaticum, Pulsatilla, Sepia, Silicea, Sulphur.*

2. *Lachesis, Phosphorus.*

3. *Aconitum, Agnus, Chelidonium, Cocculus, Drosera, Ferrum, Mercurius, Petroleum, Sabina, Valeriana, Zincum.*

4. *Ammoniacum, Aurum, Bryonia, Calcarea, Cicuta, Crocus, Digitalis, Hyoscyamus, Magnes arcticus, Magnesia muriatica, Sabadilla, Sarsaparilla, Staphysagria, Stramonium, Strontiana, Veratrum.*

5. *Arnica, Arsenicum, Belladonna, Borax, Bovista,*

Cantharis, Carbo animalis, Chamomilla, China, Colchicum, Colocynthis, Helleborus, Hepar, Ignatia, Iodium, Natrum, Nitric acid, Nux moschata, Nux vomica, Phosphoric acid., Rhododendron, Rhus, Ruta, Secale, Spigelia, Sulphuris acidum.

MENSES TOO SCANTY :—1. *Ammoniacum, Conchæ, Dulcamara, Graphites, Kali, Lachesis, Magnesia carbonica, Pulsatilla, Sulphur.*

2. *Baryta, Cocculus, Natrum muriaticum, Phosphorus.*

3. *Aconitum, Alumina, Causticum, Cuprum, Lycopodium, Magnes arcticus, Mercurius, Ruta, Sabadilla, Sarsaparilla, Sepia, Silicea, Staphysagria.*

4. *Bryonia, Carbo vegetabilis, Cicuta, Colchicum, Digitalis, Drosera, Euphrasia, Ferrum, Guajacum, Ignatia, Magnesia muriatic, Manganum, Nux vomica, Petroleum, Thuya, Valeriana, Veratrum, Zincum.*

5. *Agnus, Arnica, Asarum, Aurum, Bovista, Calcarea, Carbo animalis, Chelidonium, Crocus, Hepar, Hyoscyamus, Iodium, Ipecacuanha, Moschus, Platina, Rhododendron, Rhus, Sabina, Stramonium, Strontiana.*

MENSES TOO SHORT :—1. *Ammoniacum, Pulsatilla, Sulphur.*

1. *Ammoniacum, Pulsatilla, Sulphur.*

2. *Bryonia, Dulcamara, Phosphorus.*

3. *Conium, Graphites, Lachesis, Mercurius.*

4. *Alumina, Euphrasia, Magnesia carbonica, Natrum muriaticum, Platina, Ruta, Sabadilla.*

5. *Baryta, Bovista, Carbo animalis, Colchicum, Iodium, Ipecacuanha, Kali, Lycopodium, Magnes arcticus, Magnesia muriatica, Manganum, Moschus, Nux vomica, Rhododendron, Sarsaparilla, Silicea.*

MENSES SUPPRESSED, (MENOSTASIA):—1. *Pulsatilla*, *Sepia*, *Sulphur*.

2. *Bryonia*, *Conium*, *Dulcamara*, *Graphites*, *Kali*, *Lycopodium*, *Silicea*.

3. *Aconitum*, *Ammoniacum*, *Baryta*, *Calcarea*, *Causticum*, *Chamomilla*, *Cocculus*, *Cuprum*, *Ferrum*, *Natrum muriaticum*, *Phosphorus*, *Sabadilla*, *Staphysagria*, *Valeriana*.

4. *Agnus*, *Alumina*, *Arsenicum*, *Belladonna*, *Borax*, *Colocynthis*, *Crocus*, *Hyoscyamus*, *Ignatia*, *Lachesis*, *Magnesia carbonica*, *Magnesia muriatic.*, *Mercurius*, *Rhododendron*, *Ruta*, *Sarsaparilla*, *Veratrum*, *Zincum*.

5. *Arnica*, *Aurum*, *Carbo animalis*, *Carbo vegetabilis*, *Chelidonium*, *China*, *Colchicum*, *Digitalis*, *Drosera*, *Euphrasia*, *Guajacum*, *Helleborus*, *Iodium*, *Magnesia arcticulus*, *Manganum*, *Nitric acid*, *Nux moschata*, *Petroleum*, *Phosphoric acid*, *Platina*, *Rhus*, *Secale*, *Strontiana*, *Thuya*.

MENSTRUAL BLOOD:—

ACRID, burning, corrosive, excoriating:—1. *Kali*, *Silicea*.

2. *Bovista*, *Graphites*, *Sarsaparilla*, *Sepia*.

3. *Ammoniacum*, *Arsenicum*, *Cantharis*, *Nitrum*.

4. *Baryta*, *Carbo vegetabilis*, *Hepar*, *Rhus*, *Sulphur*, *Sulphuric acid*, *Zincum*.

BROWN.—1. *Bryonia*.

2. *Carbo vegetabilis*.

3. *Calcarea*, *Rhus*.

4. *Conium*, *Pulsatilla*.

BLACK, dark:—1. *Chamomilla*, *Crocus*, *Nux vomica*, *Pulsatilla*.

2. *Ammoniacum*, *Antimonium*, *Kreosotum*, *Lachesis*, *Magnesia carbonica*, *Nitric acid*, *Sepia*.

4. *Arnica*, *Cantharis*, *Cuprum*, *Ignatia*, *Lycopodium*, *Nux moschata*, *Phosphoric acid*, *Platina*, *Selenium*, *Stramonium*.

5. *Aconitum, Carbo vegetabilis, Cocculus, Conium, Digitalis, Drosera, Ferrum, Graphites, Ledum, Magnesia muriatic, Nitrum, Phosphorus, Secale.*

COAGULATED:—1. *Chamomilla, Platina, Rhus.*

2. *Belladonna, China, Ferrum, Hyoscyamus, Ignatia, Ipecacuanha, Pulsatilla, Sabina, Stramonium.*

3. *Arnica, Cantharis, Causticum, Conium, Crocus, Magnesia muriatica, Mercurius, Nitric acid, Phosphoric acid, Strontiana.*

4. *Bryonia, Carbo animalis, Kreosotum, Nux vomica, Secale, Sepia.*

DARK, see black.

FOUL, badly and smelling:—1. *Belladonna, Bryonia.*

2. *Carbo animalis, Chamomilla, Crocus, Sabina.*

3. *Ignatia, Silicea, Sulphur.*

4. *Arsenicum, Carbo vegetabilis, Causticum, China, Kali, Mercurius, Phosphorus, Platina, Secale.*

PALE, watery:—1. *Belladonna, Dulcamara, Hyoscyamus, Sabina.*

2. *Carbo vegetabilis, Graphites, Pulsatilla, Sulphur.*

3. *Arnica, Calcarea, Ferrum, Ledum, Magnesia australis, Phosphorus, Rhus, Secale.*

4. *Antimonium, Bryonia, Drosera, Ipecacuanha, Laurocerasus, Lycopodium, Mercurius, Nitrum, Nitric acid, Platina. Sabadilla, Strontiana, Zincum.*

5. *Ammoniacum, Arsenicum, Borax, Bovista, Cantharis, Carbo animalis, China, Digitalis, Kreosotum, Magnesia muriatic, Nitrum, Nux moschata, Sepia, Silicea, Stramonium.*

SLIMY:—1. *Cocculus.*

2. *Pulsatilla, Sulphuris acidum.*

SOUR-smelling:—*Sulphur.*

THICK:—1. *Pulsatilla.*

2. *Crocus, Cuprum, Platina.*

3. *Arnica.*

4. *Carbo vegetabilis, Fluoricum acidum, Nitrum, Nux moschata, Sulphur.*

VISCID:—1. *Crocus.*

2. *Cuprum.*

3. *Secale.*

4. *Magnesia carbonica, Magnesia muriatica.*

WATERY, see pale.

SECTION 9.

Accompanying symptoms in menstrual irregularities.—The ailments which precede, accompany or follow the catamenia, being of the utmost importance to the proper selection of a remedy, we here furnish a detailed list of all the indications resulting from such symptoms.

a GENERAL MENSTRUAL AILMENTS.

AT THE PERIOD, in general:—1. *Bryonia, Calcarea carb., Cocculus, Graphites, Nux vom., Pulsatilla, Sepia, Sulphur.*

2. *Belladonna, Coffea, Ignatia, Platina, Secale, Veratrum.*

3. *Aconitum, Ammonium carb., Ammonium mur., Carbo vegetab., Causticum, Cuprum met., Kali carb., Kreosotum, Lachesis, Lycopodium, Magnesia carb., Magnesia mur., Mercurius viv., Natrum mur., Nux mosch., Petroleum, Silicea, Zincum met.*

4. *Baryta carb., Borax, Chamomilla, Chelidonium, Conium, Phosphoric acid., Sabina, Stramonium.*

BEFORE:—1. *Calcarea carb., Cuprum met., Lycopodium, Mercurius viv., Pulsatilla, Sepia, Sulphur, Veratrum.*

2. *Ammonium carb., Baryta carb., Carbo veget., Cocculus, Conium, Kreosotum, Natrum mur., Phosphorus, Phosphori acid., Platina.*

3. *Alumina*, *Asarum*, *Causticum*, *Chamomilla*, *Ferrum met.*, *Graphites*, *Hyoscyamus*, *Jodium*, *Kali carb.*, *Lachesis*, *Magnesia carb.*, *Manganum*, *Nux mosch.*, *Silicea*, *Stannum*.

4. *Ammonium mur.*, *Belladonna*, *Borax*, *Bovista*, *Bryonia*, *Cantharis*, *Carbo anim.*, *China*, *Cina*, *Coffea*, *Crocus*, *Dulcamara*, *Hepar*, *Ignatia*, *Ipecacuanha*, *Magnesia mur.*, *Mezereum*, *Moschus*, *Muriatic acid*, *Natrum carb.*, *Nitrum*, *Nux vomica*, *Petroleum*, *Rhus toxic.*, *Ruta*, *Sabadilla*, *Sarsaparilla*, *Spigelia*, *Spongia*, *Staphysayria*, *Sulphuric acid.*, *Valeriana*, *Zincum met.*

AT THE COMMENCEMENT:—1. *Hyoscyamus*.

2. *Aconitum*, *Causticum*, *Chamomilla*, *Lycopodium*, *Phosphorus*, *Platina*, *Pulsatilla*, *Sepia*.

3. *Bryonia*, *Coffea*, *Graphites*, *Jodium*, *Ipecacuanha*, *Magnesia carb.*, *Natrum muriat.*

4. *Asarum*, *Belladonna*, *Cocculus*, *Ignatia*, *Magnesia mur.*, *Mercurius vivus*, *Moschus*, *Nitric acid.*, *Ruta*, *Sarsaparilla*, *Silicea*, *Staphysagria*.

DURING:—1. *Ammonium carb.*, *Chamomilla*, *Graphites*, *Hyoscyamus*, *Kali carb.*, *Kreosotum*, *Pulsatilla*, *Sepia*.

2. *Ammonium muriat.*, *Calcarea carb.*, *Carbo veget.*, *Cocculus*, *Coffea*, *Conium*, *Ignatia*, *Lycopodium*, *Magnesia carb.*, *Magnesia mur.*, *Nux vomica*, *Phosphorus*, *Sulphur*.

3. *Belladonna*, *Borax*, *Bovista*, *Carbo anim.*, *Causticum*, *China*, *Cuprum met.*, *Lachesis*, *Natrum carb.*, *Sabina*, *Silicea*, *Veratrum*, *Zincum*.

4. *Aconitum*, *Alumina*, *Ambra*, *Arsenicum*, *Asarum*, *Baryta carb.*, *Bryonia*, *Cannabis*, *Cantharis*, *Capsicum*, *Chelidonium*, *Crocus*, *Ferrum met.*, *Hepar*, *Jodium*, *Laurocerasus*, *Mercurius viv.*, *Moschus*, *Muriatic acid.*, *Natrum mur.*, *Nitrum*, *Nitri acid.*, *Nux mosch.*, *Petroleum*, *Phosphoric acid.*, *Platina*, *Rhodo-*

dendron, Rhus tox., Sarsaparilla, Secale, Selenium, Spongia, Stannum, Stramonium, Strontiana, Sulphuris acid.

FOLLOWING:—1. *Borax, Graphites, Kreosotum, Nux vom.*

2. *Lycopodium, Natrum mur., Phosphorus, Phosphori acid., Platina, Stramonium.*

3. *Alumina, Calcarea carb., Conium, Kali carb., Magnesia carb., Mercurius viv., Ruta, Sepia.*

4. *Ammonium carb., Bovista, Bryonia, Cantharis, Carbo anim., Carbo veget., China, Cuprum met., Jodium, Lachesis, Pulsatilla, Rhus tox., Silicea, Sulphur, Sulphuris acid., Veratrum.*

PARTICULAR AILMENTS AT THE MENSTRUAL PERIOD.

ABDOMEN DISTENDED:—*Alumina, Hepar, Kreosotum, Zincum.*

Before the menses:—*Kreosotum.*

During the menses:—1. *Zincum.*

2. *Alumina, Hepar.*

Affected with CRAMPS:—1. *Cocculus, Ignatia, Pulsatilla, Sulphur.*

2. *Chamomilla, Conium, Sepia.*

3. *Cuprum, China, Graphites, Nux vom., Platina.*

4. *Carbo veget., Hyoscyamus, Kali, Magnesia muriatica, Natrum muriaticum, Nitri acidum, Zincum.*

Before the menses:—1. *Chamomilla, Cocculus, Pulsatilla, Sulphur.*

2. *Carbo veget., Hyoscyamus, Kali.*

During the menses:—1. *Ignatia, Platina.*

2. *Cocculus, Conicum, China, Graphites, Pulsatilla, Sepia, Sulphur, Zincum.*

3. *Cuprum, Magnesia muriat., Natrum muriat., Nitric acid., Nux vom.*

PAIN in, colic:—1. *Belladonna, Calcarea, Chamomilla Cocculus, Nux vom., Pulsatilla, Sulphur.*

2. *Aconitum, Graphites, Ignatia, Phosphorus, Platina, Secale, Sepia, Veratrum.*

3. *Alumina, Ammonium, Ammonium muriat., Baryta, China, Conium, Crocus, Cuprum, Lachesis, Silicea, Zincum.*

4. *Carbo veg., Causticum, Kreosotum, Laurocerasus, Lycopodium, Magnesia carbon., Mercurius, Nitrum, Natrum, Sarsaparilla, Stannum, Stramonium, Sulphuric acid.*

Before the menses:—1. *Baryta, Belladonna, Calcarea, Chamomilla, Platina, Pulsatilla.*

2. *Alumina, Ammonium, Causticum, Graphites, Lachesis, Lycopodium, Nitrum, Phosphorus, Sepia.*

During the menses:—1. *Alumina, Ammonium, Belladonna, Calcarea, Chamomilla, Graphites, Lachesis, Phosphorus, Platina, Pulsatilla, Sepia.*

2. *Agnus, Ammonium muriat., China, Cocculus, Conium, Crocus, Ignatia, Nux vom., Secale, Silicea, Zincum.*

3. *Carbo veget., Causticum, Coffea, Kreosotum, Laurocerasus, Lycopodium, Magnesia carb., Mercurius, Natrum, Sarsaparilla, Stannum, Stramonium, Sulphur, Sulphuric acid.*

Following the menses:—*Lachesis, Pulsatilla, Veratrum.*

Heavy:—*Pulsatilla.*

Acid Mouth, during menses:— *Lycopodium.*

Anguish:—1. *Mercurius.*

2. *Cocculus, Stannum.*

3. *Belladonna, Ignatia, Phosphorus.*

Before the menses:—*Cocculus, Mercurius, Stannum.*
During the menses:—*Belladonna, Ignatia, Mercurius.*
Following the menses:—*Phosphorus.*

Appetite lost, before the menses:—*Belladonna.*

Back, pains in:—*Ammonium, Phosphorus.*

2. *Ammonium muriat., Arsenicum, Belladonna, Causticum, Lycopodium, Spongia.*

Before the menses:—*Phosphorus, Spongia.*

During the menses:—1. *Ammonium, Phosphorus.*

2. *Ammonium muriat., Arsenicum, Belladonna, Causticum, Lycopodium.*

Sweat on:—*Kreosotum.*

BREASTS PAINFUL:—1. *Conium.*

2. *Calcarea, Conium, Sanguinaria.*

Before the menses:—*Conium.*

Swollen:—*Calcarea.*

BREATHING IMPEDED:—*Cocculus.*

2. *Graphites, Lachesis, Pulsatilla, Sepia, Sulphur.*

BRUISED FEELING all over:—*Ambra, Conium, Lachesis, Spongia, Stramonium.*

BUZZING in the ears:—*Borax, Ferrum, Kreosotum, Veratrum.*

Before the menses:—*Ferrum.*

During the menses:—*Borax, Kreosotum, Veratrum.*

CATARRH, bronchiale, during the menses:—*Graphites.*

CHEEKS swollen:—*Graphites, Phosphorus, Sepia.*

CHEST affected with CRAMPS:—1. *Cocculus, Lachesis, China*

Before the menses:—*Cocculus.*

During the menses:—*China.*

CHEST, pains in:—1. *Graphites, Pulsatilla.*

2. *Kreosotum, Lachesis, Phosphorus.*

Sweat on:—*Belladonna, Kreosotum.*

COLD in head:—*Graphites.*

COLIC, see Abdomen, pain in.

CONSTIPATION:—*Kreosotum.*

CONVULSIONS:—1. *Chamomilla, Cocculus, Cuprum, Ignatia.*

2. *Aconitum, Coffea, Lachesis, Pulsatilla.*

3. *Bryonia, China, Conium, Graphites, Hyoscyamus Kreosotum, Magnesia muriatica, Natrum muriaticum, Nux vom.*

CORYZA, cold in head :—*Graphites.*

COUGH :—*Graphites, sulphur.*

CRAMPS, uterine :—1. *Chamomilla, China, Cocculus, Cuprum, Hyoscyamus, Ignatia.*

2. *Aconitum, Coffea, Lachesis, Pulsatilla.*

3. *Bryonia, Conium, Graphites, Kreosotum, Magnesia muriatic, Natrum muriatic, Nux vomica.*

DELIRIUM :—*Hyoscyamus, Lycopodium.*

DIARRHŒA :—1. *Graphites, Silicea, Veratrum.*

2. *Alumina, Ammonium, Causticum, Magnesia carbonica.*

DREAMS, many :—*Alumina, Calcarea, Causticum, Conium, Kali.*

EMOTIONS, disturbed :—*Cocculus, Lycopodium, Natrum muriatic, Pulsatilla.*

2. *Aconitum, Ammonium, Causticum, Chamomilla, Hyoscyamus, Sepia, Stannum, Stramonium, Veratrum.*

EPILEPSY :—*Sulphur.*

EPISTAXIS, see Nose-bleed.

ERUCTATIONS :—1. *Lachesis, Pulsatilla.*

2. *Graphites, Kali, Kreosotum, Magnesia carbonica, Nitri acidum.*

ERUPTIONS at vulva :—*Kali.*

EYES with RINGS :—*Phosphorus.*

Convulsed :—*Graphites, Lycopodium.*

Fatigued :—*Calcarea, Magnesia carbonica, Mercurius, Pulsatilla, Silicea, Sulphur.*

Spasms :—*China.*

FACE BLUEISH :—*Veratrum.*

PUFFED :—*China.*

HOT :—*Alumina.*

YELLOWISH :—*Causticum, Natrum muriaticum.*

PALE :—1. *Pulsatilla.*

2. *Manganum carbonica, Manganum muriatica.*

FAINTING:—*Ignatius, Nux vomica.*

FEET PAINFUL:—*Pulsatilla.*
  SWOLLEN:—*Graphites, Lycopodium.*
  FEVER:—*Phosphorus.*
  FLATULENCE:—1. *Cocculus.*
   2. *Kreosotum.*

FUROR, at the commencement of the menses:—*Aconitum.*

GASTRIC DERANGEMENTS:—1. *Nux vomica, Pulsatilla.*
  2. *Ammonium, Carbo vegitabilis, Lycopodium, Veratrum.*
  3. *Magnesia carbonica, Sulphur.*
  4. *Capsicum, Hyoscyamus, Phosphorus.*

GROINS PAINFUL:—*Argentum nitricum.*

HÆMOPTYSIS:—*Phosphorus.*

HÆMORRHOIDS:—1. *Pulsatilla.*
  2. *Lachesis.*
  3. *Cocculus, Phosphorus.*
 Before the menses:—*Lachesis, Phosphorus.*
 Following the menses:—*Cocculus, Pulsatilla.*
 Fluent:—*Ammonium muriatic, Graphites.*

HEAD, heat of:—*Calcarea, Conium, Ignatia.*
 Before the menses:—*Conium, Calcarea, Ignatia.*
 During the menses:—1. *Calcarea, Causticum.*,
 Congestion of:—1. *Mercurius.*
  2. *China, Conium, Iodium, Phosphorus, Veratrum.*
  3. *Kali, Magnesia carbonica, Sulphur.*
 Before the menses:—*Mercurius.*
 During the menses:—*Calcarea, Causticum, China, Conium, Iodium, Mercurius, Phosphorus, Sulphur, Veratrum.*

HEADACHE:—1. *Carbo, Kreosote, Lachesis, Lycopodium, Natrum muriaticum, Sulphur.*
  2. *Calcarea, Cuprum, Nux vomica, Platina.*
  3. *Alumina, Graphites, Ignatia, Kali, Magnesia carbonica, Magnesia muriatica, Natrum, Phosphorus, Pulsatilla, Sepia, Veratrum.*

4. *Ammonium muriaticum*, *Borax*, *Bovista*, *Bromine*, *Ferrum*, *Hepar*, *Hyoscyamus*, *Iodium*, *Kali bichromicum*, *Laurocerasus*, *Mercurius*, *Nitrum*, *Nux moschata*.

Before the menses:—1. *Carbo vegetabilis*, *Cuprum*, *Lachesis*, *Sulphur*.

2. *Alumina*, *Bromine*, *Calcarea*, *Ferrum*, *Hepar*, *Jodium*. *Mercurius*, *Natrum*, *Natrum muriaticum*, *Nux moschata*, *Pulsatilla*, *Silicea*, *Veratrum*.

During the menses:—1. *Carbo vegetabilis*, *Kreosotum*, *Lachesis*, *Lycopodium*, *Nux vomica*, *Platina*, *Sulphur*.

2. *Calcarea*, *Cuprum*, *Graphites*, *Ignatia*, *Kali*, *Magnesia carbonica*, *Magnesia muriatica*, *Phosphorus*, *Sepia*.

3. *Ammonium muriaticum*, *Borax*, *Carbo animalis*, *Graphites*, *Hyoscyamus*, *Natrum*, *Pulsatilla*, *Veratrum*.

Following the menses:—*Lycopodium*, *Pulsatilla*.

HEARING HARD:—*Kreosotum*.

HEART, PALPITATION of:—1. *Jodium*, *Spongia*.

2. *Alumina*, *Ignatia*, *Nitri acidum*, *Phosphorus*, *Sepia*.

HEAT, feverish:—*Carbo animalis*, *Mercurius*, *Nitri acidum*, *Nux vomica*, *Sepia*, *Sulphur*.

HOARSENESS:—*Graphites*.

HUNGER, CANINE, before the menses:—*Magnesia carbonica*.

IRRITABLE mood, before the menses:—*Kreosotum*, *Natrum muriaticum*.

ITCHING at parts:—1. *Graphites*, *Sulphur*.

2. *Hepar*, *Lycopodium*, *Petroleum*, *Zincum*.

LASSITUDE.

Before the menses:—1. *Cocculus*.

2. *Ignatia*, *Nux vomica*, *Phosphorus*.

3. *Alumina*.

During the menses:—*Calcarea*, *Causticum*, *Graphites*,

Iodium, Magnesia carbonica, Magnesia muriat., Nux vomica, Phosphorus.

Following the menses:—1. *Platina.*

2. *Alumina, Iodium, Phosphorus.*

LAUGHTER, convulsive:—*Hyoscyamus.*

LEGS WEARY:—*Kreosotum. Sulphur, Zincum.*

Painful:—*Ambra, Chamomilla, Conium, Lachesis, Spongia, Stramonium.*

Heavy:—*Baryta, Lycopodium, Pulsatilla, Zincum.*

Varicose:—*Ambra, Pulsatilla.*

LEUCORRHŒA:—1. *Alumina, Calcarea, Cocculus, Conium, Mercurius, Pulsatilla, Sepia.*

2. *Ammonium, Carbo animalis, Carbo vegetabilis, China, Graphites, Kali, Kreosotum, Lycopodium, Magnesia muriatica, Mezereum, Natrum muriaticum, Nux vomica, Petroleum, Phosphorus, Sabina, Silicea, Stannum, Sulphur, Zincum.*

3. *Aconitum, Agnus, Ambra, Anacardium, Arsenicum, Borax, Cannabis, Drosera, Hepar, Jodium, Lachesis, Nitri acidum, Ruta, Sulphuric acid.*

4. *Argentum nitricum, Belladonna, Coffea, Nitrum, Phosphoric acidum, Plumbum, Thuja, Viola tricolor.*

Before the menses:—1. *Calcarea, Lachesis.*

2. *Baryta, Carbo vegetabilis, China, Phosphorus.*

3. *Alumina, Graphites, Kreosotum, Pulsatilla, Ruta, Sepia, Sulphur, Zincum.*

During the menses:—1. *Alumina.*

2. *China, Cocculus, Graphites, Lachesis, Pulsatilla, Zincum.*

Following the menses:—1. *Alumina, Pulsatilla, Ruta, Sabina.*

2. *Bovista, Cocculus, Graphites, Kreosotum, Mercurius, Nitri acidum, Phosphoric acidum, Silicea, Sulphur.*

LIMBS PAINFUL:—1. *Conium, Phosphorus, Sepia.*

2. *Alumina*, *Arsenicum*, *Bryonia*, *Cantharis*, *Crocus*, *Graphites*, *Magnesia carbonica*, *Spongia*, *Veratrum*.

Before the menses :—*Alumina*.

During the menses :—*Alumina*, *Arsenicum*, *Cantharis*, *Crocus*, *Magnesia carbonica*, *Natrum*.

HIPS SWOLLEN :—*Phosphorus*.

LIVER, PAINS in :—1. *Pulsatilla*.

2. *Conium*, *Nux moschata*, *Phosphoric acid*.

Before the menses :—1. *Pulsatilla*.

2. *Conium*, *Nux moschata*.

During the menses :—*Phosphori acidum*, *Pulsatilla*.

LOQUACITY :—*Stramonium*.

MELANCHOLY, sad :—1. *Lycopodium*, *Natrum muriaticum*.

2. *Ammonium*, *Causticum*, *Sepia*, *Stannum*.

Before the menses :—1. *Lycopodium*, *Natrum muriaticum*.

2. *Causticum*, *Stannum*.

During the menses :—*Ammonium*, *Natrum muriaticum*, *Sepia*.

METRALGIA, uterine cramps :—*China*, *Hyoscyamus*.

MILIARY Eruption :—*Dulcamara*.

MUCUS on stomach :—1. *Nux moschata*, *Pulsatilla*.

2. *Nux moschata*.

NAUSEA, see Vomit.

NIGHTMARE, during the menses :—*Sulphuris acidum*.

NOSE-ITCHING, after the menses :—*Sulphur*.

BLEEDING :—*Lachesis*, *Sulphur*, *Veratrum*.

PAINS in the parts :—1. *China*.

2. *Belladonna*, *Conium*, *Nitric acidum*, *Platina*, *Pulsatilla*, *Silicea*.

Before the menses :—*China*, *Platina*.

Following the menses :—*China*, *Kreosotum*.

PALPITATION of Heart, see Heart.

PHOTOPHOBIA, see Eyes.

PRESSURE on PARTS:—1. *Ammonium*, *Platina*.

2. *Belladonna*, *China*, *Moschus*, *Nux moschata*, *Sepia*.

Before the menses:—*Platina*.

During the menses:—1. *Ammonium*, *Conium*, *Lachesis*.

2. *Belladonna*, *Moschus*, *Nitri acidum*, *Platina*, *Sepia*.

Following the menses:—*China*.

PYROSIS, before the menses:—*Sulphur*.

REDNESS of the Parts:—1. *Mercurius*, *Nux vomica*, *Sepia*.

2. *Aconitum*, *Belladonna*, *Calcarea*, *Carbo vegetabilis*, *Sulphur*.

RESTLESS:—*Platina*, *Sulphur*.

RUSH of BLOOD:—1. *Alumina*.

2. *Mercurius*.

3. *Cuprum*.

SALT TASTE in Mouth:—*Mercurius*.

SEMEN, body SWELLS of:—*Stramonium*.

SHIVERING:—1. *Pulsatilla*.

2. *Phosphorus*.

3. *Calcarea*, *Graphites*, *Kali*, *Lycopodium*, *Nux vomica*, *Veratrum*.

4. *Belladonna*, *Carbo animalis*, *Kreosotum*, *Magnesia carbonica*, *Natrum*.

Before the menses:—*Lycopodium*, *Pulsatilla*, *Veratrum*.

Following the menses:—*Graphites*, *Nux vomica*, *Pulsatilla*.

SIGHING:—*Stramonium*.

SIGHT BLURRED:—*Belladonna*, *Silicea*.

PALE:—*Silicea*.

SLEEP RESTLESS:—*Alumina*, *Kali*, *Natrum muriaticum*, *Sepia*.

SMALL OF BACK, PAINS IN:—1. *Calcarea, Lachesis, Pulsatilla.*

2. *Ammonium, Magnesia carbonica, Natrum, Nitrum, Sulphur.*

3. *Ammonium muriaticum, Asarum, Baryta, Bromine, Carbo vegetabilis, Hyoscyamus, Magnesia muriaticum, Phosphorus, Sarsaparilla.*

4. *Argentum nitricum, Graphites, Iodium, Kali, Kreosotum, Lycopodium, Nitri acidum, Nux moschata, Nux vomica, Platina, Sepia, Sulphuric acid.*

Before the Menses:—1. *Ammonium, Bromine, Hyoscyamus, Lachesis, Magnesia carbonica, Nux moschata, Pulsatilla.*

During the Menses:—1. *Calcarea, Lachesis.*

2. *Ammonium, Natrum, Pulsatilla, Sulphur.*

3. *Ammonium muriat., Asarum, Carbo vegetabilis, Lycopodium, Magnesia carbonica, Magnesia muriatica, Phosphorus, Sarsaparilla.*

Following the Menses:—1. *Pulsatilla.*

2. *Borax.*

SORENESSS at the parts and between the thighs:—1. *Kali.*

2. *Bovista.*

3. *Graphites, Sepia, Silicea.*

Before menses:—*Graphites, Kali, Silicea.*

During menses:—*Kali, Sepia.*

SPITTING OF BLOOD:—*Phosphorus.*

START, tendency to:—*Calcarea.*

STINGING in the parts:—*Sulphuris acidum.*

STITCH in side:—*Pulsatilla.*

STOMACH, PAINS IN, gastralgia:—1. *Lachesis, Pulsatilla.*

2. *Nux moschata, Sulphur.*

Before menses:—*Lachesis, Pulsatilla.*

During menses:—*Borax, Sarsaparilla.*

STUPOR:—*China.*

SWEAT :—1. *Belladonna, Graphites, Veratrum.*
2. *Hyoscyamus.*
3. *Kreosotum.*
Night :—*Belladonna, Graphites, Veratrum.*

TEARING in the parts :—*Phosphorus.*

TEETH, SET ON EDGE :—*Mercurius.*
Pain in :—1. *Calcarea, Carbo vegetabilis, Chamomilla.*
2. *Lachesis, Magnesia carbonica, Sepia.*
3. *Ammonium, Graphites, Kali, Laurocerasus.*
4. *Natrum muriaticum, Nitri acidum, Phosphorus, Sulphur, Sulphuric acid.*
Gritting the :—*Veratrum.*

TENESMUS :—*Pulsatilla.*

THIRST :—1. *Kali.*
2. *Belladonna, Sulphuris acidum, Veratrum.*
Before the menses :—*Kali.*
During the menses :—*Kali, Belladonna, Sulphuris acid., Veratrum.*

TONGUE, DRY :—*Mercurius.*

ULCERS WORSE :—*Graphites, Phosphorus.*

URINATE, urging to, frequent :—*Phosphorus, Pulsatilla, Sarsaparilla.*
Flow of urine :—*Hyoscyamus.*

VARICES :—*Ambra.*

VERTIGO :—
Before the menses :—1. *Lachesis, Pulsatilla, Veratrum.*
2. *Calcarea, Phosphorus.*
During the menses :—1. *Pulsatilla.*
2. *Calcarea, Veratrum.*
3. *Causticum, Phosphorus, Veratrum.*
Following the menses :—*Lachesis, Pulsatilla.*

VOMIT, desire to, nausea:—1. *Pulsatilla.*

2. *Carbo vegetabilis, Lycopodium, Nux vomica, Veratrum.*

3. *Capsicum, Cocculus.*

4. *Calcarea, Graphites, Hyoscyamus, Phosphorus, Sulphur.*

Before the menses:—1. *Cocculus.*

2. *Magnesia carbonica, Pulsatilla.*

During the menses:—1. *Carbo vegetabilis, Lycopodium, Nux vomica, Pulsatilla, Veratrum.*

2. *Borax, Calcarea, Graphites, Hyoscyamus, Phosphorus, Sulphur.*

Following the menses:—

VOMITING:—1. *Ammonium muriaticum, Carbo vegetabilis, Pulsatilla.*

2. *Kali, Kreosotum, Lycopodium, Phosphorus.*

Before the menses:—*Kreosotum, Pulsatilla.*

During the menses:—1. *Ammonium muriaticum, Carbo vegetabilis, Pulsatilla.*

2. *Ammonium, Kali, Lycopodium, Phosphorus.*

Following the menses:—*Borax, Pulsatilla.*

WEEPING mood:—*Conium, Lycopodium, Phosphorus, Platina, Zincum.*

Before the menses:—*Conium, Lycopodium, Phosphorus.*

During the menses:—*Lycopodium, Platina, Zincum.*

WOMB PAINFUL, see Metralgia:

YAWNING, frequent:—*Belladonna, Pulsatilla.*

SECTION 10.

Condition of the parts.—In treating menstrual irregularities, it is of the utmost importance to take the condition of the sexual organs into due consideration. Here follow the principal indications which the present condition of science has furnished us for this chapter :—

APHTHÆ at the parts :—*Carbo vegetabilis.*

BURNING at the parts, (vulva) :—1. *Carbo vegetabilis, Sulphur.*
2. *Ammonium, Calcarea, Cantharis.*
3. *Ambra, Bryonia, Carbo animalis, Causticum, Chamomilla, Hyoscyamus, Kali, Laurocerasus, Lycopodium, Magnes australis, Mercurius, Mezereum, Nitri acidum, Nux vomica, Petroleum, Thuja.*

In vagina :—*Chamomilla, Hyoscyamus, Lycopodium, Sulphur, Thuja.*

CONGESTION of the parts :—1. *Belladonna.*
2. *China, Hepar, Nux vomica, Secale, Sulphur.*
3. *Bryonia, Mercurius, Platina.*
4. *Crocus, Sabina, Sulphur.*

CONTRACTIVE PAIN in the parts :—1. *Nux vomica.*
2. *Ignatia, Sabina, Sepia, Thuja.*

CRAMPS in uterus :—1. *Cocculus, Ignatia.*
2. *Cicuta, Conium, Graphites, Magnesia muriaticum, Nux vomica, Pulsatilla.*
3. *Bryonia, Natrum muriaticum, Platina, Sepia, Stannum.*
4. *Argentum nitricum, Belladonna, Chamomilla, Hyoscyamus, Kreosotum, Thuja.*

DEFORMITY of uterine orifice :—*Natrum.*

DIGGING in the vulva :—*Conium.*

DISTENSION of the womb :—*Lycopodium, Magnes arcticus, Phosphorus.*

DRYNESS of vagina :—*Belladonna, Lycopodium.*

ERUPTIONS at the parts :—1. *Mercurius*, *Sepia*.
2. *Dulcamara*, *Graphites*, *Petroleum*, *Sulphur*.
3. *Angustura*, *Calcarea*, *Bryonia*, *Causticum*, *Conium*, *Kali*, *Nux vomica*, *Tartarus*.
4. *Mercurius*, *Phosphorus*, *Staphysagria*.

Pimples at the parts :—1. *Graphites*, *Mercurius*.
2. *Angustura*, *Conium*, *Kali*, *Natrum muriaticum*, *Tartarus*.

Herpes at the parts :—1. *Dulcamara*, *Petroleum*.
2. *Causticum*.

Nodes at the parts :—*Calcarea*, *Mercurius*, *Phosphorus*.

Pustules at the parts :—*Bryonia*, *Mercurius*.

FULNESS in the parts :—*Graphites*, *Staphysagria*, *Sulphur*.

HEAT at the vulva :—*China*.

HERPES at the parts :—*Carbo vegetabilis*, *Kreosotum*, *Mercurius*, *Nux vomica*, *Sepia*.

HYSTERIC BALL in uterus :—1. *Dulcamara*, *Petroleum*.
2. *Causticum*, (compare eruptions,) *Lachesis*, *Plumbum*.

INDURATION of the womb :—1. *Belladonna*, *Carbo animalis*, *Sepia*.
2. *Aurum*, *China*, *Magnesia muriatica*, *Staphysagria*.
3. *Clematis*, *Cocculus*, *Conium*, *Rhus*.

INFLAMMATION of the labia :—1. *Mercurius*, *Sepia*.
2. *Nux vomica*.
3. *Calcarea*.
4. *Aconitum*, *Belladonna*, *Nitri acidum*, *Sulphur*.

INFLAMMATION of the womb :—1. *Nux vomica*.
2. *Aconitum*, *Belladonna*, *Chamomilla*.
3. *Coffea*, *Lachesis*, *Mercurius*, *Platina*, *Rhus*, *Secale*.
4. *Bryonia*, *Cantharis*, *China*, *Ignatia*, *Pulsatilla*.

ITCHING at the parts:—*Calcarea, Carbo vegetabilis, Conium, Natrum muriaticum, Sepia, Silicea, Sulphur.*
2. *Angustura, Coffea, Kali, Kreosotum, Platina.*
3. *Ambra, Ammonium, Lachesis, Lycopodium, Mercurius.*

GNAWING at the parts:—*Kali, Lycopodium.*

LABIA irritated:—1. *Calcarea, Conium, Sepia, Silicea.*
2. *Mercurius, Nux vomica, Thuja.*
3. *Ammonium, Bryonia, Graphites, Carbo vegetabilis, Dulcamara, Hepar, Lycopodium, Natrum, Nitri acidum, Phosphorus, Pulsatilla.*

LABOR-PAINS, like:—1. *Pulsatilla.*
2. *Chamomilla, Coffea, Secale.*
3. *Arnica, Belladonna, Nux moschata, Nux vomica.*
4. *Calcarea, Cina, Iodium, Kali, Kreosotum, Opium, Sulphuris acidum.*

LEUCORRHŒA:—1. *Alumina, Calcarea, Cocculus, Conium, Mercurius, Pulsatilla, Sepia.*
2. *Ammonium, Carbo animalis, Carbo vegetabilis, China, Graphites, Kali, Kreosotum, Lycopodium, Magnesia carbonica, Magnesia muriatica, Mezereum, Natrum muriaticum, Nux vomica, Petroleum, Phosphorus, Sabina, Silicea, Stannum, Zincum.*
3. *Aconitum, Agnus, Ambra, Anacardium, Arsenicum, Borax, Cannabis, Drosera, Hepar, Iodium, Lachesis, Nitri acidum, Ruta, Sulphuris acidum.*
4. *Argentum nitricum, Belladonna, Bovista, Coffea, Manganum, Phosphori acidum, Plumbum, Thuja, Viola tricolor.*

MOLES:—*Cantharis.*

NODES of the Vulva:—*Calcarea, Mercurius, Phosphorus.*

Neck of the Womb:—*Kreosotum.*

OVARIA irritated:—1. *Belladonna, Cantharis, China, Lachesis, Mercurius.*

2. *Conium, Dulcamara, Platina, Sabina, Staphysagria, Thuja.*

3. *Aconitum, Ambra, Antimonium, Arsenicum, Asa, Aurum, Carbo animalis, Lycopodium, Mezereum, Secale, Sepia.*

4. *Carbo vegetabilis, Colocynthis, Graphites, Ignatia, Nitri acidum, Nux vomica, Sulphur, Zincum.*

PAIN at the neck of the womb, when touched:—*China, Ferrum, Kreosotum.*

At os tincæ, incisive:—*Pulsatilla.*

PIMPLES at the parts, (see Eruptions:)—1. *Graphites, Mercurius.*

2. *Conium, Kali, Natrum muriaticum, Tartarus.*

POLYPI in the womb:—1. *Calcarea.*

2. *Staphysagria, Sepia.*

3. *Nitri acidum, Thuja.*

PRESSURE on the parts:—1. *Belladonna, Chamomilla, China, Natrum, Sulphur.*

2. *Calcarea, Chininum, Platina.*

3. *Ipecacuanha, Magnesia carbonica, Moschus, Nux vomica.*

4. *Asa, Cina, Crocus, Graphites, Natrum muriaticum, Sepia, Thuja, Zincum.*

PULLING in the parts:—1. *Pulsatilla.*

2. *Moschus, Rhus, Sabina.*

3. *Lycopodium.*

PUSTULES at the parts:—*Bryonia, Mercurius.*

ROUGHNESS, heat at the parts:—1. *Kali.*

2. *Calcarea, Carbo vegetabilis, Conium, Natrum muriaticum, Sepia, Silicea, Sulphur.*

3. *Ammonium, Lycopodium, Nitri acidum.*

4. *Graphites, Kreosotum Staphysagria.*

SENSITIVENESS of the parts:—1. *China.*
2. *Mercurius, Nux vomica, Staphysagria.*
3. *Coffea, Platina, Sepia, Zincum.*

Of the neck of the womb:—*China.*

SEXUAL APPETITE increased:—1. *Belladonna, Platina, Veratrum.*
2. *China, Coffea.*
3. *Cantharis, Cina, Gratiola, Lachesis, Moschus, Nux vomica, Sulphuris acidum.*

Decreased:—*Baryta, Belladonna, Kali, Natrum muriaticum, Petroleum.*

In intercourse, painful:—*Ferrum, Kreosotum.*

Repugnant:—*Kali, Natrum muriaticum, Petroleum.*

SORENESS of the parts, and of the surrounding parts:—1. *Carbo vegetabilis, Graphites, Sepia, Sulphur.*
2. *Ammonium, Hepar, Lycopodium.*
3. *Ambra, Nitri acidum, Petroleum, Rhododendron, Thuja.*
4. *Arsenicum, Aurum, Coffea, Iodium, Kreosotum, Phosphorus.*

Pain as from:—1. *Ambra, Ferrum, Rhus, Thuja.*
2. *Chamomilla, Kali, Kreosotum, Staphysagria.*

STERILITY:—1. *Borax, Calcarea, Cannabis, Mercurius, Phosphorus.*
2. *Ammonium, Causticum, Conium, Graphites, Natrum muriat., Sulphuris acidum.*
3. *Agnus, Ferrum, Natrum, Ruta.*
4. *Cicuta, Crocus, Dulcamara, Hyoscyamus, Platina, Sepia.*

STINGING in the parts:—1. *Lycopodium, Sepia.*
2. *Kali, Kreosotum, Nitri acidum, Phosphorus, Pulsatilla, Sabina.*
3. *Alumina, Arsenicum, Belladonna, Calcarea, Conium, Graphites, Mercurius, Rhus, Staphysagria, Thuja.*

SWELLING of the parts:—1. *Nux vomica.*
2. *Belladonna, Mercurius, Sepia.*
3. *Ammonium, Bryonia, Cantharis, Carbo veget., Lachesis, Secale, Thuja.*
of the labia majora:—1. *Carbo veget., Mercurius, Sepia*
2. *Ammonium, Bryonia, Lachesis, Secale, Thuja.*
of the uterus:—1. *Nux vomica.*
2. *Belladonna, Sepia.*
3. *Angustura, Cantharis, Mercurius, Secale, Thuja.*
of the ovaria:—*Graphites, Lachesis.*
of the Vagina:—*Kali bichromicum, Mercurius.*

THROBBING in the parts:—*Alumina, Mercurius.*

ULCERS at the vulva:—1. *Sepia.*
2. *Nitri acidum, Thuja.*
3. *Graphites.*
at the neck of the womb:—1. *Nitri acidum, Thuja.*
Arsenicum, Belladonna, China, Cocculus, Mercurius, Sepia.

UTERUS irritated:—1. *Belladonna, Conium, Nux vomica, Platina, Pulsatilla, Secale, Sepia, Sulphur.*
2. *Chamomilla, Cocculus, Graphites, Hyoscyamus, Ignatia, Kreosotum, Magnesia muriat., Sabina.*
3. *Bryonia, Carbo animalis, Crocus, Ferrum, Moschus, Natrum muriat., Nux moschata, Opium, Rhus, Stannum, Thuja, Veratrum.*
4. *Arnica, Calcarea, China, Coffea, Ipecacuanha, Phosphori acidum.*

VAGINA irritated:—1. *Conium, Mercurius, Sepia, Sulphur.*
2. *Belladonna, Conium, Ferrum, Kali, Lycopodium, Nux vomica.*
3. *Arsenicum, Cantharis, China, Nitri acidum, Phosporus, Pulsatilla, Rhus, Staphysagria, Thuja.*

4. *Alumina, Capsicum, Carbo vegetabilis, Chamomilla, Graphites, Hyoscyamus, Kreosotum, Platina, Sabina, Silicea, Stannum.*

VARICES, at the parts:—*Calcarea, Carbo vegetabilis, Lycopodium, Nux vomica, Zincum,*

VESICLES, at the parts:—1. *Graphites.*

2. *Staphysagria, Sulphur.*

VULVA irritated:—1. *Calcarea, Conium, Natrum muriaticum, Sepia, Silicea.*

2. *Mercurius, Nux vomica, Thuja.*

3. *Ammonium, Bryonia, Graphites, Kali, Kreosotum, Staphysagria, Sulphur.*

4. *Agaricus, Alumina, Ambra, Cantharis, Carbo vegetabilis, Dulcamara, Hepar, Lycopodium, Magnesia carbonica, Natrum, Nitri acidum, Phosphorus, Pulsatilla.*

WIND from the vagina:—*Bromine, Lycopodium, Sanguinaria.*

ARTICLE II.

MENSTRUAL COLIC.

SECTION 11.

Nature of the malady.—Menstrual colic is generally one of the most marked symptoms of dysmenorrhœa. Its seat seems to be the uterus; it is either inflammatory or purely nervous in its character; often it resembles labor-pain, and only comes on at intervals; at other times it is continuous, and is principally felt in the loins, hips and lower limbs. It generally precedes the menstrual discharge by a few hours or days, and ceases as soon as the blood has begun to flow properly; in other cases it only makes its appearance after the courses have commenced to flow, which are sometimes interrupted in consequence of the colic, for a longer or shorter period. This colic is often accompanied by the expulsion of a kind of false membrane, after which the blood re-commences to flow. Sometimes, if the blood is arrested by the colic, the breasts swell, become more sensitive, and even painful. Few women are entirely free from these pains; some remain subject to them as long as the menstrual functions last. The most frequent and exciting causes of this colic are, a cold, especially when caused by exposure of the feet to dampness; errors in the mode of living, or the vicious and imprudent use of drugs during the menstrual flow.

SECTION 12.

Treatment.—The best remedies for these pains are, during the flow, *Belladonna, Calcarea, Chamomilla, Cocculus, Coffea, Nux vomica, Pulsatilla, Sulphur*—particularly:

Belladonna.—For pains in the abdomen, as if the parts were clutched; pains in the sides, with pulling all along the thighs; weight and pressure on the parts, as if everything would fall through; the pains come on before the appearance of the courses, with determination of blood to the head, blue before the eyes, frightful fancies and rage; red and puffed face, pains in the sides, violent thirst.

Calcarea.—Abdominal colic, with leucorrhœa; cramp-pains in the sides; colic, with shivering; swelling and painfulness of the breasts; polypi of the womb; rush of blood to the head, with vertigo and stupefaction; loss of appetite; embarrassed respiration; toothache; nausea or vomiting.

Chamomilla.—Violent colic, consequent upon profuse and premature menses, with sensitiveness of the abdomen, as if ulcerated; labor-pains; painful pressure in the sides, down to the abdomen and private parts; violent abdominal cramps, with greenish or watery diarrhœa, nausea, eructations, yellow coating of the tongue, bitter mouth; dark, coagulated blood; fainting turns, with thirst, coldness of the limbs, pale and haggard face.

Cocculus.—Abdominal cramps, colic with pressure, pressure on the chest, with restlessness, sighs; suppression or scanty menses, with black coagula; flatulence, nausea unto fainting; paralytic weakness, with oppression, cramps in the chest, anxiety, convulsive movements of the limbs; flesh-colored leucorrhœa, with bloody and purulent serum instead of the menses.

Coffea.—Distressing and maddening colic; fulness and pressure in the abdomen, as if it would burst; abdominal cramps ascending to the chest; nervousness, with restlessness, cries, and twisting of the whole body; profuse menstrual discharge, with serous mucus, voluptuous itching of the parts and excessive sexual excitement.

Nux vomica.—*Uterine cramps*, with painful pressure in the hypogastrium, down to the thighs; lameness in the sides; distention of the bowels; constipation, with ineffectual urging to stool; frequent urging to urinate, with tenesmus of the bladder; the menses are *premature* and last *too long*, reappearing several times after having seemed to cease; irascible mood.

PULSATILLA.—Colic, abdominal spasms, retarded menses; discharge of black coagula, or of a pale and serous blood; hepatic pains, gastralgia, *pains in the sides*, nausea and desire to vomit, or *sour and slimy vomiting;* megrim, vertigo; *shivering, with pale face;* leucorrhœa, weeping mood, anxiety, sadness and melancholy; weight in the bowels as from a stone; violent pressure in the lower bowels, with pulling down the thighs; numbness of the legs when sitting; violent pressure on the rectum, like urging to stool.

SULPHUR.—*Colic and abdominal cramps*, rush of blood to the head, nose-bleed, toothache, water-brash, gastralgia, itching of the parts, dyspnœa, cough, premature and profuse menses, with pale blood.

DOSE.—These different remedies may be administered as follows:—Dissolve from six to eight globules, or one or two drops, of the attenuated medicine in solution, in about ten or twelve table spoonfuls of water, and give the patient a table-spoonful of this solution every half hour, or every hour or two hours, until the pain ceases; the frequency of the dose depends upon the intensity or the frequency of the paroxysms.

SECTION 13.

Other Remedies.—If the above-mentioned remedies should prove insufficient, we may administer *Aconitum*, *Bryonia*, *Graphites*, *Ignatia*, *Phosphorus*, *Secale*, *Sepia*, *Platina*, *Veratrum.*

ACONITUM.—Distressing colic, with congestion of the head and chest; palpitation of the heart; pressive, throbbing or stinging headache; red cheeks; full and hard pulse; feverish heat, with thirst; irascible mood; vertigo or fainting turns on raising herself in bed; is most suitable to plethoric young girls, who lead a sedentary life.

BRYONIA.—Colic, with leucorrhœa, or rheumatic pains in

the limbs; pressive or burning gastralgia; pressure and fulness in the pit of the stomach; congestion of the chest and head, with short cough or nose-bleed; constipation; coldness, frequent shivering.

CUPRUM.—Abdominal cramps, ascending to the stomach and chest, with vomiting, convulsions, cries, suppression or scanty menses.

GRAPHITES.—Cutting and crampy colic, with scanty and short menses; discharge of a thick and black blood, or else pale and serous; nausea, pains in the chest, bronchial or nasal catarrh; weakness, rheumatic pains in the limbs; œdema of the feet and legs.

IGNATIA.—Contractive cramp-colic, with premature and profuse menses; discharge of black blood mixed with coagula; oppressive headache; photophobia; anxiety, palpitation of the heart, and fainting turns.

PHOSPHORUS.—Colic, as if the bowels were cut with knives, with pains in the sides, vomiting of bile, mucus and food; the menses at first delay, then become too profuse and flow too long, with weakness, rings around the eyes, loss of flesh, restlessness; stinging headache, lameness of the limbs, palpitation of the heart, spitting of blood, shivering, swelling of the gums and cheek.

PLATINA.—Cramp-colic, with painful pressure on the genital parts; the menses are premature, last too long, and are too profuse, with black and slimy blood; leucorrhœa before or after the menses; frequent urging to urinate; constipation, hard stool; anorexia; vertigo; anguish, weeping, restlessness; sleeplessness; suspicious mood.

SECALE CORNUTUM.—Tearing and cutting colic, with profuse and long menstrual flow; cold limbs, pale face, cold sweat, weakness, small and almost suppressed pulse; violent twisting of the body; cries, rolling on the ground.

SEPIA.—Cramp-colic, pressure on the parts, scanty or profuse menses; leucorrhœa, headache, lameness of the limbs, toothache, melancholy.

VERATRUM.—Colic, with nausea, vomiting, hysteric distress; labor-pains in the sides and hypogastrium; *colic with diarrhœa after the menses;* headache before the menses; icy cold hands, feet and nose; weakness, fainting turns; pale and earthy face; sense of constriction in the throat; sexual excitement.

DOSE.—These medicines are administered in the same manner as prescribed for the remedies of the previous paragraph, at the end of the list.

SECTION 14.

General Indications.—Beside the remedies mentioned in the two preceding paragraphs, we may have to resort to, 3, *Alumina*, *Ammonium*, *Ammonium muriaticum*, *Baryta*, *China*, *Conium*, *Cocculus*, *Cuprum*, *Lachesis*, *Silicea*, *Zincum*, 4, *Carbo vegetabilis*, *Causticum*, *Kreosotum*, *Laurocerasus*, *Lycopodium*, *Magnesia carbonica*, *Mercurius*, *Natrum*, *Nitrum*, *Sarsaparilla*, *Stannum*, *Stramonium*, *Sulphur*, *Sulphuric acid.*

WHEN THE COLIC SETS IN before the menses:—1. *Belladonna*, *Calcarea*, *Chamomilla*, *Platina*, *Pulsatilla.*
3. *Alumina*, *Ammonium*, *Baryta*, *Causticum*, *Graphites*, *Lachesis*, *Lycopodium*, *Nitrum*, *Phosphorus*, *Sepia.*

With the menses:—1. *Belladonna*, *Calcarea*, *Chamomilla*, *Graphites*, *Phosphorus*, *Pulsatilla*, *Sepia*, *Sulphur.*
2. *Cocculus*, *Coffea*, *Ignatia*, *Nux vom.*, *Secale.*
3. *Agnus*, *Alumina*, *Ammonium*, *Ammonium muriat.*, *China*, *Conium*, *Crocus*, *Silicea*, *Zincum.*
4. *Carbo veget.*, *Kreosotum*, *Laurocerasus*, *Lycopodium*, *Magnesia carbon.*, *Mercurius*, *Sarsaparilla*, *Stannum*, *Stramonium*, *Sulphuris acidum.*

After the menses:—*Lachesis*, *Pulsatilla*, *Veratrum.*

Moreover, if the MENSES ARE TOO LONG:—1. *Nux vomica*, *Platina*, *Secale.*
2. *Bryonia*, *Calcarea*, *Coffea*, *Ignatia*, *Phosphorus*, *Sepia.*

TOO PROFUSE:—1. *Belladonna, Calcarea, Nux vomica, Platina, Secale.*

2. *Chamomilla, Coffea, Ignatia, Phosphorus, Sepia.*

3. *Aconite, Bryonia, China, Crocus, Mercurius, Pulsatilla, Veratrum.*

PREMATURE:—*Calcarea, Chamomilla, Cocculus, Ignatia, Nux vom., Phosphorus, Platina, Sepia, Sulphur.*

RETARDED:—1. *Graphites, Pulsatilla, Sepia, Sulphur*

2. *Aconite, Calcarea, Cocculus, Phosphorus, Veratrum.*

SCANTY:—1. *Graphites, Pulsatilla, Sulphur.*

2. *Aconite, Cocculus, Phosphorus, Sepia.*

SHORT:—1. *Pulsatilla, Sulphur.*

2. *Graphites, Phosphorus, Platina.*

SUPPRESSED:—1. *Pulsatilla, Sepia, Sulphur.*

2. *Aconite, Belladonna, Bryonia, Calcarea, Chamomilla, Cocculus, Ignatia, Phosphorus, Veratrum.*

BLOOD, COAGULATED:—1. *Belladonna, Chamomilla, Ignatia, Platina, Pulsatilla.*

2. *Bryonia, Nux vomica, Secale, Sepia, Pulsatilla.*

BLACK, DARK:—1. *Chamomilla, Nux vomica, Pulsatilla.*

2. *Belladonna, Bryonia, Sepia, Sulphur.*

PALE, WATERY:—1. *Belladonna, Graphites, Pulsatilla, Sulphur.*

2. *Bryonia, Calcarea, Phosphorus, Platina, Secale.*

For further information see the Article DYSMENORRHŒA, Sections 5, 6, 7, 8, 9, 10.

ARTICLE III.

MENSTRUAL IRREGULARITIES, AND ALTERATIONS OF THE MENSTRUAL BLOOD.

WHEN THE MENSES ARE TOO COPIOUS, PREMATURE, TOO LONG, SCANTY, RETARDED, TOO SHORT, FULL. ETC.

SECTION 15.

GENERAL OBSERVATIONS.—Besides the various ailments which may occur before, after, or during the menses, and which constitute in their totality what we have termed *dysmenorrhœa*, of which a more particular description has been furnished in Sections 2–10, the menstrual flow itself is liable to irregularities, setting in before or after the regular period, and being either too copious or too scanty, too short or too long. The blood is likewise susceptible of morbid changes, as regards color, consistence, smell, etc. These irregularities may be unaccompanied by any other distress or irregularity in the menstrual functions; most frequently, however, they are the first cause of dysmenorrhœa and many other menstrual ailments. For this reason we shall furnish a more detailed account of these various sufferings than we have been able to do under the head of Dysmenorrhœa, Section 3. We shall treat in succession, 1st, of *premature* menstruation; 2nd, *profuse* menstruation; 3d, menstruation of *excessive* duration; 4th, *retarded* menstruation; 5th, *scanty* menstruation; 6th, menstruation of *insufficient duration*; 7th, of the various alterations of the menstrual blood.

Section 16.

Premature Menstruation.—The best remedies are in general,

1. *Ambra, Calcarea, Carbo vegetabilis, Chamomilla, Ignatia, Ipecacuanha, Natrum muriaticum, Nux vomica, Phosphorus, Rhus, Sabina.*

2. *Ammonium, Ammonium muriaticum, Asarum, Bovista, Cantharis, Cina, Cocculus, Colchicum, Crocus, Kali, Kreosotum, Leurocerasus, Magnes australis, Manganum, Platina, Secale, Sepia, Sulphuris acidum.*

3. *Alumina, Arnica, Asafœtida, Belladonna, Borax, Bryonia, Carbo animalis, China, Colocynthis, Hepar, Iodium, Lachesis, Ledum, Magnesia muriatica, Muriatis acidum, Natrum, Nitri acidum, Nux moschata, Phosphori acidum, Plumbum, Pulsatilla, Ruta, Silicea, Spongia, Stannum, Sulphur.*

With the following particular indications:—

Ambra.—Painful varices at the legs; *thick leucorrhœa*, with stitches in the vagina and discharges of pieces of bluish and whitish mucus; burning in the parts; excoriation-pains, violent itching and swelling of the labia.

Belladonna.—Premature and profuse menses with bright-red, foul-smelling, and coagulating blood; colic, as if every thing would fall through the vagina; throbbing headache; red and puffed face; blur before the eyes; sweat on the chest, at night, with thirst.

Calcarea.—Premature and profuse menses, with cutting in the bowels, toothache, leucorrhœa, swelling of the veins; before the menses, headache, colic, shuddering, leucorrhœa and swelling of the breasts with sensitiveness.

Carbo Vegetabilis.—Premature and profuse menses, preceded by eruptions and itching of the skin, headache or colic; cutting colic when the flow stops, with backache, lameness in the limbs, toothache, vomiting, headache.

Chamomilla.—Profuse menses, with drawing cramp-colic from the sides to the abdomen; dark coagula; thirst; cold limbs, fainting.

IGNATIA.—Menses every fortnight, with compressive cramp-pain, hardness and distention of the abdomen; hysteric symptoms; nausea with fainting; shuddering all over, with pale face; sight feeble and blurred; intolerance of light and noise.

IPECACUANHA.—The menses set in too soon without any known cause, they are too copious, the blood is bright-red and coagulates readily; weakness, restlessness and aversion to food.

NATRUM MURIATICUM.—Menses too copious and too long, preceded by irritability, melancholy and restlessness, with headache; during the menses; headache, desire to remain in bed, toothache, cramp-colic and nightly fever.

NUX VOMICA.—Profuse menses, with abdominal cramps; menses every fortnight; during the menses; vomiting, headache above the eyes, dry heat and weakness.

PHOSPHORUS.—Profuse menses, with pains in the sides, colic, swelling of the gums and cheek; during the menses; cutting in the bowels, backache, spitting of blood, palpitation of the heart and fermentation in the bowels.

RHUS TOXICODENDRON.—Profuse discharge of blood, with coagula; labor-pains; excoriation-pains in the vagina.

SABINA.—Profuse menses, with discharge of coagula; colic, labor-pains, scanty and red urine, mucous discharge from the vagina.

Moreover, if the menses break out again before their time in consequence of a violent *emotion*, give *Platina*.

If in consequence of an *exertion*, give *Arnica* and *Rhus*.

If without any *known* cause, *Ipecacuanha*.

For more precise information, see *Dysmenorrhœa*, Sections 5–10.

DOSE.—Of these different medicines give from four to six globules dry on the tongue, or one or two drops of the attenuated tincture in a teaspoonful of water or on a little sugar, a few days after the menses cease to flow, and repeat the dose every week until the next menstrual period is about to set in.

SECTION 17.

PROFUSE MENSTRUATION.—The principal remedies are:—

1. *Belladonna*, *Calcarea*. *Chamomilla*, *China*, *Ferrum*, *Ipecacuanha*, *Nux vomica*, *Platina*, *Sabina*, *Secale*, *Stramonium*.

2. *Arsenicum*, *Bryonia*, *Cantharis*, *Carbo vegetabilis*. *Coffea*, *Crocus*, *Hyoscyamus*, *Ignatia*, *Magnes australis*, *Mercurius*, *Natrum muriaticum*, *Nitri acidum*, *Nux moschata*, *Phosphorus*, *Sepia*, *Sulphur*, *Sulphuris acidum*.

3. *Aconitum*, *Agaricus*, *Ambra*, *Ammonium muriaticum*, *Antimonium*, *Borax*, *Bovista*, *Carbo animalis*, *Causticum*, *Chelidonium*, *Cina*, *Cyclamen*, *Hepar*, *Iodium*, *Kreosotum*, *Laurocerasus*, *Ledum*, *Lycopodium*, *Moschus*, *Muriatis acidum*, *Natrum*, *Nitrum*, *Phosphori acidum*, *Pulsatilla*, *Rhus*, *Ruta*, *Sambucus*, *Selenium*, *Silicea*, *Stannum*, *Veratrum*. With the following particular indications:

BELLADONNA.—Profuse and premature menses, with violent bearing-down in the genital organs; bright-red, offensive discharge, readily coagulating; pulsative headache in the temples; red and puffed face; pains in the sides.

CALCAREA.—Cutting colic, toothache and leucorrhœa during the menses; swelling and sensitiveness of the renal region before the appearance of the menses; headache, colic and shuddering; lascivious dreams; dyspnœa.

CHAMOMILLA.—Discharge of a dark-red or black blood, offensive, occasionally mixed with coagula; labor-pains, thirst, cold extremities, pale face, weakness unto fainting, blurr before the eyes, buzzing in the ears.

CHINA.—Watery and pale blood, or coagula now and then, with uterine cramps, frequent urging to urinate and painful distention of the bowels; laziness; weakness and disposition to sweat; confusion in the head and buzzing in the ears; swelling of the legs.

FERRUM.—Profuse discharge of blood which is partially thin, and partially black and coagulated, with labor-pains; vascular excitement, headache, vertigo, glowing redness of the face, full and hard pulse.

IPECACUANHA.—Copious and uninterrupted discharge of a liquid and bright-red blood, with cutting in the umbilical region, pressure on the womb and rectum, shivering, coldness, heat of the head, weakness, pale face, nausea and constant desire to lie down.

NUX VOMICA.—Menses premature and too long, with vertigo, constipation, nausea and weakness, cramp-colic frontal headache, aggravation of the symptoms in the morning.

PLATINA.—Thick and dark blood, with painful drawing in the sides down to the groin, as if the abdominal viscera were drawn down; excessive sexual excitement.

SABINA.—Discharge of dark blood, mixed with coagula, accompanied by colic and labor-pains; weakness, rheumatic pains in the limbs and head.

SECALE CORNUTUM.—Suitable to feeble, worn-out, cachectic females, with coldness of the extremities, pulse full, leaden countenance, small pulse, uneasiness and fear of death.

STRAMONIUM.—Profuse discharge of black blood, with large coagula; during the menses, drawing pains in the abdomen, thighs and limbs; talkative; the body smells of semen.

For further information concerning remedies and their indications, see *Dysmenorrhœa*, Sections 5–10.

DOSE.—The same as indicated at the end of Section 17.

SECTION 18.

MENSES OF EXCESSIVE DURATION.—The principal remedies are:—

1. *Aconitum*, *China*, *Cuprum*, *Ignatia*, *Lycopodium*, *Natrum muriaticum*, *Nux vomica*, *Platina*, *Secale*, *Sulphur*.

2. *Baryta*, *Bryonia*, *Calcarea*, *Cantharis*, *Coffea*, *Crocus*, *Ferrum*, *Kreosotum*, *Magnes australis*, *Mercurius*, *Phosphorus*, *Rhus*, *Sabina*, *Sepia*.

3. *Arsenicum*, *Asarum*, *Belladonna*, *Causticum*, *Chelidonium*, *Dulcamara*, *Kali*, *Laurocerasus*, *Stramonium*.

With the following indications:

ACONITUM.—Congestion of the head and heart, with stinging pains, full and hard pulse; blurred and bright-red blood, coagulating readily; moral and nervous excitements; feverish heat with red cheeks, or weakness, fainting turns and pale face when raising herself from a recumbent posture.

China.—Weakness, with pale face, rings around the eyes, blur before them, ringing in the ears; labor-pains; swollen feet; sleeplessness or restless sleep, with nightly headache; nervousness and irritable mood.

Cuprum.—The menses are too profuse, with abdominal cramps, congestion of the head, pressive headache at the vertex, red face and eyes, frequent nausea with vomiting, palpitation of the heart.

Ignatia.—The menses last too long, followed by hysterical symptoms, with discharge of coagula. During the menses: abdominal spasms, headache with heaviness and heat in the head, photophobia, contractive colic, anguish, palpitation of the heart, and weakness unto fainting.

Lycopodium.—Profuse menses, reappearing several times, even after having ceased to flow; before the menses: shuddering, malaise, sadness, lowness of spirits, apprehensive mood; during the menses: sour taste in the mouth, nausea.

Natrum muriaticum.—Menses last too long, with profuse discharge, headache, sadness, abdominal cramps, shivering, frequent yawning.

Nux vomica.—Premature menses; they last too long, reappear several times after having ceased to flow, with uterine cramps, frontal headache, vertigo, constipation, nausea, dyspepsia, and irritable mood.

Platina.—Profuse menses, with pressure on the parts, thick and black or else slimy and sticky blood, sexual excitement, also of the parts.

Secale.—Profuse menses, with violent cramps; all the symptoms are worse during and before the menses; tingling in the legs, weakness; nocturnal cramps in the calves and soles of the feet.

Sulphur.—When the foregoing remedies are insufficient,

with discharge of an acrid, black and corrosive blood; eruptions and tetter on the skin here and there.

For further details see Sections 5–10.

DOSE.—The same as at the close of Section 17.

SECTION 19.

RETARDED MENSTRUATION.—The principal remedies are:

1. *Causticum*, *Cuprum*, *Dulcamara*, *Graphites*, *Kali*, *Lachesis*, *Lycopodium*, *Magnesia carbonica*, *Natrum muriaticum*, *Phosphorus*, *Pulsatilla*, *Sepia*, *Silicea*, *Sulphur*.

2. *Aconitum*, *Agnus*, *Chelidonium*, *Cocculus*, *Drosera*, *Ferrum*, *Mercurius*, *Petroleum*, *Sabina*, *Valeriana*, *Zincum*.

3. *Ammonium*, *Aurum*, *Bryonia*, *Calcarea*, *Cicuta*, *Crocus*, *Digitalis*. *Hyoscyamus*, *Magnes arcticus*, *Magnesia muriatica*, *Sabadilla*, *Sarsaparilla*, *Staphysagria*, *Stramonium*, *Strontiana*, *Veratrum*.

With the following particular indications:

CAUSTICUM.—The menses are too scanty, flowing only in the day-time; melancholy, gloomy mood, pains in the sides before the menses; yellow complexion, abdominal colic and vertigo during the menses.

CUPRUM.—Abdominal spasms or general convulsions, with cries; congestion of the head; headache at the vertex; face and eyes red, or else pale, with rings around the eyes; frequent nausea with vomiting; palpitation of the heart, and cramps in the chest.

DULCAMARA.—The menstrual blood is pale, and the flow is too short; tetter at the labia; miliaria before the menses.

GRAPHITES.—Delaying menses, too scanty, with abdominal colic, weight in the abdomen and dulness of the head; heaviness of the arms and legs; abdominal cramps, pains in the chest, weakness, discharge of blood from the anus, pains in the limbs, during the menses.

KALI CARBONICUM.—Pressure towards the parts; soreness and redness around the parts and between the thighs; a good deal of heat, with thirst, and restless nights; the menstrual blood is acrid and fetid.

Lachesis.—Colic in the back, at the commencement of the menses, with abdominal cramps and throbbing headache; scanty flow, with nose-bleed, and distress.

Magnesia carbonica.—Delaying menses, with sore throat, canine hunger, pains in the stomach, nausea before the menses, which flow only at night.

Natrum muriaticum.—Menses *too late and scanty*, with rush of blood to the head; melancholy, anxiety, headache, qualmishness, blood-spitting, before the menses.

Phosphorus.—Leucorrhœa, frequent urging to urinate, weeping, before the menses; shivering, weariness, fever, stinging headache, and spitting of blood, during the menses; suitable to persons with delicate constitutions and inclining to pulmonary diseases.

Pulsatilla.—Menses at times delaying, at others premature, with black blood mixed with mucous, or pale and serous blood; nausea and vomiting, shivering, pale face, stitching colic extending to the parts; semi-lateral headache, with drawing pains extending to the face, ears and teeth; tendency to diarrhœa, leucorrhœa.

Sepia.—Delaying menses, with fainting turn, violent colic, shuddering all over, burning in the vulva, *soreness* and swelling of the parts, leucorrhœa and pressure in the abdomen, before the menses; uterine cramps and rheumatic pains in the limbs during the menses; yellow border across the nose and cheeks.

Silicea.—Delaying menses, with diarrhœa, or painful pressure above the eyes, before the menses; scanty menses; strong smell of the menstrual blood.

Sulphur.—When the other remedies fail, with headache before, during and after the menses; loss of flesh; heat in the head; weakness after eating.

For further details, see Sections 5–10.

Dose.—The same as has been indicated at the end of Section 17.

SECTION 20.

THE MENSES ARE TOO SCANTY.—Principal remedies:

1. *Ammonium*, *Conium*, *Dulcamara*, *Graphites*, *Kali*, *Lachesis*, *Pulsatilla*, *Sepia*, *Sulphur*.

2. *Baryta*, *Cocculus*, *Magnesia carbon.*, *Natrum muriaticum*, *Phosphorus*.

3. *Aconitum*, *Alumina*, *Causticum*, *Cuprum*, *Lycopodium* *Magnes arcticus*, *Mercurius*, *Ruta*, *Sabadilla*, *Sarsaparilla*, *Sepia*, *Silicea*. *Staphysagria*.

With the following particular indications:

AMMONIUM.—Menses too short, with pressure on the parts, backache, cramp-colic, toothache, violent pains in the sides, pale face, coryza and shivering.

CONIUM.—Scanty and premature menses, preceded by painful sensitiveness of the breasts. During the menses: painful abdominal cramps, bearing down on the parts, and pulling in the thighs.

DULCAMARA.—The menses are too short and scanty, with pale and serous blood; tetter at the vulva.

GRAPHITES.—Pale blood, with violent headache, nausea in the morning, labor-pains, painfulness of the varices, rheumatic pains in the limbs, uterine spasms, pains in the chest, weakness, the ulcers are worse.

KALI CARBONICUM.—Short and scanty menses, with dropsical symptoms, pale blood, soreness of the parts, abdominal colic, nausea, flatulence, etc.

LACHESIS.—Short and scanty menses, especially after the ineffectual use of Sepia, toothache which is worse in proportion as the menses flow scantily, colic, leucorrhœa, cramps in the bowels.

PULSATILLA.—Delaying and short menses, gastralgic pains, black and thick blood, or else pale and watery, flowing only at times; shivering, pale face, sadness, melancholy, weeping mood; burning cramps in the bowels, leucorrhœa.

SEPIA.—Scanty and delaying menses, with toothache, swelling of the cheeks, fainting weakness, blur before the eyes; lameness, rheumatic pains, abdominal cramps, with pressure on the parts.

SULPHUR.—When the other remedies fail, and the following symptoms occur: Pale blood, drowsiness in the day-time, abdominal cramps, convulsions, pains in the sides and bowels, itching of the parts.

For further details, see Sections 5–10, and *Amenorrhœa.*

DOSE.—The same as at the close of Section 17.

SECTION 21.

MENSES WHICH ARE TOO SHORT.—Principal remedies:

1. *Ammonium*, *Baryta*, *Conium*, *Dulcamara*, *Graphites*, *Lachesis*, *Pulsatilla*, *Sulphur.*

2. *Alumina*, *Cuprum*, *Magnesia carbonica*, *Mercurius*, *Natrum muriaticum*, *Platina*, *Ruta*, *Sabadilla.*

3. *Bryonia*, *Bovista*, *Carbo animalis*, *Colchicum*, *Iodium*, *Ipecacuanha*, *Kali*, *Lycopodium*, *Magnes arcticus*, *Magnesia muriatica*, *Manganum*, *Moschus*, *Nux vomica*, *Rhodendron*, *Sarsaparilla*, *Silicea.*

With the following particular indications:

AMMONIUM.—Menses too scanty and too pale, with colic, toothache and pains in the sides.

BARYTA.—Menses too short and too scanty, with leucorrhœa, swelling of the gums and toothache.

CONIUM.—Scanty menses and short, with painful pulling from the back to the sacrum; painful uterine spasms.

DULCAMARA.—Menses short and delaying, with pale and watery blood; scanty menses.

GRAPHITES.—Menses short and scanty, with pale blood, pains in the sides, shivering, colic and diarrhœa after the menses.

LACHESIS.—Short and scanty menses, with distress, especially at the critical age; abdominal cramps, during the menses.

PULSATILLA.—Menses short, scanty and delaying, with thick and black, or else pale and serous blood, leucorrhœa, shivering, pale face and weeping mood.

SULPHUR.—Menses too short, pale and scanty, with headache, itching at the vulva, colic, corrosive leucorrhœa.

For further details see Sections 5–10.

DOSE.—The same as at the close of Section 17.

SECTION 22.

MORBID CHANGES IN THE MENSTRUAL BLOOD.—The normal menstrual blood is red, liquid, a little sticky, almost resembling arterial blood; according to some authors, it should not coagulate, whereas others look upon the presence of coagula in the menstrual fluid as something quite natural. As a general rule the menstrual blood, as regards color, quantity, intensity of the flow, differs a good deal from one period to the other. It is successively very red, less red, pale like water, black, thick, viscous or fluid. Sometimes those changes can be traced to distinct causes, such as a keen disappointment, after which the flow becomes either more scanty or more copious, or the color of the blood changes; in spasmodic affections the blood is paler; in scrofulous persons it is scanty, paler, less consistent, or else thick and black. Among chlorotic individuals it is almost always watery, pale, causing scarcely a yellow stain. In syphilitic affections it is likewise very often discolored and pale. In eruptive, scorbutic, typhoid affections, the blood is sometimes blackish and fetid. If the blood is retained in the uterus for some time, it becomes black, thin, inodorous. In cancerous or herpetic affections, the menstrual blood has been known to possess deleterious characters, and to communicate by intercourse non-syphilitic discharges from the urethra. But in most cases it is impossible to account for the changes which take place in the menstrual blood. Hence these changes seem of very little avail in establishing a general dignosis; but they help to point out the remedy which is most adapted to some peculiar menstrual irregularity. Here follow the various therapeutic indications which we are enabled to offer in reference to this subject:

BLOOD ACRID, burning, excoriating, smarting:—1. *Kali, Silicea.*
2. *Bovista, Graphites, Sarsaparilla, Sepia.*
3. *Ammonium, Arsenicum, Cantharis, Nitrum.*
4. *Baryta, Carbo veget., Hepar, Rhus, Sulphur, Sulphuris acidum, Zincum.*

BLACK, dark:—1. *Chamomilla, Crocus, Nux vomica, Pulsatilla.*
2. *Ammonium, Antimonium, Kreosotum, Lachesis, Magnesia carbon., Nitri acidum, Sepia.*
3. *Aurum, Belladonna, Bryonia, China, Sulphuris.*
4. *Arnica, Cantharis, Cuprum, Ignatia, Lycopodium, Nux moschata, Phosphorus acidum, Platina, Selenium, Stramonium.*
5. *Aconite, Carbo veget., Cocculus, Conium, Digitalis, Drosera, Ferrum, Graphites, Ledum, Magnesia muriatica, Nitrum, Phosphorus, Secale.*

COAGULATED:—1. *Chamomilla, Platina, Rhus.*
2. *Belladonna, China, Ferrum, Hyoscyamus, Ignatia, Ipecacuanha, Pulsatilla, Sabina, Stramonium.*
3. *Arnica, Cantharis, Causticum, Crocus, Magnesia muriat., Mercurius, Nitrum, Nitri acidum, Phosphori acidum, Strontiana.*
4. *Bryonia, Carbo animalis, Kreosotum, Nux vomica, Secale, Sepia.*

FETID:—1. *Belladonna, Bryonia.*
2. *Carbo animalis, Chamomilla, Crocus, Sabina.*
3. *Ignatia, Silicia, Sulphur.*
4. *Arsenicum, Carbo veget., Causticum, China, Kali, Mercurius, Phosphorus, Platina, Secale.*

PALE, watery:—1. *Belladonna, Dulcamara, Hyoscyamus, Sabina.*
2. *Carbo veget., Graphites, Pulsatilla, Sulphur.*
3. *Arnica, Calcarea, Ferrum, Ledum, Magnes australis, Phosphorus, Rhus, Secale.*

4. *Antimonium, Bryonia, Drosera, Ipecacuanha, Laurocerasus, Lycopodium, Mercurius, Nitrum, Nitri acidum, Platina, Sabadilla, Strontiana, Zincum.*
5. *Ammonium, Arsenicum, Borax, Bovista, Cantharis, Carbo animalis, China, Digitalis, Kreosotum, Magnesia, Nux moschata, Sepia, Silicea, Stramonium.*

SLIMY:—1. *Cocculus.*
2. *Pulsatilla, Sulphuric acidum.*

LOUR:—*Sulphur.*

THICK:—1. *Pulsatilla.*
2. *Crocus, Cuprum, Platina.*
3. *Arnica.*
4. *Carbo veget., Nitrum, Nux moschata, Sulphur.*

VISCOUS:—1. *Crocus.*
2. *Cuprum.*
3. *Secale.*
4. *Magnesia Carbon., Magnesia muriatica.*

For further details see Sections 5–10.

ARTICLE IV

AMENORRHŒA.

SECTION 23.

GENERAL OBSERVATIONS.—By amenorrhœa we understand, in common with other authors, a menstrual suppression, which may occur between the periods of pregnancy and nursing, from the age of pubescence to the critical age at a later period. According to the functions of the organs which preside over the process of menstruation, a suppression may be owing to two distinct circumstances, namely:

1st. *Deficient exhalation or secretion*, in which case the menstrual blood is not furnished or secreted by the exhalants.

2d. *Deficient excretion*, in which case the blood is indeed regularly secreted, but its discharge from the womb is prevented by some cause or other.

Either of these cases may occur from the period when the first menses were to appear; or else it may only occur as an accidental derangement in females who had already menstruated. With reference to these conditions we distinguish:

1. *Primitive amenorrhœa*, also termed *menstrual retention* or *anæmia*, such as occurs in young girls at the age of pubescence and afterwards.

2. *Secondary amenorrhœa*, or *menstrual suppression*, as may set in suddenly in consequence of some accident or morbid cause, or else developing itself gradually, and causing a more or less complete suspension of the menstrual flow in females who had already menstruated.

But howsoever distinct these various conditions may be in a physiological aspect, pathologically and symptomatically they are so nearly related to each other that they cannot well be treated separately without plunging into endless repetitions. Whatever may be the nature of amenorrhœa in a given case, and independently of its primary or secondary origin, the symptoms, so far from being the same in every case, may present, on the contrary, an endless variety, and the same symptoms may occur in one form as well as in another.

This shows that the symptoms ought to be presented independently of the various forms of amenorrhœa where they occur, so much more as these symptoms may be classed under two distinct categories, namely: such as denote *inflammation*, and such as denote *weakness;* upon which distinction several authors have founded the division of amenorrhœa in

a, *Sthenic* amenorrhœa, with inflammatory symptoms; and

b, *Asthenic* amenorrhœa, with symptoms of debility or anæmia.

We will treat of these various forms in the following order:

1st. Of the *symptoms* of amenorrhœa generally.

2nd. Of the *causes* of amenorrhœa.

3rd. *Course* and *complications.*

4th. *Diagnosis* and *prognosis.*

5th. *Treatment* of the various forms of amenorrhœa.

SECTION 24.

SYMPTOMS OF AMENORRHŒA.—What strikes us most in the condition of females attacked with amenorrhœa, is the *sthenic*, *asthenic* or purely *local* character of the symptoms, denoting either general *hyperæmia* or *anæmia*, or a *local engorgement;* so far as a rational treatment of amenorrhœa is concerned, these differences are of the utmost importance. *Sthenic* or *inflammatory* amenorrhœa, which is peculiar to sanguineous constitutions, attacks more particularly young girls of a rose-colored and warm skin, with tendency to perspire, swelling of the sub-cutaneous veins, etc. The most frequent uterine symptoms in such cases are: distress in the hypogastrium and the umbilical region, extending sometimes to the sides and at other times to the vagina and thighs, and consisting either of a simple heaviness or of violent, cutting or boring colic, with uterine cutting pains, swelling of the abdomen, tumefaction of the labia majora and minora, heat in the vagina, with discharge of mucus; loss of appetite, nausea, eructations, vomiting, constipation, dysuria, swelling of the breasts, with or without secretion of milk, dyspnœa, palpitation, febrile movements, general lassitude, pain in the limbs or joints, redness of the face, congested state of the eyes, headache, vertigo, buzzing in the ears, drowsiness, or sleep disturbed by dreams; pains in the stomach, diarrhœa, fainting turns, neuralgic pains in the breasts or thighs, etc. In primary amenorrhœa, the symptoms of abdominal congestion generally disappear, one after another, in a few days, and return again with increased intensity at the next period; whereas, in secondary amenorrhœa, when the menses are suppressed by some sudden cause, a real metritis may develope itself, together with many other symptoms, such as—general anasarca, partial dropsy, mental derangement, hysteria, paralysis, epilepsy, convulsions, tonic spasms, aphonia, loss of memory, etc. In *asthenic amenorrhœa*, which most generally occurs in lymphatic young girls, that have not yet menstruated, the symptoms of uterine congestion are almost wanting; but there occur, on the other hand, a good many symptoms of constitutional derangement, such as discoloration of the skin, flabby and bloated flesh, dull and languid look, headache in the back part of the head, buzzing in the ears, small and frequent pulse, lassitude, aversion to exercise, taste for strange things to eat, nausea, vomiting, chlorotic symptoms. In amenorrhœa caused by obstructions in the passage from the uterus and through the vagina, we have, besides the abovementioned sympathetic symptoms of sthenic amenorrhœa, which may all be present again, several local symptoms, such as an enlargement, increasing from below upwards, and extending from the pubes to the umbilicus; at each successive period it grows larger and larger, so that it sometimes simulates pregnancy, especially if the breasts swell at the same time. When the blood accumulates in large quantity in the uterus, it gradually compresses the rectum, bladder, the sacral plexus, the sciatic nerves, impeding stool and the urinary emission, and causing a tingling in the lower extremities, pains in the groins, colic, uterine cramps, sensitiveness of the hypogastrium, and a variety of other sympathetic symptoms, resembling those of sthenic amenorrhœa.

Section 25.

Causes of Amenorrhœa.—We have stated above that menstrual suppression may arise, first: from *deficient secretion* of blood in the womb; and secondly, from *retention* of the secreted blood in the cavity of the uterus, or in the vagina. In the former case, where the menstrual blood is not secreted in sufficient quantity to be expelled from the womb, the causes of this deficiency generally exist anteriorly to the period of pubescence, and are inherent in the constitution of the girl. These causes are:—first: a nervous constitution; second, a robust or plethoric constitution; third, a weakly or cachectic constitution; fourth, a lymphatic, flabby constitution, with white skin and tendency to grow fleshy. Among the direct causes we have to notice, atrophy of the uterus or ovaria, deficient development, functional weakness, or entire absence of the uterus. Primary amenorrhœa is sometimes owing to organic affections and visceral lesions in other parts of the body, such as pulmonary phthisis, chlorosis, scrofula, etc. Hence we see that the causes which prevent the first appearance of the menses, in young girls, are generally of a constitutional character, and predispose the person for such a difficulty. This remark likewise, applies to *secondary* or accidental amenorrhœa, which develops itself gradually, slowly, or incompletely, for the same causes which prevent the first menstrual flow in young girls, afterwards operate to gradually arrest the menses after they have made their appearance. It is different in *sudden* menstrual suppressions; here *occasional causes* play the chief part. Among them we distinguish in the first place low dwellings, badly lighted, cold, wet and insalubrious; extreme changes of temperature; the requirements of fashion and gallantry, in consequence of which, dashing women sometimes expose themselves half covered to the air, and at other times load themselves with unnecessary garments. The improper use of corsets, cold baths, washes, astringent injections, stimulating food or insufficient nourishment, may likewise occasion the suppression. Changes of locality and occupation, and the functions to which females may have to attend, are likewise exciting causes.

A sedentary mode of life, like that of the seamstress, nun, etc., or excessive exercise, like that of dancers, singers, servants, etc., induce amenorrhœa as readily as a change from the country to a large city, admission to an hospital, a boarding-school or convent, a fatiguing journey, standing behind the counter, or any other radical change in the condition of young girls. Complete abstemiousness or sexual excesses, may likewise occasion amenorrhœa. Exposure to cold air when sweating, cold drinks or washes, ice-cream, loss of blood, sudden acute diseases, intense pain, odors, considerable changes in one's mode of life, fatigue, emetics, purgatives, abuse of drugs either in domestic practice or under treatment; all such causes may likewise induce menstrual suppression. The same may be said of sudden emotions, such as anger, sudden joy, fright, etc. In some cases amenorrhœa is only a symptomatic and sympathetic condition, caused by some other affection, such as pulmonary tubercles, chronic laryngitis, epilepsy, chlorosis, carcinoma, arthritis, diseases of the womb, ovaries, brain, heart, stomach, lungs, breasts, etc. As regards amenorrhœa from *deficient excretion*, it is always produced by mechanical difficulties which prevent the free discharge of blood, such as malformation of the parts, closing of the vulva, obstruction of the mouth of the womb by mucous secretions, membranes across the vagina, etc.

Section 26.

Course, Complications and Terminations.—Considered in itself, amenorrhœa runs a continuous course, except that, in the sthenic variety, when the suppression took place suddenly, there occurs about the period when the menses ought to appear, an aggravation of all the general and local symptoms. As regards the duration of amenorrhœa, it is exceedingly variable; accidental amenorrhœa may last but a very short time, whereas primary amenorrhœa, and such as is depending upon some other organic affections, may run a very long course. As regards complications, we find almost every form of disease mentioned by the various authors as resulting from the gradual or sudden suppression of the menses. Such are pulmonary phthisis, asthma, chlorosis, heart-disease, cancer, pains in the stomach, dyspepsia, piles, megrim, hysteria, hypochondria, various moral and mental affections, chorea, convulsions, nervous diseases, lesions of the lymphatic system, phlegmasiæ, disorganizations, rheumatisms, gout, various eruptions and ulcerations, herpes, styes, erysipelas, cutaneous diseases, ophthalmia, toothache, catarrhal discharges, hæmorrhages from other organs. However, although many of these diseases are undoubtedly caused by amenorrhœa, yet it is well known at this day that they, on the contrary, cause the suppression. Such are all chronic affections, such as phthisis, cancer, plethora, chlorosis, anæmia, general weakness, heart-disease, chronic rheumatism, gout, paralysis, etc. But it is different as regards the mucous discharges, vicarious hæmorrhages, inflammatory congestions, leucorrhœa, mucous diarrhœa, otorrhœa, bronchial catarrh, blind or fluent piles, ophthalmia, otitis, stomachitis, megrim and the other forms of neuralgia or neurosis that develope themselves as consequences of sudden amenorrhœa. These symptoms are real complications of amenorrhœa, and disappear again as soon as the discharge returns, whereas, in all cases where amenorrhœa is a symptom of some other disease, the flow can only be restored by removing the disease which causes the suppression.

Section 27.

Diagnosis and prognosis.—The existence of amenorrhœa is known by the evidence of the fact; but what we have particularly to ascertain is, whether the suppression arises from the retention of the menstrual blood, or from deficient secretion of this fluid in the womb. Retention often simulates pregnancy; but when the menses have been suppressed for several months, the absence of the uterine *souffle*, and of the beating of the fœtal heart, will enable us to establish a correct diagnosis. It is likewise easy to know whether amenorrhœa is caused by an imperforate hymen, a simple inspection of the vulva being sufficient to convince ourselves of this fact. If the obstacle to the discharge of the menstrual blood is situated higher up in the vagina, we have to institute a fuller exploration of the parts, which is unfortunately not always practicable; the touch through the rectum, or the introduction of a probe into the vagina, are sometimes sufficient to obtain a good diagnosis. If no mechanical difficulty whatever opposes the passage of the blood from the womb, the amenorrhœa is evidently caused by deficient secretion, in which case we have to determine whether the disorder arises from a simple delay, or from constitutional weakness, or from some other peculiar irregularity or morbid condition. In diagnosing this difficulty, the physician may be guided by the age of the patient, influences of climate, her mode of life, poverty or wealth, education, etc. In Paris, the first menses generally appear at the age of fourteen; in the country they generally appear later; in capitals and manufacturing towns at an earlier period. Young girls who are exposed to misery and starvation, menstruate later than those of the middle classes; the young ladies of wealth and fashion menstruate soonest. This shows that, without a careful examination of all the surrounding circumstances, we may mistake a natural delay for an actual suppression. At the critical period a most natural cessation of the menstrual flow may likewise be mistaken for amenorrhœa. If there is reason to apprehend the existence of pregnancy, we had better, in case of doubt, wait some months before we make up any diagnosis, until the beating of the fœtal heart can be heard. Lastly, in order to decide whether amenorrhœa is *symptomatic* or *idiopathic*,—in other words, whether it is caused by, or results from the concomitant affections, it will be sufficient, in most cases, to ascertain whether the suppression has preceded or followed the alteration of the general health, or whether in case of *primary* amenorrhœa, the young girl is suffering from one of those affections which generally induce absence of the menstrual secretion, such as: chlorosis, phthisis, scrofula, diseases of the uterus, etc. As regards *prognosis*, it differs a good deal, and depends entirely upon the causes of the irregularity. As a general rule *sthenic* amenorrhœa yields more speedily to remedial agents than *asthenic* amenorrhœa, and a *sudden* suppression is often removed very easily. A mechanical retention of the menses is not at all dangerous when caused by an imperforate hymen; but if such a retention should be caused by adhesion of the parietes of the vagina or uterus, it may lead to fatal results.

SECTION 28.

TREATMENT, PRINCIPAL REMEDIES:—It is of particular importance, in the treatment of amenorrhœa, to ascertain whether the absence of the menstrual discharge is owing to constitutional or accidental causes, in other words, whether it is an idiopathic or sypmtomatic condition. In the latter case, it becomes absolutely necessary to treat the disease of which amenorrhœa is a symptom. In the present instance we shall, therefore, treat only of *idiopathic* amenorrhœa, especially when caused by some accidental circumstance; as regards *primary* absence of the menstrual flow, it will be treated of in detail in the next article, under the head of *amœnia* of young girls. However we shall here give all the phenomenal indications which may possibly occur in amenorrhœa; and likewise in order to meet those cases where the diagnosis might be more or less doubtful. The principal remedies for amenorrhœa are:

1. *Conium*, *Dulcamara*, *Graphites*, *Kali*, *Lycopodium*, *Pulsatilla*, *Sepia*, *Silicea*, *Sulphur*.

2. *Aconitum*, *Ammonium*, *Baryta*, *Bryonia*, *Calcarea*, *Causticum*, *Chamomilla*, *Cocculus*, *Cuprum*, *Ferrum*, *Natrum muriaticum*, *Phosphorus*, *Sabadilla*, *Valeriana*.

3. *Alumina*, *Arsenicum*, *Belladonna*, *Borax*, *China*, *Iodium*, *Mercurius*, *Natrum*, *Nux moschata*, *Opium*, *Platina*, *Sabina*, *Staphysagria*, *Veratrum*, *Zincum*.

4. *Agnus*, *Arnica*, *Aurum*, *Carbo animalis*, *Carbo veget.*, *Colchicum*, *Colocynthis*, *Crocus*, *Digitalis*, *Drosera*, *Euphrasia*, *Guajacum*, *Helleborus*, *Hyoscyamus*, *Ignatia*, *Lachesis*, *Magnesia carbon.*, *Magnesia muriat.*, *Manganum*, *Nitri acidum*, *Petroleum*, *Phosphoric acidum*, *Rhododendron*, *Rhus*, *Ruta*, *Sarsaparilla*, *Secale*, *Stramonium*, *Strontiana*.

With the following particular indications:

CONIUM.—Chlorotic symptoms and hysteria; the breasts are flabby and shrivelled, or else hard and painful; nervous prostration, weakness with involuntary laughing and weeping; exhaustion after the shortest walk; anxiety and sadness; abdominal and uterine cramps, with distention of the bowels, and lancinating pains; hardness of the neck of the uterus; stinging in the parts; itching of the vulva; leucorrhœa with uterine cramps or colic; painful pimples at the pubes; abstemiousness.

DULCAMARA.—Suppression in consequence of a cold, or in females affected with tetter at the parts or on other parts of skin; the breasts are engorged and hard; scrofulous constitution, with glandular engorgements; warts on the hands; disposition to cold in the head and other mucous discharges; tendency to urticaria; frequent sore throat.

GRAPHITES.—Occasional show of the menses, but they are too pale and short, with abdominal cutting pains, uterine cramps, hysteric spasms, rheumatic pains in the limbs; œdema of the feet and hands; tetter or erysipelatous affections; hysteric headache; nausea; pains in the chest; weakness; leucorrhœa, sterility, piles, chlorosis.

KALI CARBONICUM.—One of our best remedies, for primary or secondary amenorrhœa, especially when the following symptoms are present; dyspnœa, palpitation of the heart; frequent erysipelatous eruptions; alternate paleness and redness of the face; febrile heat, with thirst and restless sleep; abdominal cramps, with sour eructations; swelling of the cheek, with stinging and swelling of the gums; leucorrhœa; smarting redness and soreness of the parts and between the thighs; irritation of the vagina during cöit; disposition to pulmonary phthisis; organic disease of the heart.

LYCOPODIUM.—Chlorotic symptoms, sadness, weeping; hysteric headache; sour mouth and vomiting; swelling of the feet; headache with pain in the sides and colic; frequent fainting turns; leucorrhœa; swelling and pressure in the pit of the stomach; drawing and tensive pains in the abdomen; the menses are suppressed by the least fright; frequent shivering; milky leucorrhœa; burning in the vagina during an embrace; bearing-down on the groin; *dryness of the vagina;* passage of wind from the vagina.

PULSATILLA.—One of our best remedies for amenorrhœa, when caused by exposure to dampness and cold, or by getting the feet wet, with the following symptoms; *semilateral headache*, with stitches through the face and teeth; pale complexion; vertigo with buzzing in the ears; stinging and wandering toothache; frequent cold in the head; dyspnœa and oppression after the least emotion; *palpitation of the heart;* coldness of the hands and feet; mucous diarrhœa; leucorrhœa; stomach ache, with nausea and vomiting; continual shuddering with yawning and stretching; swelling of the feet; gentle disposition, with tendency to sadness; freckles in the face.

SEPIA.—Almost as important a remedy for amenorrhœa as Pulsatilla, especially when accompanied by leucorrhœa or by the following symptoms; hysteric headache or megrim, frequently; toothache, with sensitiveness of the nerves; delicate constitution; delicate, white and tender skin; pale complexion, or yellowish spots in the face; nervous weakness, with disposition to perspire; alternate shuddering and heat; melancholy, sad mood, weeping; frequent cold in the head; lameness and soreness of the limbs; frequent colic and pain in the sides.

Silicea.—Melancholy, anguish in the epigastrium, with thought of suicide; soreness and redness of the parts; blur before the eyes, diarrhœa; weak chest, with pthisicky disposition, pressive headache above the eyes; constipation, hard stool; smarting, acrid, corrosive leucorrhœa, with abdominal colic and cutting pains; itching of the vulva.

Sulphur.—Pressive and tensive headache, especially at the occiput; congestion of the head, with throbbing and buzzing in the brain; pale and sickly face, with red spots on the cheeks and rings around the eyes; excessive appetite, with loss of flesh; pressure, fulness and weight in the stomach, hypochondria and abdomen; piles; mucous diarrhœa, or else constipation, with ineffectual urging to stool; leucorrhœa, with itching of the parts; hysteria and chlorotic symptoms; dyspnœa; tendency to take cold; weariness after talking; irascible mood, or sad and weeping disposition.

Dose.—Give from four to six globules dry on the tongue, or one or two drops of the attenuated tincture on sugar, or in a spoonful of water, the morning after the day when the menses should have made their appearance, and repeat this dose every week until the flow sets in. In acute cases of sudden suppression, one or two drops of the attenuated remedy may be mixed in ten table-spoonfuls of water, and a table-spoonful of this solution may be given every five or six hours, until the discharge returns. If it does not return in a day or two, discontinue the medicine, and resume it again a few days before the next period.

Section 29.

Other Remedies.—To the above-mentioned remedies, which will be found sufficient in most cases, we will subjoin a few more, which will likewise be found indicated by the symptoms in some cases:

Aconitum.—Frequent congestion of the head or chest, with stitching or throbbing pains, and beating of the heart; pressive headache; red face; pulse full and hard; frequent attacks of heat, with thirst; irascible mood; fainting and vertigo on raising one's head in a recumbent posture; the symptoms are aggravated by motion and heat, eased by cold. Is particularly suitable to plethoric young girls of a sanguine temperament, and leading a sedentary life.

Ammonium carbonicum.—Pains in the sides, toothache and shivering; pale face, frequent coryza, violent tearing colic; cutting colic, with pressure on the parts; profuse, acrid and corrosive leucorrhœa; soreness of the parts and between the thighs; scrofulous symptoms, impetiginous eruptions, with swelling of the glands and earache; scorbutic symptoms.

Baryta.—Toothache, with swelling of the gums; colic, with heaviness of the limbs; scrofulous symptoms; retarded development and growth, in young girls; weakness, leucorrhœa, pains in the breasts.

Bryonia.—Vascular excitement, frequent congestion of the head or chest, with nose-bleed and dry cough; frequent coldness and shuddering, sometimes alternating with dry heat; constipation; pressive gastralgia or colic.

Calcarea.—Frequent congestion of the head, with vertigo; burning pains in the forehead, or pulsative headache; buzzing in the ears; painful pressure in the hypochondria, even the pressure of the clothes is unpleasant to bear; colic and cutting in the bowels, down to the thighs, especially at the time when the menses should appear; fatigue and heaviness in the whole body, especially the legs.

Causticum.—In cases where *Ammonium* seems indicated, but has no effect; hysteric symptoms, cutting colic; uterine cramps; yellowish complexion; gloomy melancholy, vertigo; backache; stinging in the breasts; profuse leucorrhœa, with colic; soreness of the parts; aversion to intercourse.

Chamomilla.—Suppression in consequence of suppressed sweat; cramp-colic, peevish mood, quarrelsome, irascible; yellowish complexion, redness of one cheek and paleness of the other; cramps in the stomach, with dyspnœa and wind; diarrhœa, with colic and cutting pains; fainting turns; nausea, desire to vomit, with yellowish tongue and bitter mouth; distress in the sides.

Cocculus.—Leucorrhœa in the place of the menses, with abdominal cramps, hysteric symptoms, pressure on the chest, oppression, uneasiness and anguish, with sadness and frequent sighs; weakness, so that she is almost unable to speak; nervous symptoms; discharge of a few drops of black blood.

Cuprum.—Congestion of the head; feverish headache on the top of the head; redness of the face and eyes, or else full face with rings around the eyes; frequent nausea and vomiting; abdominal cramps; convulsions and cries; palpitation of the heart and cramps in the chest.

Ferrum.—Weariness and weakness with trembling, loss of flesh and desire to remain seated or lying; congestion of the head, with pulsative headache; buzzing and pricking in the brain; pale and leaden face, with margins around the eyes, or red face and eyes; pressure in the shoulder and head; œdematous swelling of the face, hands and feet; lassitude in the legs and other chlorotic symptoms.

Natrum muriaticum.—Chlorotic, phthisicky, or scrofulous symptoms; pimples and itching at the vulva; falling off of the hair; congestion of the head, headache; irascible mood; uneasiness and melancholy; stinging and tearing in the teeth; cramp-colic; blood-spitting; nocturnal fever with thirst and sleeplessness; aversion to intercourse; leucorrhœa.

Phosphorus.—Suppression in young persons who generally menstruate pretty copiously, with leucorrhœa; frequent desire to urinate; weeping mood; toothache; abdominal colic; violent backache; *spitting of blood;* lameness of the limbs; congestion of the chest and head; *vicarious hæmorrhage* from the anus, urethra or other organs.

Sabadilla.—Sometimes useful in cases where *Pulsatilla, Sepia* or *Sulphur* seem indicated, but do not produce any effect.

Valeriana.—Suitable to nervous or hysteric females who have drank much chamomile-tea.

Dose.—The same as at the close of Section 28.

SECTION 30.

REMEDIES THAT ARE RARELY INDICATED.—If none of the previously-named remedies suffice, we may have recourse to the following:

ALUMINA, if *Calcarea* seems indicated, but remains ineffectual; restless sleep, with dreams and headache, heat in the face, palpitation of the heart on waking; leucorrhœa with weakness; uterine cramps.

ARSENICUM.—Prostration; pale face with margins around the eyes; desire for acids, coffee, brandy; sexual excitement; corrosive leucorrhœa; fainting turns.

BELLADONNA, suitable to plethoric girls, with congestion of the head and chest; throbbing headache; heat in the head; red and bloated face; numbness of the legs when sitting; anguish about the heart; burning thirst; cramp-pains in the sides and back.

BORAX.—Suppression in females who generally menstruate sufficiently; weight on the chest, dyspnœa, buzzing in the ears, throbbing in the head, etc.

CHINA.—Pale face, rings around the eyes, pressive headache at night; pressure at the stomach after eating; dyspepsia; loss of flesh; weakness; restless sleep, with anxious and fatiguing dreams; abdominal and pulmonary spasms; nymphomania; nervousness.

IODIUM.—Frequent palpitation of the heart; pale face, alternating sometimes with redness; out of breath on going up stairs; weariness in the legs, chlorotic symptoms.

MERCURIUS.—Congestion of the head, with dry heat and vascular excitement; leucorrhœa; œdematous swelling of the hands, feet and face; pale face; sickly look; weakness and trembling after the least work; sad or peevish; contrary mood.

NATRUM CARBONICUM.—Frequent headache; hysteric or chlorotic symptoms; disposition to sadness, with apathy; physical and mental weakness, with heaviness in the limbs, aversion to motion; irascible mood.

NUX MOSCHATA.—Suppression, with spasms and other hysteric symptoms, tending to sleep and fainting; prostration after the least effort; mucus on the stomach; fitful mood.

OPIUM.—Suppression with congestion of the head which feels heavy; red and hot face; drowsiness; convulsive twitchings.

PLATINA.—Sudden suppressions in females who are ordinarily regular, with spasmodic colic; constipation; hard stool; anguish; uneasiness; weeping.

SABINA.—Sudden suppression, followed by a thick and fetid leucorrhœa.

STAPHYSAGRIA.—Sensitiveness of the parts, with cramp-pains; itching of the parts; blotches and vesicles at the labia.

VERATRUM.—Amenorrhœa, with nervous headache and hysteric ailments; pale, leaden face, frequent nausea with vomiting and cold hands, feet and nose; weakness, fainting turns, sexual excitement.

For further information and details, see Sections 5–10, and the following:

DOSE.—The same as at the close of Section 28.

SECTION 31.

PARTICULAR INDICATIONS.—We here subjoin a few particular indications regarding the different forms of Amenorhœa, and the ailments which sometimes accompany the cessation of the menstrual flow.

a. FOR THE DIFFERENT SPECIES OF AMENORRHŒA.

AMENORRHŒA, primary, from the period of pubescence:—

1. *Pulsatilla*, *Sulphur*.
2. *Causticum*, *Graphites*, *Kali*.
3. *Conium*, *Ferrum*, *Magnesia carbon.*, *Natrum muriat.*, *Petroleum*, *Sabina*, *Sepia*.
4. *Agnus*, *Ammonium*, *Chelidon.*, *Cocculus*, *Digitalis*, *Dulcamara*, *Silicea*, *Veratrum*.

5. *Aconite, Aurum, Bryonia, Calcarea, Cicuta, Crocus, Cuprum, Drosera, Guajacum, Hyoscyamus, Lachesis, Magnesia muriat., Mercurius, Phosphorus, Sabadilla, Sarsaparilla, Spigelia, Staphysagria, Stramonium, Strontiana, Veratrum, Zincum.*

From EXCESSIVE VITALITY, with sthenic or inflammatory character:—1. *Aconite, Belladonna, Bryonia, Calcarea, Nux vomica, Opium, Platina, Sabina, Sulphur.*

2. *Chamomilla, Ipecacuanha, Crocus, Mercurius, Natrum muriaticum, Phosphorus.*

From CONSTITUTIONAL WEAKNESS, with asthenic character:—1. *Arsenicum, China, Conium, Graphites, Iodium, Natrum, Pulsatilla, Sepia, Sulphur.*

2. *Ammonium, Baryta, Calcarea, Cocculus, Dulcamara, Ferrum, Kali, Magnesia carbon.*

3. *Alumina, Causticum, Cuprum, Lycopodium, Mercurius, Sabadilla, Silicea, Staphysagria, Veratrum.*

AMENORRHŒA SYMPTOMATIC.

With CEREBRAL symptoms:—*Ammonium, Belladonna, Bryonia, Causticum, Cuprum, Mercurius, Nux vomica, Opium, Sepia, Sulphur, Zincum.*

Chlorosis:—1. *Belladonna, Calcarea, Cocculus, Ferrum, Lycopodium, Nitri acidum, Platina, Pulsatilla, Sulphur.*

2. *China, Conium, Helleborus, Kali, Nux vomica, Phosphorus, Plumbum, Sepia, Spigelia.*

3. *Arsenicum, Digitalis, Graphites, Mercurius, Phosphoricum acidum, Staphysagria, Valeriana.*

4. *Baryta, Carbo animalis, Carbo vegetabilis, Causticum, Ignatia, Oleander, Sabina, Sulphuris acidum, Zincum.*

With HEART AFFECTIONS:—1. *Calcarea, Kali, Natrum muriaticum, Pulsatilla, Spigelia, Sulphur.*

2. *Aconitum, Arsenicum, Aurum, Iodium, Lycopodium, Phosphorus, Sepia, Veratrum, Zincum.*

3. *Belladonna, Carbo vegetabilis, Causticum, Chamomilla, China, Cuprum, Graphites, Mercurius, Natrum, Nitri acidum, Nux moschata, Nux vomica, Platina, Sabina, Secale, Sulphuris acidum.*

With EPILEPSY:—1. *Belladonna, Calcarea, Cuprum, Hyoscyamus, Sulphur.*

2. *Arsenicum Chamomilla, Cocculus, Kali, Lachesis, Lycopodium Natrum muriaticum, Nitri acidum, Nux vomica, Sepia, Silicea.*

3. *Conium, Magnesia carbonica, Opium, Platina, Rhus, Secale, Stramonium.*

With GASTRIC affections:—1. *Arsenicum, Bryonia, Calcarea, Nux vomica, Phosphorus, Pulsatilla, Sulphur, Veratrum.*

2. *Aconitum, China, Cocculus, Kali, Lycopodium, Natrum muriaticum, Rhus, Sepia, Silicea.*

3. *Alumina, Baryta, Belladonna, Carbo vegetabilis, Chamomilla, Conium, Cuprum, Ferrum, Graphites, Hyoscyamus, Iodium, Mercurius, Platina, Plumbum, Sabadilla, Sabina, Secale, Staphysagria, Sulphuris acidum, Valeriana, Zincum.*

With GOUT, symptoms of:—1. *Belladonna, Bryonia, Kali, Mercurius, Rhus, Sabina, Staphysagria.*

2. *Agnus, Baryta, Calcarea, Causticum, China, Cocculus, Ferrum, Graphites, Hyoscyamus, Natrum muriaticum Phosphorus, Pulsatilla, Sepia, Sulphur, Zincum.*

3. *Alumina, Carbo vegetabilis, Chamomilla, Dulcamara, Iodium, Lycopodium, Nux moschata, Nux vomica, Sabadilla, Secale, Silicea.*

Chronic LARYNYSTIS:—1. *Iodium, Nux vomica, Phosphorus, Pulsatilla.*

2. *Aconitum, Belladonna, Carbo vegetabilis, Causticum, Chamomilla, Lachesis, Rhus, Sabadilla, Sulphur, Veratrum, Zincum.*

3. *Alumina*, *Ammonium*, *Arsenicum*, *Calcarea*, *China*, *Cocculus*, *Conicum*, *Graphites*, *Hyoscyamus*, *Kali*, *Magnesia muriatica*, *Mercurius*, *Natrum muriaticum*, *Phosphori acidum*, *Sabina*, *Sepia*.

Mammæ, affection of:—1. *Bryonia*, *Chamomilla*, *Conium*, *Phosphorus*, *Silicea*.

2. *Arsenicum*, *Belladonna*, *Calcarea*, *Graphites*, *Pulsatilla*, *Sulphur*.

3. *Iodium*, *Lycopodium*, *Mercurius*, *Nitri acidum*, *Rhus*, *Sabina*, *Sepia*.

Uterus:—1. *Belladonna*, *Chamomilla*, *Kali*, *Platina*, *Pulsatilla*, *Sabina*, *Sepia*.

2. *Carbo animalis*, *Conium*, *Crocus*, *Ferrum*, *Nux vomica*, *Opium*, *Rhus*, *Secale*, *Sulphur*.

3. *Calcarea*, *China*, *Cocculus*, *Graphites*, *Hyoscyamus*, *Kreosotum*, *Magnesia muriatica*, *Natrum muriaticum*.

Ovaria:—1. *Staphysagria*.

2. *Carbo animalis*, *China*, *Lachesis*, *Lycopodium*, *Secale*, *Sepia*, *Zincum*.

3. *Aconitum*, *Carbo vegetabilis*, *Graphites*, *Mercurius*, *Nitri acidum*, *Nux vomica*, *Sulphur*, *Thuja*.

Pulmonary:—1. *Calcarea*, *China*, *Conium*, *Kali*, *Lycopodium*, *Phosphorus*, *Sepia*, *Silicea*.

2. *Ferrum*, *Kreosotum*, *Mercurius*, *Natrum*, *Phosphoric acid*, *Rhus*, *Staphysagria*.

3. *Arsenicum*, *Cocculus*, *Pulsatilla*, *Sabina*, *Sulphur*.

Schirrous or cancerous of uterus, or breasts:—1. *Carbo animalis*, *Graphites*, *Kreosotum*.

2. *Arsenicum*, *Belladonna*, *China*, *Cocculus*, *Conium*, *Dulcamara*, *Mercurius*, *Nitri acid.*, *Sepia*, *Silicea*, *Staphysagria*, *Thuja*.

Secondary:—1. *Pulsatilla*, *Sepia*, *Sulphur*.

2. *Aconitum*, *Bryonia*, *Conium*, *Dulcamara*, *Graphites*, *Kali*, *Lycopodium*, *Silicea*.

3. *Ammonium*, *Arsenicum*, *Baryta*, *Belladonna*, *Cal carea*, *Chamomilla*, *Cocculus*, *Cuprum*, *Ferrum*, *Natrum muriaticum*, *Phosphorus*.
4. *Alumina*, *Borax*, *Bovista*, *China*, *Mercurius*, *Nux moschata*, *Opium*, *Platina*, *Sabadilla*, *Sabina*, *Staphysagria*, *Stramonium*, *Valeriana*, *Veratrum*, *Zincum*.

By some emotion:—1. *Aconitum*, *Coffea*, *Lycopodium*.
2. *Opium*, *Platina*, *Veratrum*.

By exposure, a cold:—1. *Aconitum*.
2. *Nux moschata*, *Pulsatilla*.
3. *Belladonna*, *Dulcamara*, *Sepia*, *Sulphur*.

By exposure to dampness, wet feet, etc.:—1. *Pulsatilla*.
2. *Nux moschata*.
3. *Calcarea*.

AMENORRHŒA, SECONDARY.

Of young girls who generally menstruate COPIOUSLY:—
1. *Aconitum*, *Belladonna*, *Bryonia*, *Calcarea*, *Nux vomica*, *Opium*, *Platina*, *Sabina*, *Sulphur*.
2. *Chamomilla*, *Crocus*, *Mercurius*, *Natrum muriaticum*, *Phosphorus*.

Of FEEBLE, cachectic females:—1. *Arsenicum*, *China*, *Conium*, *Graphites*, *Iodium*, *Natrum*, *Pulsatilla*, *Sepia*, *Sulphur*.
2. *Ammonium*, *Baryta*, *Cocculus*, *Dulcamara*, *Ferrum*, *Kali*, *Magnesia carbonica*.
3. *Alumina*, *Causticum*, *Cuprum*, *Lycopodium*, *Mercurius*, *Sabadilla*, *Silicea*, *Staphysagria*.

SLOW and gradual:—1. *Ammonium*, *Conium*, *Dulcamara*, *Graphites*, *Kali*, *Lachesis*, *Magnesia carbon.*, *Pulsatilla*, *Sulphur*.
2. *Baryta*, *Cocculus*, *Natrum muriaticum*, *Phosphorus*.
3. *Arnica*, *Alumina*, *Cuprum*, *Lycopodium*, *Mercurius*, *Ruta*, *Sabadilla*, *Sepia*, *Silicea*, *Staphysagria*.

4. *Bryonia*, *Carbo vegetabilis*, *Cicuta*, *Colchicum*, *Digitalis*, *Ferrum*, *Ignatia*, *Magnesia muriatic*, *Nux vomica*, *Thuja*, *Valeriana*, *Veratrum*, *Zincum*.

(See above: *Symptomatic Amenorrhœa, and Primary Amenorrhœa.*)

SECTION 32.

B. ACCOMPANYING SYMPTOMS OF AMENORRHŒA.—By these symptoms we mean all such ailments as may follow menstrual suppression or primary absence of the menstrual flow, as a necessary consequence of such irregularities, not as having been instrumental in producing such suppression. Here follows a list of the principal of such ailments, together with their remedies.

ALIENATION, MENTAL derangement:—1. *Belladonna*, *Hyoscyamus*, *Lachesis*, *Nux vomica*, *Opium*, *Pulsatilla*, *Stramonium*, *Veratrum*.
2. *Arsenicum*, *Calcarea*, *Crocus*, *Cuprum*, *Mercurius*, *Platina*, *Rhus*, *Silicea*, *Sulphur*.
3. *Aconitum*, *Lycopodium*, *Nux moschata*, *Sepia*.

ANASARCA, general:—1. *Arsenicum*, *China*, *Kali*.
2. *Graphites*, *Helleborus*, *Lycopodium*, *Sulphur*.
3. *Bryonia*, *Dulcamara*, *Ferrum*, *Phosphorus*, *Sepia*.
4. *Aconitum*, *Belladonna*, *Iodium*, *Pulsatilla*, *Sabina*.

APHONIA, loss of voice:—*Baryta*, *Belladonna*, *Causticum*, *Sulphur*.
2. *Carbo veget.*, *Mercurius*, *Phosphorus*.
3. *Lachesis*, *Natrum muriat.*, *Platina*, *Pulsatilla*, *Veratrum*.

APPETITE, lost:—1. *Arsenicum*, *Bryonia*, *China*, *Mercurius*, *Nux vomica*, *Pulsatilla*, *Sulphur*.
2. *Aconitum*, *Ammonium*, *Belladonna*, *Calcarea*, *Lachesis*, *Lycopodium*, *Natrum muriat.*, *Platina*, *Rhus*, *Sepia*, *Silicea*.
3. *Baryta*, *Cocculus*, *Conium*, *Iodium*, *Nux moschata*, *Opium*, *Veratrum*.

ARTICULATIONS, pains in the :—1. *Belladonna, Bryonia, Kali, Mercurius, Pulsatilla, Rhus, Sabina, Staphysagria.*

2. *Agnus, Baryta, Calcarea, Causticum, China, Cocculus, Ferrum, Graphites, Hyoscyamus, Natrum, Natrum muriat., Phosphorus, Pulsatilla, Sepia, Sulphur, Zincum.*

3. *Alumina, Carbo veget., Chamomilla, Dulcamara, Iodium, Lycopodium, Nux moschata, Nux vomica, Sabadilla, Secale, Silicea.*

ASCITES :—*Arsenicum, China, Belladonna, Kali, Sulphur.*

2. *Aconitum, Bryonia, Dulcamara, Iodium, Mercurius, Sepia.*

3. *Cuprum, Lycopodium, Pulsatilla.*

ASTHMA :—*Aconitum, Arsenicum, Belladonna, Bryonia, Cuprum, Ferrum, Nux vomica, Phosphorus, Pulsatilla, Sulphur.*

2. *Ammonium, Carbo veget., Hyoscyamus, Kali, Lachesis, Stramonium, Zincum.*

3. *Calcarea, Chamomilla, Cocculus, Dulcamara, Opium, Silicea, Veratrum.*

BRONCHITIS :—1. *Graphites.*

2. *Aconitum, Belladonna, Bryonia, Chamomilla, Mercurius, Nux vomica, Pulsatilla, Rhus, Sulphur.*

3. *Arsenicum, China, Dulcamara, Hyoscyamus, Lachesis, Phosphorus.*

4. *Calcarea, Sepia, Silicia, Staphysagria, Veratrum.*

BUZZING IN EARS :—1. *Belladonna, Graphites, Nux vomica, Pulsatilla, Sulphur.*

2. *Bryonia, Calcarea, Conium, Kali, Lachesis, Lycopodium, Mercurius, Natrum muriat., Platina, Sepia.*

3. *Aconitum, Ammonium, Aurum, Cocculus, Dulcamara, Iodium, Magnesia carbonica, Nitri acidum, Petroleum, Phosphorus, Sabadilla, Silicea, Veratrum.*

CEPHALALGIA congestive : — 1. *Aconitum, Belladonna, Bryonia, Lachesis, Mercurius, Nux moschata, Opium, Pulsatilla, Sulphur.*

2. *Alumina, Chamomilla, China, Dulcamara, Kali, Lycopodium, Nitri acidum, Phosphorus, Sepia, Silicea.*

3. *Calcarea, Crocus, Natrum, Natrum muriaticum, Veratrum.*

HYSTERIC :—1. *Cocculus, Magnesia carbon., Phosphorus, Platina, Sepia, Valeriana, Veratrum.*

2. *Aurum, Hepar, Ignatia, Magnesia muriat., Nitri acidum.*

3. *Chamomilla, Rhus, Ruta.*

Nervous, megrim :—1. *Calcarea, China, Colocynthis, Pulsatilla, Sanguinaria, Sepia.*

2. *Bryonia, Ignatia, Nux vomica, Rhus, Veratrum.*

3. *Aconitum, Arnica, Arsenicum, Belladonna, Chamomilla, Nitri acidum, Silicea, Sulphur.*

CHLOROSIS :—1. *Belladonna, Calcarea, Cocculus, Ferrum, Lycopodium, Nitri acidum, Platina, Pulsatilla, Sulphur.*

2. *China, Conium, Helleborus, Kali, Nux vomica, Phosphorus, Plumbum, Sepia, Spigelia.*

3. *Arsenicum, Digitalis, Graphites, Mercurius, Phosphori acid., Staphysagria, Valeriana.*

4. *Baryta, Carbo animalis, Carbo vegetabilis, Ignatia, Oleander, Sabina, Sulphuris acid., Zincum.*

CHOREA :— 1. *Belladonna, Causticum, Cuprum, Ignatia, Nux vomica.*

2. *Hyoscyamus, Stramonium, Zincum.*

3. *Arsenicum, China, Dulcamara, Iodium, Pulsatilla, Sepia, Silicea.*

4. *Rhus, Sabina, Sulphur.*

COLIC, intestinal :—1. *Belladonna, Calcarea, Chamomilla, Cocculus, Nux vomica, Pulsatilla, Sulphur.*

2. *Aconitum, Graphites, Ignatia, Phosphorus, Platina, Secale, Sepia, Veratrum.*

3. *Alumina, Ammonium, Baryta, China, Conium, Crocus, Cuprum, Lachesis, Silicea, Zincum.*

Uterine; cramps in uterus:—1. *Chamomilla, China, Cocculus, Cuprum, Hyoscyamus, Ignatia.*
2. *Aconitum, Coffea, Lachesis, Pulsatilla.*
3. *Bryonia, Conium, Graphites, Kreosotum, Magnesia muriatica, Natrum muriat., Nux vomica.*

CONGESTIONS OF BRAIN:—1. *Aconitum, Belladonna, Bryonia, Mercurius, Nux vomica, Opium, Pulsatilla, Sulphur.*
2. *Alumina, Chamomilla, China, Dulcamara, Kali, Lycopodium, Nitri acidum, Phosphorus, Sepia, Silicea.*
3. *Calcarea, Crocus, Natrum muriat., Veratrum.*

CHEST:—1. *Aconitum, Belladonna, Nux vomica, Phosphorus, Sulphur.*
2. *Aurum, China, Mercurius.*
3. *Ammonium, Carbo vegetabilis, Cocculus, Ferrum, Iodium, Nitri acidum, Pulsatilla, Rhus, Sepia.*

CONSTIPATION, costiveness:—1. *Bryonia, Calcarea, Cocculus, Lycopodium, Nux vomica, Opium, Silicea, Staphysagria, Sulphur.*
2. *Alumina, Belladonna, Carbo vegetabilis, Conium, Dulcamara, Graphites, Kali, Mercurius, Nitri acidum, Phosphorus, Platina, Sabadilla, Sarsaparilla, Sepia, Sulphuris acidum, Veratrum, Zincum.*
3. *Aconitum, Ammonium, Antimonium, Arsenicum, Baryta, China, Colchicum, Colocynthis, Iodium, Lachesis, Magnesia carbon., Magnesia muriat., Natrum muriat., Pulsatilla, Rhus, Sabina, Stramonium.*

CONVULSIONS, general:—1. *Belladonna, Chamomilla, Cuprum, Hyoscyamus, Opium, Sepia, Stramonium.*
2. *Arsenicum, Bryonia, Calcarea, Causticum, Conium, Ignatia, Kali, Lycopodium, Mercurius, Natrum muriat., Platina, Secale, Silicea, Strontiana, Sulphur.*

3. *Alumina, Carbo vegetabilis, Dulcamara, Iodium, Magnesia carbonica, Manganum, Natrum, Petroleum, Phosphorus, Phosphori acidum, Rhododendron, Rhus, Veratrum.*

DIARRHŒA:—1. *Chamomilla, China, Mercurius, Phosphorus, Phosphori acid., Pulsatilla, Rhus, Sulphur, Veratrum.*

2. *Aconite, Arsenicum, Bryonia, Calcarea, Conium, Digitalis, Hyoscyamus, Lachesis, Nitri acid., Sepia, Silicea.*

3. *Alumina, Antimonium, Baryta, Belladonna, Carbo veget., Cocculus, Colocynthis, Cuprum, Drosera, Dulcamara, Ferrum, Graphites, Ignatia, Iodium, Lycopodium, Nux moschata, Nux vomica, Opium, Petroleum, Sabadilla, Sabina, Secale, Staphysagria, Valeriana, Zincum.*

DYSPNŒA, oppressed breathing:—*Bryonia, Nux vomica, Pulsatilla, Sulphur.*

2. *Arnica, Calcarea, Carbo veget., Mercurius, Natrum, Rhus, Sepia, Silicea.*

3. *Ammonium, Arsenicum, Baryta, Belladonna, Conium, Drosera, Ferrum, Graphites, Hyoscyamus, Ignatia, Kali, Lycopodium, Phosphorus, Staphysagria, Veratrum.*

DYSPEPSIA:—1. *Aconite, Arsenicum, Belladonna, Bryonia, Cuprum, Nux vomica, Phosphorus, Pulsatilla, Sepia, Sulphur, Veratrum.*

2. *Calcarea, Carbo veget., Chamomilla, Cocculus, Ignatia, Kali, Lycopodium, Opium, Platina, Rhus, Zincum.*

3. *Arnica, Aurum, Conium, Ferrum, Hepar, Mercurius, Nux moschata, Sabadilla, Silicea, Staphysagria.*

DYSURIA, difficulty of urinating:—1. *Aconite, Belladonna, Dulcamara, Mercurius, Nux vomica, Pulsatilla, Sulphur.*

2. *Arsenicum, Baryta, Causticum, Graphites, Kali, Nux moschata, Phosphorus, Rhus, Sabina, Staphysagria.*

3. *Arnica, Aurum, Colocynthis, Digitalis, Hepar, Phosphori acidum, Ruta, Sarsaparilla.*

ECCHYMOSIS:—1. *Arsenicum, Bryonia, Rhus.*

2. *Belladonna, Nux vomica, Phosphorus, Secale, Silicea.*

3. *Arnica, Hyoscyamus, Stramonium, Sulphuris acid.*

EPILEPSY:—1. *Belladonna, Calcarea, Cuprum, Hyoscyamus, Sulphur.*

2. *Arsenicum, Chamomilla, Cocculus, Kali, Lachesis, Lycopodium, Nitri acidum, Nux vomica, Sepia.*

3. *Conium, Opium, Platina, Rhus, Secale, Stramonium.*

EPISTAXIS:—1. *Bryonia, Lycopodium.*

2. *Aconite, Belladonna, China, Mercurius, Nux vom., Phosphorus, Pulsatilla, Rhus, Sulphur.*

3. *Arnica, Crocus, Ferrum, Kreosotum, Nitri acidum, Sabina, Secale.*

4. *Ammonium, Arsenicum, Baryta, Calcarea, Carbo veget., Drosera, Dulcamara, Sepia, Silicea.*

ERUCTATIONS:—1. *Belladonna, Bryonia, Cocculus Conium, Mercurius, Nux vomica, Phosphorus, Pulsatilla, Sepia, Sulphur, Veratrum.*

2. *Alumina, Baryta, Calcarea, China, Graphites, Kali, Lycopodium, Natrum, Rhus, Sabadilla, Silicea, Staphysagria, Valeriana.*

3. *Antimonium, Arsenicum, Carbo animalis, Carbo veget., Dulcamara, Ferrum, Ignatia, Ruta, Sulphuris acidum, Zincum.*

ERUPTIONS, cutaneous:—*Arsenicum, Calcarea, Lycopodium, Rhus, Sepia, Silicea Sulphur.*

2. *Aconite, Ammonium, Baryta Bryonia, Conium, Dulcamara Graphites, Kali, Mercurius, Natrum muriat., Pulsatilla, Staphysagria.*

3. *Antimonium, Carbo vegetabilis, Chamomilla, Helleborus, Ignatia, Natrum, Nitri acidum, Nux vomica, Petroleum, Sulphuris acidum, Veratrum, Zincum.*

ERYSIPELAS:—1. *Aconitum, Belladonna, Graphites, Mercurius, Rhus.*

2. *Ammonium, Arsenicum, Bryonia, Calcarea, Iodium, Lycopodium, Phosphorus, Sulphur.*
3. *Arnica, Baryta, Carbo animalis, Carbo vegetabilis, Hepar, Hyoscyamus, Natrum, Petroleum, Pulsatilla, Silicea, Stramonium.*

EYES INJECTED, red:—

BLEEDING:—1. *Belladonna, Nux vomica.*
2. *Calcarea, Carbo vegetabilis, Chamomilla.*
3. *Arnica, Cuprum, Ruta.*

FACE, PALE:—1. *Arsenicum, China, Pulsatilla, Sepia, Sulphur.*
2. *Bryonia, Cocculus, Conium, Cuprum, Ferrum, Kali, Lycopodium, Nux vomica, Phosphorus, Platina, Rhus, Secale, Silicea, Veratrum.*
3. *Ammonium, Antimonium, Belladonna, Calcarea, Chamomilla, Helleborus, Ignatia, Magnesia muriat., Nitri acidum, Petroleum, Phosphori acidum, Sabina, Staphysagria, Zincum.*

RED:—1. *Aconitum, Belladonna, Bryonia, Chamomilla, China, Nux vomica, Opium.*
2. *Cocculus, Ferrum, Hyoscyamus, Ignatia, Lycopodium, Mercurius, Platina, Pulsatilla, Rhus, Sabadilla, Stramonium, Sulphur, Valeriana, Veratrum.*
3. *Ammonium, Arsenicum, Baryta, Calcarea, Conium, Cuprum, Dulcamara, Kali, Natrum, Phosphorus, Sepia, Silicea, Staphysagria.*

FAINTING:—1. *Aconitum, Chamomilla, China, Nux vomica, Sepia, Stramonium.*
2. *Arsenicum, Bryonia, Cocculus, Ferrum, Hyoscyamus, Nux moschata, Opium, Phosphorus, Silicea, Veratrum.*
3. *Belladonna, Calcarea, Carbo vegetabilis, Colocynthis, Digitalis, Ignatia, Kali, Mercurius, Pulsatilla, Rhus, Sabadilla, Sulphur.*

FEVER:—1. *Aconitum, Belladonna, Bryonia, Mercurius, Nux vomica, Phosphorus, Pulsatilla, Rhus.*

2. *Aurum*, *Chamomilla*, *Kali*, *Sulphur*, *Veratrum*.
3. *China*, *Cocculus*, *Nitri acidum*, *Opium*, *Phosphorus*, *Secale*, *Sepia*.

GASTRALGIA, pain in stomach:—*Belladonna*, *Calcarea*, *Cocculus*, *Nux vomica*, *Pulsatilla*, *Sulphur*.
2. *Ammonium*, *Bryonia*, *Chamomilla*, *China*, *Conium*, *Graphites*, *Lachesis*, *Lycopodium*, *Nux moschata*, *Phosphorus*, *Sepia*, *Silicea*.
3. *Carbo animalis*, *Carbo vegetabilis*, *Cuprum*, *Digitalis*, *Ferrum*, *Hyoscyamus*, *Ignatia*, *Kali*, *Magnesia carbonica*, *Natrum muriaticum*, *Petroleum*, *Staphysagria*.

GUMS, SWOLLEN:—1. *Aconitum*, *Belladonna*, *Calcarea*, *Causticum*, *China*, *Nux vomica*, *Staphysagria*, *Sulphur*.
2. *Chamomilla*, *Graphites*, *Rhus*, *Sepia*.
3. *Ammonium*, *Baryta*, *Nitri acid.*, *Phosphorus*, *Silicea*.

BLEEDING:—1. *Calcarea*, *Mercurius*, *Sulphur*.
2. *Arsenicum*, *Carbo vegetabilis*, *Iodium*, *Silicea*, *Zincum*.
3. *Carbo animalis*, *Magnesia muriatica*, *Nux vomica*, *Phosphorus*, *Sepia*, *Staphysagria*.

GOUT:—1. *Belladonna*, *Bryonia*, *Kali*, *Mercurius*, *Rhus*, *Sabina*, *Staphysagria*.
2. *Agnus*, *Baryta*, *Calcarea*, *China*, *Cocculus*, *Ferrum*, *Graphites*, *Hyoscyamus*, *Natrum*, *Phosphorus*, *Pulsatilla*, *Sepia*, *Sulphur*, *Zincum*.
3. *Alumina*, *Carbo vegetabilis*, *Chamomilla*, *Dulcamara*, *Iodium*, *Lycopodium*, *Nux vomica*, *Sabadilla*, *Secale* *Silicea*.

HÆMATEMESIS:—1. *Ferrum*, *Phosphorus*.
2. *Aconitum*, *China*, *Nux vomica*, *Pulsatilla*, *Sepia*, *Sulphur*.
3. *Arnica*, *Arsenicum*, *Belladonna*, *Calcarea*, *Causticum*, *Chamomilla*, *Cuprum*, *Hyoscyamus*, *Ipecacuanha*, *Mercurius*, *Nitri acidum*, *Rhus*, *Silicea*.

HÆMATURIA:—1. *Pulsatilla*, *Sepia*.
2. *Dulcamara*, *Zincum*.
3. *Aconitum*, *Calcarea*, *Mercurius*, *Phosphorus*, *Sulphur*,

HÆMOPTYSIS:—1. *Ferrum*, *Phosphorus*, *Pulsatilla*, *Sulphur*.
2. *Aconitum*, *Arsenicum*, *Belladonna*, *Bryonia*, *Calcarea*, *China*, *Mercurius*, *Rhus*, *Sabina*, *Sepia*, *Zincum*.
3. *Ammonium*, *Arnica*, *Conium*, *Crocus*, *Cuprum*, *Drosera*, *Hepar*, *Hyoscyamus*, *Ipecacuanha*, *Kali*, *Natrum muriaticum*, *Nitri acidum*, *Nux moschata*, *Nux vomica*, *Opium*, *Sabadilla*, *Silicea*, *Sulphuris acidum*.

HÆMORRHOIDS:—1. *Arsenicum*, *Calcarea*, *Nux vomica*, *Pulsatilla*, *Sulphur*.
2. *Ammonium*, *Graphites*, *Kali*, *Lycopodium*, *Phosphorus*.
3. *Antimonium*, *Carbo vegetabilis*, *Colocynthis*, *Nitri acidum*,
4. *Alumina*, *Cuprum*, *Ferrum*.

HYPOCHONDRIA:—1. *Nux vomica*, *Sepia*, *Sulphur*.
2. *China*, *Natrum*.
3. *Belladonna*, *Chamomilla*, *Conium*, *Lachesis*, *Natrum muriaticum*, *Phosphorus*, *Phosphori acidum*, *Pulsatilla*, *Staphysagria*, *Veratrum*, *Zincum*.

HYSTERIA:—1. *Conium*, *Nux moschata*, *Nux vomica*, *Pulsatilla*, *Sulphur*.
2. *Belladonna*, *Calcarea*, *Cocculus*, *Platina*, *Sepia*, *Silicea*.
3. *Agnus*, *Aurum*, *Bryonia*, *Chamomilla*, *China*, *Hyoscyamus*, *Ignatia*, *Iodium*, *Magnesia muriatica*, *Nitri acidum*, *Phosphorus*, *Plumbum*, *Staphysagria*, *Stramonium*, *Valeriana*, *Veratrum*.

LEUCORRHŒA:—1. *Calcarea*, *Cocculus*, *Conium*, *Mercurius*, *Pulsatilla*, *Sepia*.

2. *Alumina*, *Ammonium*, *China*, *Graphites*, *Kali*, *Lycopodium*, *Natrum muriaticum*, *Nux vomica*, *Phosphorus*, *Sabina*, *Silicea*, *Sulphur*, *Zincum*.

3. *Aconitum*, *Agnus*, *Arsenicum*, *Carbo animalis*, *Carbo vegetabilis*, *Drosera*, *Iodium*, *Kreosotum*, *Lachesis*, *Magnesia carbonica*, *Magnesia muriatica*, *Nitri acidum*, *Petroleum*.

JAUNDICE:—1. *Aconitum*, *China*, *Mercurius*, *Sulphur*.

2. *Chamomilla*, *Nux vomica*.

3. *Arsenicum*, *Belladonna*, *Calcarea*, *Cuprum*, *Pulsatilla*, *Rhus*.

4. *Aurum*, *Bryonia*, *Carbo vegetabilis*, *Cocculus*, *Conium*, *Digitalis*, *Hepar*, *Iodium*. *Magnesia muriatica*, *Nitri acidum*, *Opium*, *Phosphorus*, *Secale*, *Sepia*, *Veratrum*.

INDOLENCE, aversion to motion:—1. *Aconitum*, *Arsenicum*, *Nux vomica*, *Sepia*.

2. *Baryta*, *Cocculus*, *Lycopodium*.

3. *Alumina*, *Belladonna*, *Bryonia*, *Digitalis*, *Dulcamara*, *Ignatia*, *Mercurius*, *Phosphorus*, *Zincum*.

MAMMÆ diseased:—1. *Bryonia*, *Chamomilla*, *Conium*, *Phosphorus*, *Silicea*.

2. *Arsenicum*, *Belladonna*, *Calcarea*, *Graphites*, *Pulsatilla*, *Sulphur*.

3. *Iodium*, *Mercurius*, *Nitri acidum*, *Rhus*, *Sabina*, *Sepia*.

MANIA furor:—1. *Belladonna*, *Veratrum*.

2. *Arsenicum*, *Hyoscyamus*, *Mercurius*, *Opium*, *Stramonium*.

3. *Baryta*, *Cocculus*, *Colchicum*, *Crocus*, *Cuprum*, *Kali*, *Lachesis*, *Phosphorus*, *Sabadilla*, *Secale*.

METRITIS, etc.:—1. *Belladonna*, *Nux vomica*, *Pulsatilla*, *Sabina*, *Sepia*.

2. *Chamomilla*, *China*, *Cocculus*, *Conium*, *Platina*, *Secale*, *Sulphur*.

3. *Calcarea, Carbo animalis, Crocus, Ferrum, Graphites, Hyoscyamus, Kali, Kreosotum, Magnesia muriatica, Opium.*

MELANCHOLIA:—1. *Arsenicum, Pulsatilla.*

2. *Causticum, Graphites, Natrum, Nux vomica, Platina, Rhus, Sepia, Silicea, Sulphur, Veratrum.*

3. *Aurum, Belladonna, Calcarea, Cocculus, Cuprum, Helleborus, Hyoscyamus, Ignatia, Lachesis, Mercurius, Phosphorus, Phosphori acidum, Stramonium, Zincum.*

MEMORY weakened or lost:—1. *Lachesis, Nux moschata, Staphysagria, Sulphur.*

2. *Arsenicum, Belladonna, Bryonia, Opium, Rhus, Sepia, Silicea, Veratrum.*

3. *Alumina, Baryta, Calcarea, Conium, Graphites, Helleborus, Hepar, Hyoscyamus, Ignatia, Kreosotum, Zincum.*

NAUSEA:—1. *Chamomilla, Nux nomica, Pulsatilla, Rhus, Sepia, Silicea, Sulphur, Veratrum.*

2. *Aconitum, Arsenicum, Belladonna, Bryonia, Calcarea, China, Cocculus, Conium, Cuprum, Graphites, Kali, Mercurius, Natrum muriaticum, Phosphorus, Sabadilla, Sepia, Valeriana.*

3. *Agnus, Ammonium, Antimonium, Carbo vegetabilis, Digitalis, Dulcamara, Ipecacuanha, Magnesia muriatic., Nitri acidum, Phosphori acidum, Staphysagria, Sulphuris acidum.*

NEUROSIS:—1. *Belladonna, Cuprum, Hyosyamus, Opium, Stramonium.*

2. *Arsenicum, Calcarea, Conium, Ignatia, Mercurius, Platina, Silicea, Sulphur.*

NYMPHOMANIA:—1. *Phosphorus, Platina, Veratrum.*

2. *Belladonna, China, Hyoscyamus, Mercurius, Nux vomica, Pulsatilla, Stramonium, Sulphur,*

ODONTALGIA:—1. *Bryonia, Chamomilla, China, Natrum, Sepia, Staphysagria, Zincum.*

2. *Belladonna, Kali, Nux moschata, Nux vomica, Phosphorus, Pulsatilla, Rhus.*
3. *Alumina, Ammonium, Baryta, Calcarea, Carbo vegetabilis, Hyoscyamus, Kreosotum, Magnesia muriatica, Platina, Sabadilla, Sabina Sulphur.*

OPTHALMIA.—1. *Aconitum, Belladonna, Calcarea, Chamomilla, Mercurius, Nux vomica, Phosphorus, Pulsatilla, Rhus, Sepia, Sulphur.*
2. *Arsenicum, China, Dulcamara, Graphites, Silicea, Valeriana.*
3. *Antimonium, Arnica, Digitalis, Ferrum, Hyoscyamus, Ignatia, Nitri acidum, Phosphori acidum, Staphysagria, Veratrum.*

OTALGIA, ear-ache:—1. *Belladonna, Chamomilla, Mercurius, Pulsatilla, Sulphur.*
2. *China, Dulcamara, Nux vomica, Platina.*
3. *Antimonium, Arnica, Bryonia, Calcarea.*

PAINS in the limbs or joints:—1. *Aconitum, Bryonia, Mercurius, Nux vomica, Pulsatilla.*
2. *Arnica, Belladonna, Carbo vegetabilis, Chamomilla, China, Phosphorus, Sulphur, Veratrum.*
3. *Arsenicum, Ferrum, Ignatia, Nux moschata, Rhododendron, Sepia.*

PALPITATION of the heart:—1. *Aconitum, Calcarea, China, Iodium, Mercurius, Phosphorus, Pulsatilla, Sepia, Sulphur.*
2. *Arsenicum, Belladonna, Bryonia, Cuprum, Kali, Natrum, Nux vomica, Rhus, Silicea, Veratrum, Zincum.*
3. *Alumina, Ammonium, Antimonium, Arnica, Aurum, Baryta, Carbo vegetabilis, Chamomilla, Digitalis, Ferrum, Graphites, Ignatia, Nux moschata, Phosphori acid., Platina, Sabina, Secale.*

PARALYSIS of various parts:—1. *Belladonna, Cocculus, Dulcamara, Pulsatilla, Secale, Silicea.*

2. *Aconitum, Calcarea, Causticum, Nux vomica, Phosphorus, Sepia, Sulphur, Zincum.*
3. *Alumina, Arsenicum, Baryta, Conium, Graphites, Hyoscyamus, Kali, Mercurius, Nitri acidum, Nux moschata, Ruta, Stramonium.*

RHEUMATISM :—1. *Aconitum, Bryonia, Mercurius, Nux vomica, Pulsatilla.*
2. *Arnica, Belladonna, Carbo vegetabilis, Chamomilla, China, Lachesis, Phosphorus, Rhus, Sulphur, Veratrum.*
3. *Antimonium, Arsenicum, Ferrum, Ignatia, Nux moschata, Rhododendron, Sarsaparilla, Sepia.*

SCIATICA :—1. *Pulsatilla, Sepia.*
2. *Belladonna, Bryonia, Calcarea, Chamomilla, Lycopodium, Nux vomica.*
3. *Arsenicum, Graphites, Mercurius, Rhus, Staphysagria, Sulphur.*

STOOLS BLOODY, discharge of blood from anus :—1. *Ammonium, Arsenicum, Mercurius, Phosphorus, Sepia, Sulphur.*
2. *Belladonna, Calcarea, Conium, Nux vomica, Pulsatilla.*
3. *Ammonium, Carbo vegetabilis, Cuprum, Ferrum, Kali, Platina, Sabina, Valeriana, Zincum.*

SLEEP, RESTLESS :—1. *Arsenicum, Baryta, China, Silicea, Sulphur.*
2. *Alumina, Belladonna, Bryonia, Calcarea, Chamomilla, Ferrum, Kali, Nux vomica, Phosphorus, Pulsatilla, Sabadilla, Sabina, Sepia.*
3. *Aconitum, Aurum, Colocynthis, Conium, Dulcamara, Ignatia, Mercurius, Nitri acidum, Ruta, Secale, Staphysagria, Valeriana, Veratrum.*

SOMNOLENCE :—1. *Nux vomica, Phosphorus, Pulsatilla.*
2. *Aconitum, Arsenicum, Belladonna, Bryonia, Calcarea, Conium, Kali, Nux moschata, Opium, Sepia, Sulphur, Veratrum.*

3. *Alumina, Antimonium, Baryta, China, Cocculus, Cuprum, Hyoscyamus, Lachesis, Mercurius, Phosphori acidum, Rhus, Secale, Silicea, Staphysagria, Stramonium, Zincum.*

SWEAT, BLOODY :—1. *Calcarea, Lycopodium, Nux vomica.*
2. *Arnica, Chamomilla, China, Lachesis, Nux moschata.*

ULCERATIONS :—1. *Arsenicum, Lycopodium, Mercurius, Pulsatilla, Silicea, Sulphur,*
2. *Belladonna, Bryonia, Calcarea, Conium, Phosphorus, Sepia, Staphysagria.*
3. *Aconitum, Baryta, Carbo vegetabilis, Causticum, Chamomilla, China, Graphites, Natrum, Nitri acidum, Phosphori acidum, Sabina, Secale.*

ULCERS BLEEDING a good deal :—1. *Arsenicum, Graphites, Phosphorus.*
2. *Kali, Lachesis, Lycopodium, Mercurius, Pulsatilla, Silicea, Sulphur.*
3. *Belladonna, Carbo vegetabilis, Conium, Iodium, Sabina, Secale, Sepia, Zincum.*

VAGINA, irritated :—1. *Calcarea, Kali, Sepia.*
2. *Belladonna, China, Ferrum, Lycopodium, Mercurius, Nux vomica, Pulsatilla, Sulphur.*
3. *Arsenicum, Cocculus, Conium, Graphites, Lycopodium, Platina, Sabina, Secale, Staphysagria.*

VERTIGO :—1. *Belladonna, Calcarea, Phosphorus, Pulsatilla.*
2. *Aconitum, Bryonia, Causticum, Nux vomica, Pulsatilla, Sepia, Silicea, Sulphur, Valeriana, Veratrum, Zincum.*
3. *Arnica, Chamomilla, Cocculus, Cuprum, Ferrum, Graphites, Kali, Mercurius, Natrum, Nux moschata, Opium, Phosphori acidum, Rhus, Secale, Staphysagria, Stramonium.*

VESICLES, BLOODY :—1. *Arsenicum, Secale.*
2. *Aurum, Bryonia, Sulphur.*

VOMITING :—1. *Arsenicum, Bryonia, Chamomilla, Cuprum, Ferrum, Nux vomica, Pulsatilla, Silicea, Sulphur, Veratrum.*
2. *Belladonna, Calcarea, China, Phosphorus, Secale, Sepia.*
3. *Aconitum, Antimonium, Drosera, Dulcamara, Graphites, Hyoscyamus, Ignatia, Ipecacuanha, Lycopodium, Mercurius, Opium, Stramonium.*

VULVA swollen, inflamed :—1. *Mercurius, Nux vom., Sepia.*
2. *Aconitum, Ammonium, Belladonna, Bryonia, Calcarea, Nitri acidum, Secale, Sulphur.*

WOUNDS BLEEDING a good deal :—1. *Lachesis, Phosphorus.*
2. *Mercurius, Pulsatilla, Sulphur.*
3. *Carbo vegetabilis, Natrum muriaticum, Phosphori acidum, Rhus, Sulphuris acidum, Zincum.*

For further details see: *Indications and accompanying symptoms of Dysmenorrhœa*, Section 10.

ARTICLE V.

AMÆNIA OF YOUNG GIRLS

AT THE AGE OF PUBESCENCE, AND AILMENTS WHICH SOMETIMES ACCOMPANY THE FIRST APPEARANCE OF THE MENSES.

SECTION 33.

SYMPTOMS.—In the chapter on amenorrhœa, we have said all that we have to say concerning the causes, symptoms, and the various forms of *primary* amenorrhœa, occurring at the age of pubescence, and consisting in a non-appearance of the first menstrual discharge. We shall therefore dispense with any further remarks on this point, so much more as it is exceedingly difficult to determine whether the delay in the appearance of the first menses is not rather a natural occurrence than a morbid condition of the organism. There are cases, however, where symptoms develope themselves which are evidently caused by the retarded appearance of the first menses, and which almost always disappear again as soon as the menstrual functions have fairly begun, and continue regularly to take place at the right period. It is to this condition, and to its treatment, that we will here devote a few lines. We have likewise stated that the age when the first menses appear is not the same in different persons, and that it depends upon differences of constitution, climate, education, mode of life, condition in society, national usages, etc. All that remains for us to do, is, therefore, simply to treat of the accidents which sometimes accompany the appearance of the first menses. The most frequent ailment, at the commencement of menstruation in young girls, is *menstrual colic,* which may either take place in the bowels or in the womb. Sometimes it is so trifling that it is scarcely noticed by the patient; at others so violent that the patient utters cries, and becomes convulsed. It may last a few days only, or several months, and even years, always recurring at the period when the menses set in. In some cases this colic is complicated with pains in the sides and in the sciatic nerve. The most important ailments are the general concomitant symptoms. Many young girls, at this period, are affected with more or less headache, either continually or at intervals, in one side of the head only or in the whole head. In others, the mental and moral faculties become altered, being either duller or keener than usual; sometimes even a furious mania or inclination to suicide setting in. The appetite is sometimes morbidly excited and altered, the patients manifesting a desire for coal, clay, chalk, sand, etc., or for acid things, green fruit, etc. Deafness is likewise met with, and, in some females, attacks of catalepsy, hysteria, epilepsy, and other nervous and spasmodic affections. The circulation is likewise deranged. We meet with vertigo, drowsiness, general heaviness, redness of and ascension of heat to the face, dyspnœa, palpitation of the heart, and other symptoms that seem to point to some organic affection of the heart. We likewise meet with opthalmia and other affections of the eyes, which are sometimes very obstinate; or with vicarious hæmorrhages from different organs, such as gums, nose, lips, and even from the uterus, from which latter organ a bloody discharge sometimes takes place every eight days, or every two, five or six weeks, until the menstrual discharge becomes quite regular. The pulse of these young females is generally fuller, more developed, and febrile movements are frequently present. They may co-exist with colic and pains in the sides, and give rise to a slight form of metritis. In other young girls we meet with leucophlegmasia, general dropsy, or partial œdema. We ought likewise to mention a dry, nervous cough, which continues all the time, and is very fatiguing, and which might give rise to the belief that there are tubercles in the lungs, but which is generally of little consequence, although it is undoubtedly true that pulmonary and laryngeal phthisis developes itself very frequently at the age of pubescence. The digestive functions are likewise disturbed; besides morbid and strange changes in the appetite for particular things, the patients are attacked with nausea, vomiting, gastralgia, and especially with a species of tympanitis, that is sometimes characterized by an intermittent type. The skin is likewise the seat of a variety of morbid appearances: vesicles, pustules and blotches break out in large numbers, especially in the face. Not unfrequently copious sweats break out, with rapid and excessive emaciation, weakness, lameness and distress in the limbs, and all the other symptoms which sometimes set in with amenorrhœa, and which have been described in the preceding article.

SECTION 34.

TREATMENT.—However efficacious our remedies for any form of menstrual disorder may be, they will be found of little avail, unless we institute a mode of life suitable to the condition of the patient. Unfortunately this is not always possible. The requirements of fashion, of society, and even of coquetry, are so imperious, and the character of our young ladies is so frivolous, and their mothers are so condescending, that it is really wonderful that the number of our fashionable victims is not much larger than it really is. Sometimes we see them lightly clad, exposing themselves to the keenest winds and to all sorts of atmospheric inclemencies; at others they are loaded with a heap of unnecessary garments required by fashion; then they will drink ice-water at the very moment when they are heated by the exciting dance, or they will cool themselves by sitting in a cold current of air; is it to be wondered under these circumstances, that pulmonary phthisis should attack so many girls, even at the age of sixteen or twenty, or that, at any rate, their nerves should become shattered, and the menstrual functions should never assume a regular development? And to cap the climax of folly, the young girls are frequently deluged with strong drinks, beer, wine, and even brandy, in the vain hope that these stimulating beverages will restore the strength that had been wasted by fashionable excesses. And what are we to say of the premature use of corsets, of the abuse of cold bathing, of stimulating food, and of the dainty luxuries which the capricious taste of our young ladies cannot do without? These are some of the causes which delay the first appearance of the menses, and induce the whole train of symptoms that sometimes accompany this state of anæmia, Hence, if we wish to afford relief to our patient, we have in the first place to regulate her diet and general habits. Next to this precaution we may derive benefit from the use of the following remedies:

1. *Causticum*, *Graphites*, *Kali*, *Pulsatilla*, *Sulphur*.

2. *Arsenicum*, *Belladonna*, *Bryonia*, *Cocculus*, *Conium*, *Ferrum*, *Lachesis*, *Lycopodium*, *Magnesia carbonica*, *Natrum muriaticum*, *Petroleum*, *Phosphorus*, *Sabina*, *Sepia*, *Veratrum*.

3. *Agnus*, *Ammonia*, *Chelidon.*, *Digitalis*, *Dulcamara*, *Silicea*, *Valeriana*.

4. *Aconite*, *Aurum*, *Calcarea*, *Cicuta*, *Crocus*, *Drosera*, *Guajacum*, *Hyoscyamus*, *Magnesia muriatic.*, *Mercurius*, *Sabadilla*, *Sassafras*, *Spigelia*, *Staphysagria*, *Stramonium*, *Strontia*, *Zincum*.

With the following particular indications:

CAUSTICUM.—If the patient is very melancholy, with hysteric symptoms, etc. (See this remedy under Amenorrhœa.)

GRAPHITES.—When there are herpetic and other symptoms on the skin, the patient is sad, chlorotic, etc. (See Amenorrhœa.)

KALI.—Tendency to pulmonary phthisis, dyspepsia, palpitation of the heart, etc. (See Amenorrhœa.)

PULSATILLA.—Suitable to young girls of gentle disposition, with pains in the sides, colic, vertigo, congestion of the head, megrim, pale face, buzzing in the ears, dyspepsia, depression of spirits, frequent palpitation of the heart, etc.

Sulphur.—When none of the other remedies helps, the patient is disposed to religious reveries, etc.

Arsenicum.—Pale and bloated face in the morning on rising, with swelling of the feet in the evening; sensation of heat in the body, followed by great weakness.

Belladonna.—Vertigo when standing, redness of the eyes and face, photophobia, nose-bleed.

Bryonia.—Frequent nose-bleed, stinging pain in the head, congestion of the chest, gastralgia.

Cocculus.—Nervous symptoms, sadness, contractive and pinching colic in the hypogastrium, oppression, hysteric spasms.

Conium.—Hysteric or chlorotic spasms, hard and painful breasts, nervous weakness, and prostration after the least walk.

Cuprum.—Convulsions of the limbs and spasms of the internal organs; cramps in the calves, nausea and vomiting.

Ferrum.—Chlorotic symptoms, emaciation, aversion to motion, frequent congestion of the head.

Lachesis.—Dyspnœa and frequent attacks of suffocation; nose-bleed; the symptoms are worse after sleeping.

Lycopodium.—Chlorotic symptoms; the nose-bleed yields neither to *Lachesis* nor to *Bryonia.*

Magnesia carbonica.—Intestinal colic, uterine cramps, acidity and vomiting.

Natrum muriaticum.—Hysteric symptoms, sadness, constant weeping.

Petroleum.—Scrofulous symptoms, breaking out on the skin.

Phosphorus.—Irritable to delicate girls, disposed to pulmonary phthisis, with short and dry cough, dyspepsia, rheumatic pains.

Sabina.—Irritable to robust, plethoric girls, with frequent nose-bleed, uterine colic, etc.

Sepia.—Sometimes after *Pulsatilla*, when this medicine is ineffectual, with yellow spots in the face, and a yellow streak across the nose.

VERATRUM.—Continual coldness of the hands and feet, with disposition to diarrhœa.

For further information and details, see *Amenorrhœa*, Sections 23–32.

DOSE.—Give a dose of the appropriate remedy every three or four days, morning and evening, the dose may consist of six globules, dry on the tongue, or of one or two drops of the attenuated solution on sugar, or in a spoonful of water.

ARTICLE VI.

MENOSPASIS, OR CRITICAL AGE,

AND AILMENTS WHICH ARE INCIDENTAL TO A CESSATION OF THE MENSTRUAL FUNCTIONS AT THAT PERIOD.

SECTION 35.

SYMPTOMS.—The age when menstruation ceases entirely, is not the same with all women. At an average it is between forty and fifty, generally forty-five or six in France, and somewhat later in cold, but earlier in warm climates. In females with weak constitutions the menses may likewise cease to flow at an earlier period. This cessation is not, however, depending upon the earlier or retarded appearance of the first menses; it seems agreed that, the more children a woman has had, the longer the menstrual flow is disposed to continue. If nothing untoward occurs, the intervals between the menstrual periods become more and more prolonged, until the menses cease entirely. In many cases this change takes place without any unpleasant sensations or local disorders. The most frequent and the least dangerous symptom is an irregular return of the menstrual flow, every week, or every two or three weeks, or every two, three, four or six months, and being more or less irregular as regards quantity or quality of the menstrual blood. Serious and alarming hæmorrhages frequently set in, especially among plethoric and nervous women, or such as have indulged in sexual excesses. Sometimes these hæmorrhages alternate with whitish or yellowish leucorrhœa, which often has a fetid smell, is acrid and extremely copious. This leucorrhœa may continue long after the menstrual discharge has entirely ceased to appear. At this period we likewise meet not unfrequently with colic, uterine cramps, pains in the sides, weight in the loins, or distressing itching of the parts. In some cases the abdomen swells as during pregnancy, with sympathetic development of the breasts, until the swelling suddenly disappears after the expulsion of a mole, or after the emission of a quantity of gas, or after an hæmorrhage, or a profuse discharge of serum. With reference to the *general* symptoms, we notice sometimes congestions of the head, hæmoptysis, bloody urine, piles, nose-bleed, and other vicarious hæmorrhages; pulmonary phthisis likewise takes a fresh development, and frequently terminates fatally. In other cases we meet with diarrhœa, weakness of the stomach, flatulence, vomiting and other derangements of the digestive canal, which are sometimes accompanied by consumption and profuse sweats. Some women complain at this period of attacks of rheumatism of the shoulder or thigh, or of a considerable swelling of the joints; others experience attacks of hysteria, hypochondria and even nymphomania; others again are attacked with various eruptions, such as tetter at the genital organs, acne rosacea or erysipelas. The most distressing maladies which break out at this period and often terminate fatally, are ulcers and polypi of the uterus, and carcinoma of this organ and of the breasts. These various ailments do not always set in; in many females the critical change takes place so slowly and gradually, that they are not aware of any particular transformation which the organic life is undergoing. Their health becomes more vigorous and durable than before.

Section 36.

Treatment.—If no important difficulties set in, we ought not to prescribe remedies for every little distress that may show itself in conjunction with the critical change. It is of more importance to attend to a proper and simple diet, which should consist in plain and nourishing food, without being either stimulating or heating. Coffee, tea, strong spices, and domestic drugs, and decoctions, are never more hurtful than at this period. An exclusively sedentary life and too much exercise are alike hurtful. Every day the patient should take exercise in the open air. Keen and windy weather and over-heated apartments are to be avoided. The patient should be clad agreeably to the states of the weather, temperature, season. So far as remedies are concerned by means of which the various ailments incidental to a critical suppression of the menses are combated, they are the same as those which have been recommended for *Amenorrhœa*, Section 34, except that, according to the symptoms, we may have to accord a preference to: 1. *Pulsatilla*, *Lachesis*: 2. *Bryonia*, *Cocculus*, *Ignatia*, *Sepia*, *Sulphur*, these remedies being peculiarly adapted to the ailments incidental to the critical period. For further details we refer the reader to the articles *Amenorrhœa*, and *Metrorrhagia*, *Cancer of the womb*, *Diseases of the breasts*, *Leucorrhœa*, etc., which will be found in subsequent parts of this work.

ARTICLE VII.

ABNORMAL CHANGES OF THE MENSTRUAL BLOOD.

Section 37.

Symptoms.—A noteworthy symptom, which not unfrequently occurs during amenorrhœa and menstrual irregularities, is hæmorrhage or congestion, which often occurs in place of the menses and seems to supply the deficiency in the normal secretion. Such an hæmorrhage may take place from any orifice of the body. In young girls it mostly occurs in the superior organs, whereas, at the critical age, it generally takes place from the lower organs. In plethoric and nervous females, such hæmorrhages are more frequent than in young girls or lymphatic individuals. They likewise attack more readily the organs which are naturally predisposed for this kind of derangement—for instance, organs where hæmorrhages had taken place previously, or which had been more or less affected during the menstrual flow. Thus, hæmorrhages may take place from the socket of a tooth, if a female should have it pulled at the critical period; nasal hæmorrhage may set in in consequence of violent sneezing; vomiting of blood in consequence of violent straining, etc. These vicarious hæmorrhages may either be preceded by local symptoms in the region where they are to take place, or by general symptoms resembling those which used to occur previous to the appearance of the menses; sometimes they set in without any precursory symptoms. Ordinarily they occur one or two days before the menses generally set in, and they either last as long as these habitually lasted, or else they continue a few days longer, or break out after the period for the menstrual appearance is past. If hæmorrhage takes place while the menses are flowing, this flow is generally very scanty, whereas an abnormal hæmorrhage is copious and prolonged. These various vicarious hæmorrhages are very apt to take place repeatedly from the same organ, until the critical change is completed; though it sometimes occurs that hæmorrhages from different organs take place in the same patient. In some, milk flows from the breasts, or a serous liquid from the ear; whereas, in others again, there is no hæmorrhage, but simply a congested condition of the organ. As we stated above, these hæmorrhages may occur from any orifice or tissue of the body; but the tissue which is most frequently affected, is the *mucous membrane*, giving rise to nose-bleed, spitting or vomiting of blood, bloody stool, piles, bloody urine, hæmorrhage from the mucous lining, conjunctiva or corner of the eye, or from the mouth, gums and teeth. Not unfrequently such hæmorrhages occur from the external integuments of the body, from former sores, cicatrices, or from recent wounds, cuts, excoriations, flea-bites, or other injuries of the external parts. They likewise take place from the sound skin, in the arm-pits, breasts, cheeks, tips of the fingers, etc. As regards duration, the hæmorrhage may consist in a simple show of blood for a few hours, or it may continue for six or eight days, and even longer; sometimes a simple effervescence and congestion of the parts may take place, without any sanguineous secretion. If once existing, the hæmorrhage is very apt to occur again at the next catamenia, unless cured by a rational treatment. These vicarious changes do not seem to be very dangerous; even hæmorrhages from important and vital organs, such as the lungs, may continue for a long time without producing organic alterations; the same remark applies to hæmorrhages from the mouth or rectum; hæmorrhages from the stomach, bladder, and smaller intestines, do not seem, however, to be without danger if they last too long; hæmorrhages from the bladder often cause great debility.

SECTION 38.

TREATMENT.—Although most authors look upon these vicarious hæmorrhages as something useful and desirable, and advise even to favor them by various means, yet we have no hesitation in laying down an opposite principle of practice. It is true that, in retention or primary absence of the menstrual discharge in the case of plethoric females, the ailments arising from such a condition generally disappear as soon as a vicarious hæmorrhage from some other part of the body, or from the uterus, takes place, and it would be the height of absurdity to undertake to suppress such an hæmorrhage by the revulsive means of the old school. But our school possesses remedies which not only tend to arrest the hæmorrhage but likewise to restore the menstrual discharge, and it is perfectly proper to administer one of these remedies, agreeably to the existing indications. By this means we avoid all risk of improper interference with drugs, especially if we first content ourselves with a minute dose—a few globules of the 15th to the 30th attenuation—and do not repeat the dose until we are sure that the remedy has been well chosen. In this way the hæmorrhage will gradually cease and give way to a normal restoration of the menstrual flow. The best remedies for these various hæmorrhages are:

For hæmorrhage from the CONJUNCTIVA or simple CONGESTION of the EYES:—

1. *Belladonna, Calcarea, Chamomilla, Lachesis, Nux vomica, Ruta.*
2. *Aconitum, Bryonia, China, Mercurius, Phosphorus, Sepia.*
3. *Arnica, Arsenicum, Graphites, Pulsatilla, Silicea, Sulphur.*

For NASAL hæmorrhage, epistaxis:—

1. *Bryonia, Lachesis, Lycopodium.*
2. *Aconitum, Belladonna, China, Mercurius, Nux vomica, Phosphorus, Pulsatilla, Rhus, Sulphur.*

3. *Arnica, Crocus, Ferrum, Nitri acidum, Sabina, Secale.*
4. *Ammonium, Arsenica, Baryta, Calcarea, Carbo vegetabilis, Drosera, Dulcamara, Sepia, Silicea.*

For hæmorrhage from the MOUTH, GUMS or TEETH:—

1. *Calcarea, Mercurius, Sulphur.*
2. *Arsenicum, Carbo vegetabilis, Iodium, Silicea, Zincum.*

Carbo animalis, Magnesia muriat., Natrum muriat., Nux vomica, Phosphorus, Sepia, Staphysagria.

For PULMONARY hæmorrhage:—

1. *Ferrum, Phosphorus, Pulsatilla, Sulphur.*
2. *Aconitum, Arsenicum, Belladonna, Bryonia, Calcarea, China, Lycopodium, Mercurius, Rhus, Sabina, Secale, Sepia, Zincum.*
3. *Ammonium, Arnica, Conium, Crocus, Cuprum, Drosera, Dulcamara, Hepar, Hyoscyamus, Ipecacuanha, Kali, Natrum muriat., Nitri acidum, Nux moschata, Nux vomica, Opium, Sabadilla, Silicea, Sulphuric acid.*

For VOMITING of blood:—

1. *Ferrum, Phosphorus.*
2. *Aconitum, China, Nux vomica, Pulsatilla, Sepia, Sulphur.*
3. *Arnica, Arsenicum, Belladonna, Calcarea, Chamomilla, Cuprum, Drosera, Hyoscyamus, Ipecacuanha, Lycopodium, Mercurius, Nitri acidum, Rhus, Silicea.*

For hæmorrhage from the INTESTINES, anus:—

1. *Ammoniacum, Carbo vegetabilis, Mercurius, Phosphorus, Sepia.*
2. *Conium, Lachesis.*
3. *Calcarea, Platina, Pulsatilla, Sabina, Stramonium, Valeriana, Zincum.*

For PILES:—1. *Aconitum, Belladonna, Phosphorus.*

2. *Calcarea, China, Mercurius, Pulsatilla, Sepia, Sulphur.*

3. *Ammoniacum, Carbo vegetabilis, Cuprum, Ferrum, Kali, Lachesis, Nitri acidum.*

For HÆMATURIA:—1. *Pulsatilla, Sepia.*

2. *Dulcamara, Lycopodium, Zincum.*

3. *Aconitum, Calcarea, Mercurius, Phosphorus, Sulphur.*

In order to select the right remedy for one or the other of these various kinds of hæmorrhage, we ought of course to consider all the other symptoms which may have been developed in the sick organism, and likewise the character of the amenorrhœa or dysmenorrhœa, with which the patient is affected. We refer the reader to the articles *Amenorrhœa* and *Dysmenorrhœa*, Sections 9–10 and 28–32, where we have furnished the necessary indications as completely as possible.

ARTICLE VIII.

METRORRHAGIA;

OR, FLOODING BETWEEN THE MENSTRUAL PERIODS.

SECTION 39.

CAUSES.—By metrorrhagia we understand every discharge of blood from the uterine vessels, which either exceeds the natural limit of the catamenia, or else takes place abnormally at a period when the menses are not expected. The condition of the uterus having much to do with the character of these hæmorrhages, it is of importance to inquire into the state of this organ, both during pregnancy and at other periods; but inasmuch as the former condition will be treated of in a special chapter, we here confine ourselves to a consideration of hæmorrhages from the unimpregnated uterus. Sometimes such an hæmorrhage is no more than increased menstruation; at other times, however, it is a morbid discharge of blood occurring between the menstrual periods. In the former of these two cases, excessive menstruation, the blood may flow too long, too profusely, too frequently, or it may flow continually. The causes which may determine such an hæmorrhage, are the same as those which tend to exercise the normal menstrual flow; most frequently, however, such metrorrhagia occurs either during the first menstrual periods, or at the critical age, although it may likewise occur at any period between these two extremes. Women who have been guilty of sexual excesses, of onanism, or who have increased the sensitiveness of the uterus by any other cause, or who have borne many children, are particularly liable to this derangement. In many cases metrorrhagia is induced by a stimulating diet, abuse of spirits, coffee, drugs, warm baths; also by fatigue, excessive walking, riding on horseback, standing erect, or by compression of the body by means of corsets, tight dresses, or by exciting the parts by lascivious novels, thoughts or conversations, or finally by the use of abortive means. According to some authors atmospheric influences have something to do with metrorrhagia; women who inhabit high districts, and are less exposed to atmospheric pressure, are less subject to metrorrhagia than persons who live more near the level of the sea. The most frequent determining causes of metrorrhagia, are: excessive sexual intercourse, sudden emotions, such as fright, anger, intense joy; violent exercise, such as: running, leaping, dancing, riding in a carriage or on horseback; violent commotion of the body, falling upon the feet or nates, blows on the abdomen or pelvis; straining in consequence of coughing, sneezing, vomiting; irritating or warm injections in the vagina, cauterization of the neck of the uterus, application of leeches to the uterus, use of pessaries, warm sitz-baths, sinapisms to the lower limbs, etc. In many cases metrorrhagia is only a symptom, for instance, when it depends upon diseases of the uterus, chronic metritis, hydatids or moles in the uterus, polypi, carcinomatous ulceration, displacement of the womb, etc. Bilious affections, worms in the intestines or other inflammatory or gastric irritations may occasion uterine hæmorrhage. Beside these *active* hæmorrhages, there are others which might be regarded as passive; these occur in women of feeble, cachectic or scorbutic constitutions, in consequence of a weakening mood of life, depressing passions, long sickness, excessive nursing of infants at the breast, etc.

Section 40.

Symptoms and Course.—Uterine hæmorrhage may take place as soon as the cause begins to operate, or in a few days only. In the latter case, precursory symptoms generally indicate a congestion towards the uterus; but in either case the hæmorrhage may set in with so much violence, that the life of the patient may be endangered thereby. Accidental hæmorrhage occurs much less frequently than an hæmorrhage which is occasioned by predisposing causes, and sets in gradually by a successive increase of the quantity, duration and frequency of the menstrual periods. The precursory symptoms of metrorrhagia are sometimes a simple malaise with slight colic, whereas, at other times, the symptoms are much more marked, such as: swelling of the breasts, tension in the hypochondria, heaviness, heat and pain in the sacral and hypogastric regions; constipation, general lassitude, febrile pulse, pale face, cold extremities, shuddering, heat and itching of the parts; after the first appearance of blood these symptoms first seem to abate; but, if the flow becomes a little more copious, a fainting sensation is experienced in the region of the stomach, with paleness of the face and lips, feeble pulse, blur before the eyes, buzzing in the ears, weakness of hearing, embarrassed and stertorous breathing; death. In nervous females most of these symptoms may develope themselves before the hæmorrhage has become very profuse; most cases are accompanied by a violent headache, especially in the occipital region, which sometimes continues even after the cessation of the hæmorrhage. If the hæmorrhage, although feeble in itself, continues too long or occurs too frequently, the digestive functions become deranged, the patient becomes excessively weak, pale, with rings around the eyes, œdema of the feet and legs, nervous distress, and collection of serum in the peritoneal and pleural cavities. These latter symptoms generally only set in after the hæmorrhage from the active had changed to the passive form, in which case the blood is pale, serous or blackish. The course of metrorrhagia varies a great deal; as a general rule, the more copious the flow, the less it will last. In young girls, at the age of pubescence, the metrorrhagia is but trifling, and frequently consists only in a sero-sanguineous discharge which only lasts a few days, and is generally accompanied by a sensation of heat and swelling in the vagina and vulva, and followed by debility, paleness of the face, rings around the eyes, flabbiness of the flesh, lassitude in the limbs.

At the critical period metrorrhagia generally lasts longer. Somtimes it sets in suddenly like a flood; at other times, the blood flowes scantily; in most cases the flow stops in a few days, and recommences again after an interval of two or more days. Chronic metrorrhagia may continue for several years; the discharge of blood is generally little, and either continues all the time or at short intervals, during which the patients are generally troubled with leucorrhœa.

Section 41.

Diagnosis and Prognosis.—Metrorrhagia cannot possibly be mistaken for the menstrual discharge; but the quantity of the discharge, its duration and weakness caused by it, may serve to render our diagnosis still more certain. Moreover, the blood in metrorrhagia is always more coagulable than the menstrual blood, and which sometimes comes off in large coagula in consequence of the accumulation of the blood in the vagina; it is only in cases of chronic cachexia or of exhaustion by previous hæmorrhages, that the blood may have become very thin and destitute of fibrin or cruor. It is particularly important to know the character of the metrorrhagia, whether it is *idiopathic* or symptomatic, depending upon other preexisting diseases of the uterus or other organs. In this case the diagnosis can only be established after an attentive examination of the other organs, and particularly of the uterus and its appendages. In order to distinguish between *active* and *passive* metrorrhagia, we have to bear in mind that the passive form is almost always chronic; but it attacks principally lymphatic constitutions and such as had been weakened by previous causes; that it is not accompanied by any sign of reaction, and that the blood is watery and impoverished, whereas active metrorrhagia is almost always preceded or accompanied by symptoms of general or local reaction, runs a rapid course, attacks principally robust women of strong constitutions, and the blood is highly coagulable. The prognosis depends upon the age, constitution and strength of the patient, upon the causes which have produced the disease, upon the quantity of the blood which is discharged and upon the length of time that the disease has lasted; in the case of girls at the age of pubescence, as well as in the case of women at the critical period, metrorrhagia is scarcely ever a serious disease; nor is it any more so in the case of robust women, when the accident is owing to some sudden cause, and the discharge is not excessive; but profuse, rapid metrorrhagia which is accompanied by sudden prostration, is always dangerous and may terminate fatally; chronic metrorrhagia is likewise more or less dangerous, especially if it has occurred more than once and the constitution has been deeply affected in consequence; in the case of lymphatic, nervous or debilitated females, such hæmorrhages are particularly dangerous. If the metrorrhagia is occasioned by the presence of a polypus, moles, ulcer or uterine cancer, or by chronic metritis or any other morbid condition of the uterus, the prognosis always depends upon the primary disease, and the hæmorrhage cannot be radically cured unless the disease is cured likewise.

SECTION 42.

TREATMENT.—The first thing to be done in any kind of metrorrhagia is to regulate the diet and regimen of the patient, and to remove all influences that tend to keep up the hæmorrhage. The patient should at once be placed in an horizontal position, the pelvis being slightly raised by means of a pillow placed underneath; hair-mattrasses or spring-beds should be preferred to feather beds which are too soft and too warm; the patient should be covered only slightly, and be kept in a cool rather than a warm room; care, however, should be taken to keep the extremities warm; at the same time the patient's mind should be kept perfectly quiet, and all disturbing emotions should be carefully avoided; all mental exertions of any kind should be avoided; these precautions having been taken, we may administer one of the following remedies:—

9

1. *Belladonna, Calcarea, China, Ferrum, Ipecacuanha, Nux vomica, Sabina.*
2. *Arnica, Bryonia, Chamomilla, Crocus, Hyoscyamus, Lycopodium, Mercurius, Nitri acidum, Phosphorus, Platina, Pulsatilla, Secale, Sepia, Stramonium, Sulphur.*
3. *Aconitum, Antimonium, Arsenicum, Cantharis, Carbo vegetabilis, Coffea, Iodium, Nux moschata, Silicea, Sulphuris acid.*
4. *Arnica, Borax, Capsicum, Carbo animalis, Cina, Cocculus, Cuprum, Ignatia, Kreosotum, Natrum, Plumbum, Rhus, Ruta, Sambucus, Zincum.*

Giving particularly for ACUTE metrorrhagia:—

1. *Belladonna, Chamomilla, Crocus, Ipecacuanha, Platina, Sabina.*
1. *Aconitum, Arsenicum, Calcarea, Cannabis, China, Coffea, Hyoscyamus, Kreosotum, Mercurius, Nux moschata, Nux vomica, Phosphorus, Secale.*

For CHRONIC metrorrhagia :—

1. *Belladonna, Calcarea, Nux vomica, Platina, Sabina, Secale, Stramonium.*
2. *Arsenica, Bryonia, Carbo vegetabilis, China, Kreosotum, Nitri acidum, Phosphorus, Sepia, Sulphuric acid.*
3. *Ambra, Ammonium, Acid muriaticum, Borax, Bovista, Carbo animalis, Hepar, Iodium, Ledum, Lycopodium, Natrum, Nitrum, Phosphori acid., Pulsatilla, Selenium, Silicea, Stannum, Sulphur.*

For ACUTE metrorrhagia :—

1. *Aconitum, Belladonna, Chamomilla, Platina, Rhus, Sabina.*
2. *Arnica. Bryonia, Calcarea, Carbo vegetabilis, Ferrum, Hyoscyamus, Ignatia, Ipecacuanha, Nux vomica, Phosphorus, Pulsatilla, Sepia, Silicea, Veratrum.*
3. *Cantharis, Carbo animalis, Causticum, Conium, Crocus, Kreosotum, Mercurius, Nitri acidum, Strontiana.*

For PASSIVE metrorrhagia:—

1. *Calcarea, China, Ferrum, Hyoscyamus, Ipecacuanha, Pulsatilla, Secale, Sulphur.*
2. *Arnica, Carbo vegetabilis, Crocus, Lachesis, Nitri acidum, Nux moschata, Nux vomica, Phosphori acidum, Pulsatilla, Veratrum.*

For HÆMORRHAGE of GIRLS AT THE AGE OF PUBESCENCE:—

1. *Calcarea, Ferrum, Sabina.*
2. *Bryonia, Crocus, Hyoscyamus, Mercurius, Phosphorus, Pulsatilla, Sepia, Stramonium, Sulphur.*
3. *Aconitum, Cocculus, Cuprum, Silicea, Zincum.*

For hæmorrhage at the CRITICAL AGE:—

1. *Belladonna, Calcarea, Pulsatilla, Secale.*
2. *Antimonium, Bryonia, Conium, Ignatia, Sepia, Sulphur.*
3. *China, Ferrum, Conium, Ipecacuanha, Nux vomica, Sabina.*

For hæmorrhage caused by a VIOLENT EMOTION:—

1. *Platina.*
2. *Aconitum, Bryonia, Chamomilla, Coffea, Nux vomica.*
3. *Belladonna, China, Cocculus, Crocus, Ferrum, Hyoscyamus, Mercurius, Phosphorus, Pulsatilla, Sepia, Stramonium, Sulphur.*

For hæmorrhage produced by CONCUSSION, a blow, fall, etc.:—

1. *Arnica, Pulsatilla.*
2. *Bryonia, Phosphorus, Rhus, Ruta, Sulphur.*
3. *Calcarea, Chamomilla, Crocus, Hyoscyamus, Mercurius, Nux vomica, Phosphori acid., Silicea.*

For SYMPTOMATIC metrorrhagia, depending upon some prior affection of the uterus and its appendages, we refer the reader to the articles on, UTERUS, FOREIGN BODIES IN THE UTERUS, ULCERS, CARCINOMA, etc.

Section 43.

Symptomatic indications of the above mentioned remedies.

Belladonna—If the blood is neither too light-colored nor too dark, with violent dragging and tensive pains in the abdomen, sense of constriction or pressing asunder; painful pressure on the parts as if everything would issue from the vulva; pains in the small of the back as if the sacrum were broken; red face with headache, vertigo, throbbing of the carotids, and great vascular excitement.

Calcarea—Especially in the case of plethoric girls of full habit, with pains in the small of the back, profuse discharge of a bright-red blood, abdominal colic, congestion of the head.

China.—When the blood is discharged at intervals, with uterine cramps, colic, frequent desire to urinate and painful tension in the abdomen; or, if much blood has already been lost, *even in the most serious cases,* with heaviness of the head, vertigo, dulness of the senses, coldness of the extremities, pale face, fainting turns, convulsive starting of the body.

Ferrum.—Profuse discharge of thin blood which is partly black and coagulated, with pains in the small of the back and labor-pains; vascular excitement, vertigo, glowing redness of the face, full and hard pulse; or pale and watery blood, with pale face, weakness, fainting turn, rapid prostration although the quantity of blood lost is not large.

Ipecacuanha—Profuse and continual discharge of a thin and bright-red blood, with cutting pains in the umbilical region, pressure on the uterus and rectum; shivering and coldness of the body, heat of the head, fainting weakness, pale face, nausea, desire to remain in bed.

Nux vomica—For chronic metrorrhagia when the hæmorrhage returns from the least cause, with scanty discharge, bearing-down colic, pains in the small of the back as if broken, painful weight and tightness in the hypochondria, frequent urging to urinate, constipation with ineffectual desire to go to stool; irritable and angry mood.

SABINA.—Discharge of a dark blood mixed with coagula, accompanied by abdominal pains, and labor-pains in the small of the back; weakness, rheumatic pains in the limbs and head; irritation of the womb, increased sexual desire, increase of the discharge from the least emotion, red urine, painful urination, mucous discharge from the vagina.

ARNICA.—The hæmorrhage is caused by a strain, a false step, a concussion, with discharge of bright-red blood mixed with coagula; nausea in the pit of the stomach, warmth about the head and cold extremities.

BRYONIA—Often after CROCUS, if this remedy has not been sufficient, with profuse discharge of a dark-red blood, violent dragging pains in the small of the back; distensive pain in the temples, pressure in the abdomen, nausea, vertigo, fainting turn.

CHAMOMILLA.—Discharge of a dark-red or black blood, badly smelling and mixed with coagula; the discharges take place at intervals, colic like labor-pain; violent thirst, cold extremities, pale face, fainting weakness, blur before the eyes and buzzing in the ears.

CINNAMOMUM—For metrorrhagia in consequence of a false step, effort, strain, fall or other concussion, if *arnica* proves ineffectual and the sexual desire is very much excited.

CROCUS.—Black and viscous blood, mixed with coagula, after the ineffectual use of *Chamomilla*, *China* or *Ferrum*, with movements in the abdomen as from a ball or fetus; yellowish or livid complexion, great weakness, sadness, uneasiness.

HYOSCYAMUS.—Labor-pains, with dragging pains in the loins, small of the back and limbs; heat all over, with full and hurried pulse; swelling of the veins of the hands and feet; restlessness, intense liveliness of disposition, trembling; or, numbness of the extremities, dulness of the senses, blur before the eyes, delirium, twisting of the tendons, and convulsive shaking of the limbs alternating with tetanic stiffness of the body.

Lycopodium—After *Calcarea*, especially suitable to girls and women of gentle disposition, in chronic metrorrhagia with scanty discharge, compressive headache, nausea, violent pains in the small of the back, weakness.

Mercurius.—Metrorrhagia at the critical age, with vascular excitement, congestion of the head, swelling of the labia, violent colic, painful swelling of the breasts, itching of the vulva.

Nitri acidum.—Chronic metrorrhagia from the least cause, and even without any perceptible cause, itching and soreness of the vulva; heat and dryness of the parts; colic and headache; weakness.

Phosphorus.—Frequent metrorrhagia with profuse discharge, colic, toothache, sexual excitement, shivering, cold extremities, palpitation of the heart, lameness of the extremities.

Platina.—Thick and dark-colored blood, with drawing pains down to the groin, sensation as if the internal organs were drawn down, excitement of the parts and of the sexual instinct.

Pulsatilla.—Occasional flow, recurring after an interval with renewed violence, or black blood mixed with coagula, accompanied by labor-pains; also suitable to women at the critical age.

Secale cornutum—Adapted to exhausted and cachectic females, with cold extremities, pale or livid face, small and almost suppressed pulse, uneasiness and dread of death.

Sepia.—Induration of the neck of the uterus, with spasmodic colic, painful pressure on the parts with stitches through the parts.

Stramonium.—Profuse discharge of black blood mixed with coagula; drawing pains in the limbs, thighs and abdomen, talkative mood, lascivious thoughts and smell of the whole body as of semen.

Sulphur—In chronic metrorrhagia, with discharge of a thick, black, acrid and corrosive blood; or frequent scanty discharges of blood; almost every day, ceasing only at short intervals.

For further indications, see the articles *Dysmenorrhœa*, Sections 5–10; *Menstrual Irregularities*, Sections 16–21, and *Morbid Changes of the Menstrual Blood*, Section 22.

Dose.—Dissolve six globules, or one or two drops of the liquid preparation in ten table-spoonfuls of water, and give the patient a table-spoonful of this solution every ten minutes, or every half hour or hour, until the hæmorrhage is arrested; in passive or chronic metrorrhagia the medicine may be given morning and evening, or three or four times a day, according to the gravity of the case.

ARTICLE IX.

LEUCORRHŒA.

Section 44.

Symptoms.—We understand by leucorrhœa, a catarrhal discharge from the mucous membrane of the vagina, or of the uterus and its appendages, without regard to color. This discharge which may be more or less copious, often constitutes the only symptom; in most cases it is white or colorless, scarcely leaving any stains upon the linen, but stiffening it and coming off under friction in the shape of a fine powder or of little scales. At other times it has a slightly yellow or greenish yellow tinge; as regards consistence, it varies from that of a thin serum to the consistence of milk or cream, or even of an albuminous or viscous fluid. The quantity of the discharge varies likewise; at times it is a mere exudation, at others the discharge is so copious that the woman has to wear a bandage as during the catamenial flow. There are even cases where the leucorrhœal discharge resembles a perfect flooding. In *idiopathic* or *catarrhal* leucorrhœa, the liquid discharge is what is termed *mild*, and does not irritate or excoriate the parts; but when the leucorrhœal discharge is merely a symptom indicative of violent phlegmasia, or depending upon organic lesions of the uterus or its appendages, the discharge becomes acrid, corrosive, fetid, brownish or greenish, and finally assumes a malignant color and quantity. In most cases the leucorrhœal discharge proceeds both from the vagina and from the uterine cavity; the discharge from the vagina is generally thin, white, of the consistence of milk or cream; the discharge from the uterine cavity, on the contrary, is thicker, more viscid, albuminous, flocculent, and has an alkaline reaction, whereas the vaginal secretion is always acid. If the discharge proceeds both from the vagina and uterus, the two are always found mixed up together. As a general rule, the leucorrhœal discharge is more copious at the time of the menses than at any other period; in other cases the discharge continues all the time, although varying in quantity. It may even occur before the first menses have made their appearance, especially in the case of fair, lymphatic or scrofulous girls; sometimes this leucorrhœa ceases as soon as menstruation has set in, whereas, in other cases, the first menses are delayed by the leucorrhœal discharge. According to some authors the leucorrhœa intermits during the menses; but this assertion is not borne out by experience. In some females the leucorrhœal discharge sets in several days or a week before the menses, and ceases as soon as these set in; in other cases the leucorrhœa only shows itself after the cessation of the menstrual discharge; sometimes, again, a leucorrhœal discharge takes place instead of the menses which remain absent. If the leucorrhœa is but slight and not too frequent, the general health of the female is not much affected by it, except some general debility and a gnawing at the stomach; but, if the discharge becomes more copious or continues all the time, the patient experiences pains and a heaviness in the epigastrium, paroxysms of factitious hunger with fainting, nausea and vomiting, irregular and capricious appetite, sometimes with desire for strange things not belonging to the class of ailments; digestion becomes slow and difficult, and is often followed in its train by headache, vertigo, laziness and slowness of motion, pains in the limbs, especially between the shoulder-blades. After a season the patient grows thin, with pale, thin or bloated face, livid or discolored skin, dull eyes surrounded by margins, languid looks, inability to perform the least exercise without being attacked with palpitation of the heart or losing her breath; the intellectual and moral faculties are weakened. Cases of this kind, where leucorrhœa produces such a perfect state of exhaustion, are indeed rare, although some of these symptoms are always more or less complained of by women of an enfeebled constitution, whenever the leucorrhœal discharge is at all unusually copious and lasting.

Section 45.

Causes.—In most cases leucorrhœa is the result of an hereditary predisposition, especially in the case of fair women with a cachectic, feeble, lymphatic or lymphatico-nervous constitution, soft flesh and pale skin. No age is exempt from this affection; it has been noticed even in children of eight, six, four and two years old; but it occurs more characteristically between the age of fifteen and forty-five. In cold and damp regions, leucorrhœa is quite common; women who move from the country to a large city, are very often attacked with leucorrhœa; recently-built houses, or houses situated in narrow and deep valleys or in marshy and damp districts, likewise engender a predisposition to leucorrhœa. Some authors speak of epidemic leucorrhœa, which they pretend broke out in spring and fall-seasons that were colder and wetter than usual. According to some observers a predisposition for leucorrhœa is likewise induced by insufficient clothing, exposure of the neck and shoulders to the cold air, compression of the body by corsets, abuse of warm baths, warm injections, and washes, etc. Feculent food, fish, crabs and oysters, watery or acid fruits, milk, new beer, cider, hard water, the excessive use of tea and coffee, abuse of purgatives or emmenagogues, are likewise supposed to pave the way for leucorrhœa; let us not forget to mention among the causes of this disease depressing passions, chagrin, grief, etc. As regards the various modes of life and professions, we are not yet sufficiently possessed of facts in order to enable us to measure the influence which they exercise over this disorder; but onanism, excessive sexual intercourse, foreign bodies in the vagina, such as pessaries, sponges, etc., are undoubtedly productive of leucorrhœa. In some cases leucorrhœa results from some prior disease, such as scrofula, chlorosis, vaginitis, displacements of the womb, menstrual irregularities, confinement, miscarriage, pregnancy, dentition, chronic gastritis, intestinal worms, constipation and even pulmonary phthisis. A most frequent or, at any rate, a very frequent cause of leucorrhœa is a certain metastasis developing itself in consequence of a sudden suppression of the perspiration, habitual sweat of the feet, piles, diarrhœa, milky secretion, suppurations of long standing, ulcer or issue, and even of a cold in the head, bronchial expectoration or vomiting. To this category likewise belong retrocessions of the gout, of an eruption, an old tetter or any other exanthem.

Section 46.

Diagnosis, prognosis, and terminations.—Leucorrhœa may be easily confounded with catarrhal inflammation of the vagina or uterus. In order to prevent such a mistake, all that we have to do is to bear in mind that, in catarrhal inflammations of the vagina and uterus, symptoms of local inflammations are always present, such as pain, heat, tension of the affected parts, aggravation of the symptoms by walking or by any other fatiguing exercise; and that the discharge, which, in simple leucorrhœa, is mild and white, in catarrhal inflammations on the contrary, is yellow, greenish and more or less acrid and corrosive. Moreover, the mucous membrane of the vagina, which, in simple leucorrhœa, preserves its natural aspect, in a case of inflammation looks more or less red, injected, swollen. Discharges resulting from the presence of polypus, engorgements of the neck of the uterus, cancers and ulcerations, are readily distinguished from the white and mucous secretions occurring in simple leucorrhœa; they are, according to circumstances, purulent, colored, bloody, fetid, etc.; the other local symptoms and an examination of the organs will banish all doubt. Much greater is the difficulty of distinguishing a non-contiguous leucorrhœa from a venereal discharge caused by the presence of chancrea or gonorrhœa. If gonorrhœa is present, the mucous lining of the vagina is always more or less inflamed; and, if the leucorrhœa, is caused by chancres, they can easily be discovered by a careful exploration of the parts. It behooves us moreover to distinguish between *active* or *sthenic* and *passive* or *asthenic* leucorrhœa; the former which is owing to an acute irritation of the mucous lining, occurs in robust women in consequence of onanism or sexual abuses, or from some other irritating cause; whereas the latter results from weakness of the parts, and is met with in feeble, cachectic or lymphatic women, in whom it is caused by debilitating influences. As regards *prognosis*, leucorrhœa is scarcely ever in itself a serious disease; it is only when it becomes excessive and permanent, that it may weaken the constitution and pave the way for serious maladies. Leucorrhœa is a very tedious malady and difficult to cure, unless we make an exception in favor of intermittent leucorrhœa, and of that which is induced by gastric or other local irritations. If depending upon some deep-seated organic disorder, or kept up by an unnatural mode of living, mental excitement, etc., the disease is exceedingly obstinate; the older the patient, the more enfeebled and the more lymphatic her disposition, the more difficult the cure. If leucorrhœa continues after the period when the menses have permanently ceased to flow, it becomes a very serious disorder. In some cases, on the contrary, for instance in girls at the age of pubescence, the leucorrhœal discharge disappears almost of itself; in other women it ceases after their first confinement, or during pregnancy, or even after their first cohabitation. A change of locality from a damp to a dry region of country sometimes effects a cure; in other cases a cure is wrought by the breaking out of a sweat, a catarrh, a diarrhœa, vomiting, bronchial irritation, ptyalism or hæmorrhage. Lastly, it is here as in other affections, the prognosis depends a good deal upon the treatment; under allœopathic treatment a number of cases remain unimproved, whereas, under homœopathic treatment, the most obstinate and apparently incurable cases sometimes disappear as if by magic.

Section 47.

Treatment.—Preventive and even hygienic means are just as important in the treatment of leucorrhœa as in that of amenorrhœa or any other menstrual irregularity. It is absolutely necessary to the cure of leucorrhœa that the patient should live in a dry and open country, away from stagnant water, in a healthy habitation; that she should be properly clad, fed; and that coffee, tea, injections, warm baths, cathartics and all other disturbing causes by the presence of which the discharge might be kept up, should be carefully removed. Having attended to the regimen, the following remedies will be found efficient in arresting the disorder:—

1. *Pulsatilla*, *Sepia*, *Alumina*, *Calcarea*, *Kreosotum*, *Mercurius.*
2. *Ammonium*, *Bovista*, *Carbo vegetabilis*, *China*, *Cocculus*, *Conium*, *Ferrum*, *Graphites*, *Phosphorus*, *Sabina*, *Silicea*, *Sulphur.*
3. *Arsenicum*, *Borax*, *Cantharis*, *Carbo animalis*, *Chamomilla*, *Iodium*, *Kali*, *Mezereum*, *Natrum*, *Nitri acidum*, *Phosphori acidum*, *Ruta*, *Stannum*, *Sulphuris acid.*

4. *Aconitum*, *Agnus*, *Ambra*, *Anacardium*, *Baryta*, *Belladonna*, *Bryonia*, *Cannabis*, *Coffea*, *Drosera*, *Guajacum*, *Hepar*, *Ignatia*, *Manganum*, *Nitrum*, *Nux moschata*, *Nux vomica*, *Petroleum*, *Platina*, *Plumbum*, *Ranunculus*, *Sarsaparilla*, *Secale*, *Senega*, *Squilla*, *Strontiana*, *Viola tricolor*, *Zincum*.

With the following particular indications.

ALUMINA, for leucorrhœa before or after the menses; *frequent*, *acrid* and profuse leucorrhœa, with heat and soreness of the parts, and relief from the use of cold washes; *discharge of a flesh colored liquid*, after the menses or between the menstrual periods, especially at night, or in the afternoon, when walking or sitting; *transparent*, *mucous leucorrhœa*, stiffening the linen; watery, yellowish and mucous leucorrhœa; itching at the vulva in consequence of the discharge.

CALCAREA.—Leucorrhœa *before the menses;* mucous or milky leucorrhœa, at intervals and when urinating; *leucorrhœa* with heat and itching of the vulva.

KREASOTUM.—Whitish leucorrhœa, preceded by pains in the small of the back, with heat in the face; white leucorrhœa, smelling like rye; acrid, yellowish-white leucorrhœa causing red spots, with itching at the vulva; yellowish leucorrhœa, with weakness of the legs; flesh-colored leucorrhœa, having a foul smell; discharge of blood and mucous from the vagina, in the morning on rising; *mild* or *acrid leucorrhœa*, always with great weakness.

MERCURIUS.—*Mild* or *acrid leucorrhœa*, *whitish*, *purulent and corrosive leucorrhœa;* greenish leucorrhœa, especially in the evening, with itching of the parts at night; *discharge of mucous and purulent flocks from the vagina.*

PULSATILLA.—Watery, acrid and burning leucorrhœa; *milky* leucorrhœa, sometimes without smell, and at times with swelling of the vulva, flowing especially after the menses; *mucous*, *thick* and *white* leucorrhœa, especially when lying down, or before and during the menses, with abdominal cramps.

Sepia.—Leucorrhœa with stinging in the womb, pulling in the abdomen, itching in the vagina and at the vulva, or distention and heaviness of the abdomen, leucorrhœa after urinating or after making an effort to vomit, *acrid* leucorrhœa, with pain when walking; leucorrhœa with discharge of fetid mucous flocks; *yellowish*, watery leucorrhœa; *mucous* leucorrhœa; milky leucorrhœa, only in the day-time, with burning pain and soreness of the parts; puriform or muco-sanguineous leucorrhœa; discharge of a reddish-green liquid from the vagina during pregnancy.

Moreover:

Ammonium.—Acrid, corrosive leucorrhœa; watery discharge from the uterus; burning, watery leucorrhœa.

Bovista.—Leucorrhœa after the menses; viscid, albuminous leucorrhœa, or greenish, acrid, corrosive.

Carbo-vegetabilis.—Leucorrhœa before the menses; watery, white leucorrhœa; corrosive, greenish leucorrhœa.

Causticum.—Leucorrhœa at night; leucorrhœa preceded by abdominal cramps, with emission of flatulence, pulling and lameness of the small of the back, and painful flatulence in the bowels.

China.—Leucorrhœa before the menses, with painful pressure on the groin and anus; *bloody leucorrhœa*, and discharge of small black coagula of fetid, purulent matter, with distressing itching and painful contraction in the inner organs.

Cocculus.—*Leucorrhœa instead of the menses or between the periods;* flesh-colored leucorrhœa, with discharge of a purulent and sanious liquid; discharge of bloody mucous during pregnancy.

Conium.—*Acrid*, *gnawing*, corrosive leucorrhœa; acrid, burning, mucous leucorrhœa; thick, milky, leucorrhœa with labor-pains. Before the discharge, *pinching colic*, or lameness in the small of the back. Afterwards, lassitude and hoarseness with cough and expectoration.

Ferrum.—*Milky*, gnawing and corrosive leucorrhœa, also before the menses, with discharge of mucous shreds from the vagina.

GRAPHITES.—White mucous leucorrhœa, also with weakness in the small of the back; thin, light-coloured leucorrhœa, with distention of the abdomen.

LYCOPODIUM.—Leucorrhœa at intervals; also preceded by cutting colic; rose-coloured leucorrhœa before full-moon.

PHOSPHORUS.—Mucous leucorrhœa; acrid and blistering leucorrhœa; viscid leucorrhœa in the place of the menses.

SABINA.—Leucorrhœa with amenorrhœa; *itching* and milky leucorrhœa; *jelly-like, yellowish, ichorous* and fetid leucorrhœa, with flesh-coloured discharge every fortnight.

SILICEA.—Smarting leucorrhœa, especially after eating acids; watery leucorrhœa, after urinating, or after colic around the navel.

SULPHUR.—Leucorrhœa before the menses; *leucorrhœa preceded by cutting colic or pinching around the navel*, watery or yellowish; corrosive leucorrhœa, burning or smarting like salt.

ALSO:

ARSENICUM.—Leucorrhœa when standing; *acrid, corrosive*, thick and yellowish leucorrhœa.

BORAX.—Albuminous leucorrhœa, with sensation as if hot water were running down the thighs; *corrosive* leucorrhœa, also like starch.

CANTHARIS.—Acrid, burning leucorrhœa; discharge of bloody mucus after the menses.

CARBO ANIMALIS.—Yellowish, burning leucorrhœa.

CHAMOMILLA.—Yellowish, smarting leucorrhœa; acrid and watery discharge from the vagina after a meal.

IODIUM.—Chronic leucorrhœa, flowing particularly at the period of the menses, with soreness of the thighs.

KALI CARBONICUM.—Yellowish leucorrhœa, also with itching of the parts.

MAGNESIA CARBONICA.—*Chronic leucorrhœa;* also particularly when walking or sitting, preceded by uterine cramps.

MAGNESIA MURIATICA.—*Leucorrhœa after stool* or after urinating, also *preceded by uterine cramps;* leucorrhœa between the periods, followed by bloody discharge.

MEZEREUM.—Chronic *malignant* leucorrhœa.

NATRUM CARBONICUM.—Leucorrhœa preceded by colic and cutting pain in the bowels; putrid leucorrhœa.

NATRUM MURIATICUM.—Leucorrhœa preceded by cramps, contraction in the abdomen; acrid leucorrhœa, with yellowish compression; yellowish leucorrhœa, especially when walking; profuse mucous, white and transparent leucorrhœa; leucorrhœa with headache, colic, mucous diarrhœa.

NITRI ACIDUM.—Mucous, filamentous, flesh-colored leucorrhœa; mucous and greenish leucorrhœa after the menses; fetid, brownish leucorrhœa.

PHOSPHORI ACIDUM.—Yellowish, and purulent leucorrhœa after the menses.

RUTA.—Acrid, gnawing leucorrhœa, after the menses.

STANNUM.—Yellowish, debilitating leucorrhœa.

SULPHURIS ACIDUM.—Painless leucorrhœa; *acrid burning* leucorrhœa; bloody mucus from the vagina.

ALSO:

ACONITUM.—Profuse, yellowish, viscid leucorrhœa; bloody leucorrhœa.

AMBRA.—*Chronic* leucorrhœa; thick, mucous leucorrhœa, preceded by stitches in the vagina; discharge of blueish mucus from the vagina.

AMMONIA MURIATICUM.—Leucorrhœa with distention of the abdomen; brownish leucorrhœa after urinating.

ANACARDIUM.—Itching leucorrhæa, with soreness of the parts.

ANTIMONIUM CRUDUM.—Acrid, stinging water from the vagina.

BARYTA.—Mucous leucorrhœa, with palpitation of the heart, fainting weakness.

BELLADONNA.—Leucorrhœa with colic, alternating sometimes with metrorrhagia.

CAPSICUM.—Fetid leucorrhœa.

COFFEA.—Profuse discharge of mucus from the vagina, with frequent discharge of blood, itching and excitement of the parts.

COPAIVA.—Bloody and mucous leucorrhœa; thick, purulent leucorrhœa, with constant pressure on the vagina.

DROSERA.—Leucorrhœa, with colic like labor-pains, during the suppression of the menses.

HEPAR SULPHURIS.—Leucorrhœa with smarting of the vulva.

IGNATIA.—Puriform, acrid, gnawing leucorrhœa, preceded by uterine cramps.

LACHESIS.—Leucorrhœa before the menses, a greenish mucus, with scanty and short menses.

NITRUM.—White leucorrhœa, with lameness in the small of the back.

NUX VOMICA.—*Fetid*, *yellowish* or mucous leucorrhœa.

PETROLEUM.—Leucorrhœa with voluptuous dreams.

PLATINA.—Albuminous leucorrhœa, only in the day-time.

SARSAPARILLA.—Mucous leucorrhœa when walking.

TABACUM.—Flesh-coloured leucorrhœa, a fortnight after the menses.

TARTARUS EMETICUS.—Viscid, white, mucous leucorrhœa.

ZINCUM.—Mucous leucorrhœa, especially after stool; leucorrhœa preceded by cutting in the bowels, gnawing, or pinching in the epigastrium; thick leucorrhœa, morning and evening, before and during the menses.

DOSE.—Of the appropriate remedy give the patient six globules or one or two drops of the attenuated remedy on sugar or in a spoonful of water, morning and evening.

SECTION 48.

PARTICULAR INDICATIONS.—We shall here give only the symptomatic indications that refer exclusively to idiopathic leucorrhœa, depending upon a catarrhal state of the vagina and uterus. We shall say nothing of symptomatic leucorrhœa, depending upon organic diseases of the uterus and its appendages, such as, polypi, ulcerations, scirrhus, cancer, etc.; for in all such cases of leucorrhœa, it is these diseases that have to form the main object of the treatment. For the treatment of these affectious we refer the reader to the chapters where they have been treated with full details. Here follow the symptomatic indications of idiopathic leucorrhœa, or leucorrhœa resulting from a simple, catarrhal or inflammatory condition of the vaginal and uterine mucous membrane:—

For COPIOUS LEUCORRHŒA:—1. *Ammonium*, *Graphites*, *Lachesis*, *Natrum muriaticum*.

2. *Aconitum*, *Alumina*, *Carbo vegetabilis*, *Causticum*, *Magnesia muriatica*, *Phosphorus*, *Phosphoric acid*, *Sepia*, *Silicea*.

OBSTINATE:—1. *Alumina*, *Borax*, *Calcarea*, *Iodium*, *Kreosotum*, *Mercurius*, *Mezereum*, *Pulsatilla*, *Sepia*.

2. *Carbo vegetabilis*, *China*, *Cocculus*, *Conium*, *Ferrum*, *Graphites*, *Lycopodium*, *Phosphorus*, *Sabina*, *Silicea*, *Sulphur*.

SIMPLE:—1. *Calcarea*, *Pulsatilla*, *Sepia*.

2. *Ammoniacum*, *Borax*, *Graphites*, *Silicea*, *Stannum*, *Sulphur*.

3. *Arsenicum*, *Carbo vegetabilis*, *Ferrum*, *Natrum*, *Nitrum*, *Nitri acidum*, *Nux vomica*, *Sabina*, *Zincum*.

4. *Ambra*, *Belladonna*, *Bryonia*, *Cantharis*, *Carbo animalis*, *Cocculus*, *Conium*, *Ferrum*, *Guaiacum*, *Mercurius*, *Phosphorus*, *Plumbum*, *Senega*, *Sulphuris acid*.

INFLAMMATORY, with vaginitis or catarrhal metritis:—

1. *Alumina*, *Ferrum*, *Mercurius*, *Phosphorus*.

2. *Arsenicum*, *Bovista*, *Carbo vegetabilis*, *Conium*, *Iodium*, *Sepia*, *Silicea*.

3. *Ammoniacum*, *Chamomilla*, *Ignatia*, *Lycopodium*, *Pulsatilla*, *Ruta*, *Sulphuris acidum*.

4. *Antimonium*, *Calcarea*, *Cannabis*, *Cantharis*, *Carbo animalis*, *China*, *Hepar*, *Kali*, *Nitri acidum*, *Thuja*.

STHENIC or active:—1. *Calcarea*, *Carbo vegetabilis*, *Ferrum*, *Mercurius*, *Phosphorus*, *Pulsatilla*, *Sepia*, *Silicea*, *Sulphur*.

2. *Arsenicum*, *Chamomilla*, *Cocculus*, *Coffea*, *Iodium*, *Phosphorus*, *Sabina*.

ASTHENIC or passive :—1. *China, Cocculus, Ferrum, Pulsatilla, Sulphur.*

2. *Arsenicum, Carbo vegetabilis, Conium, Graphites, Kali, Natrum, Phosphorus, Sepia, Stannum.*

For leucorrhœa BEFORE the MENSES :—1. *Calcarea, Lachesis.*

2. *Baryta, Carbo vegetabilis, China, Phosphorus.*

3. *Graphites, Pulsatilla, Ruta, Sepia, Sulphur, Zincum.*

DURING the menses :—1. *Alumina.*

2. *China, Cocculus, Graphites, Lachesis, Pulsatilla, Zincum.*

FOLLOWING the menses :—1. *Alumina, Pulsatilla, Ruta, Sabina.*

2. *Bovista, Cocculus, Graphites, Kreosotum, Mercurius, Nitri acidum, Silicea, Sulphur.*

In PLACE of the menses :—1. *Calcarea, Conium, Mercurius, Pulsatilla, Sepia.*

2. *Alumina, China, Graphites, Kali, Natrum, Nux vomica, Phosphorus, Sabina, Silicea, Sulphur, Zincum.*

3. *Aconitum, Agnus, Arsenicum, Carbo animalis, Carbo vegetabilis, Drosera, Iodium, Lachesis, Magnesia carbonica, Nitri acidum, Petroleum.*

With reference to the character of the leucorrhœal discharge :—

Leucorrhœa, ALBUMINOUS :—*Borax, Bovista, Platina.*

BLOODY :—1. *China, Cocculus.*

2. *Arsenicum, Nitri acidum.*

3. *Lycopodium, Sepia, Silicea, Sulphuris acid.*

4. *Alumina, Calcarea, Cantharis, Conium, Tartarus.*

BLUEISH :—*Ambra.*

BURNING:—1. *Calcarea, Pulsatilla.*

2. *Conium, Kreosotum.*

3. *Cantharis, Carbo animalis, Kali, Sulphuric acid.*

4. *Arsenicum, Borax.*

LEUCORRHŒA, BROWNISH :—*Cocculus*, *Nitri acidum*.

CORROSIVE, acrid:—1. *Alumina*, *Ferrum*, *Mercurius*, *Phosphorus*.

2. *Arsenica*, *Carbo vegetabilis*, *Conium*, *Iodium*, *Sepia*, *Silicea*.

3. *Ammoniacum*, *Chamomilla*, *Ignatia*, *Lycopodium*, *Pulsatilla*, *Ruta*, *Sulphur*.

4. *Borax*, *Calcarea*, *Cantharis*, *Carbo animalis*, *China*, *Hepar*, *Kali*, *Lachesis*, *Magnesia*, *Natrum muriaticum*, *Nitri acidum*, *Thuja*.

FETID :—1. *Kreosotum*, *Sabina*.

2. *Natrum*, *Nux vomica*.

3. *China*, *Nitri acidum*, *Sepia*.

4. *Capsicum*, *Sabina*.

FLESH-COLORED :—1. *Cocculus*.

2. *Alumina*, *Calcarea*, *Lycopodium*, *Nitri acidum*, *Phosphorus*, *Sabina*, *Sepia*, *Silicea*.

3. *Baryta*, *Carbo vegetabilis*, *China*, *Conium*, *Tartarus*.

GREENISH .—1. *Sepia*.

2. *Bovista*, *Mercurius*.

3. *Carbo vegetabilis*, *Nitri acidum*, *Pulsatilla*.

ITCHING :—1. *Calcarea*.

2. *Alumina*, *Mercurius*.

3. *Sabina*, *Sepia*.

4. *Arsenicum*, *Chamomilla*, *China*, *Conium*, *Ferrum*, *Kali*, *Phosphorus*, *Silicea*, *Sulphur*.

MILKY :—1. *Calcarea*, *Pulsatilla*.

2. *Silicea*.

3. *Carbo vegetabilis*, *Ferrum*, *Sulphur*.

4. *Conium*, *Lycopodium*, *Natrum muriaticum*, *Phosphorus*, *Sabina*, *Sepia*.

MUCOUS :—1. *Borax*, *Pulsatilla*.

2. *Graphites*, *Natrum*, *Stannum*, *Sulphur*.

3. *Alumina*, *Ambra*, *Bovista*, *Carbo vegetabilis*, *Conium*, *Mercurius*, *Nitri acidum*, *Nux vomica*, *Sabina*, *Sepia*, *Zincum*.

4. *Arsenicum, Belladonna, Bryonia, Cantharis, Carlo animalis, China, Ferrum, Guajacum, Phosphorus, Senega, Thuja.*

PURULENT:—1. *Cocculus, Mercurius, Sabina.*
2. *China, Sepia.*
3. *Copaiva, Nitri acidum.*

REDDISH:—1. *Cocculus.*
2. *Calcarea, Nitri acidum, Phosphorus, Sabina, Sepia, Silicea.*
3. *Baryta, Carbo vegetabilis, China, Tartarus.*

THICK:—1. *Pulsatilla.*
2. *Sabina.*
3. *Arsenica, Zincum.*
4. *Ambra, Borax, Bovista, Carbo vegetabilis, Conium, Sepia.*

VISCID:—1. *Borax, Stannum.*
2. *Bovista, Sabina.*
3. *Aconitum, Phosphorus, Tartarus.*

WATERY:—1. *Graphites, Pulsatilla, Sepia.*
2. *Alumina, Carbo animalis, Carbo vegetabilis, Silicea, Sulphur.*
3. *Chamomilla, China, Kreosotum, Mercurius, Nitrum, Tartarus.*

WHITE:—1. *Calcarea, Pulsatilla.*
2. *Silicea.*
3. *Carbo vegetabilis, Ferrum, Mercurius, Sulphur.*
4. *Borax, Conium, Graphites, Nitrum, Phosphorus, Sabina, Sepia, Sulphur, Sulphuris acidum.*

YELLOWISH:—*Sepia.*
2. *Kreosotum, Sabina.*
3. *Carbo animalis, Carbo vegetabilis, Chamomilla, Nux vomica.*
4. *Aconitum, Alumina, Mercurius, Stannum, Sulphur.*

With reference to the existing causes:—

After COIT:—*Natrum.*

At INTERVALS:—*Calcarea, Silicea.*

At FULL-MOON:—*Lycopodium.*

During a WALK:—*Strontiana.*

MOTION:—*Magnesia carbonica.*

At NIGHT:—*Ambra, Natrum muriaticum.*

After STOOL:—*Zincum.*

When URINATING or after:—1. *Carbo vegetabilis, Silicea.* 2. *Calcarea.*

Leucorrhœa in the secondary symptoms in general:—

1. *Kreosotum, Mercurius, Sepia.*
2. *Alumina, Calcarea, Cocculus, Kali, Lycopodium, Pulsatilla, Silicea.*
3. *Arsenica, Carbo animalis, Ferrum, Magnesia, Natrum, Phosphorus, Sulphur, Sulphuris acidum, Zincum.*
4. *Ambra, Ammoniacum, Antimonium, Baryta, Belladonna, Borax, Bovista, Cannabis, Cantharis, Carbo vegetabilis, Causticum, Chamomilla, China, Copaiva, Drosera, Graphites, Hepar, Iodium, Nitrum, Nitri acidum, Phosphori acidum, Platina, Ruta, Sabina, Secale, Stannum, Thuja.*

With DISTENTION of abdomen:—*Graphites, Sepia.*

With CEPHALGIA:—*Natrum muriaticum.*

Leucorrhœa with COLIC:—1. *Magnesia muriatica.*

2. *Ignatia, Lycopodium, Magnesia carbonica.*
3. *Causticum, Conium, Drosera, Pulsatilla, Sepia, Silicea, Sulphur, Zincum.*
4. *Alumina, Ammonia muriatica, Belladonna, Kali, Mercurius, Natrum, Natrum muriaticum.*

With uterine CRAMPS:—1. *Magnesia muriatica.* 2. *Causticum, Ignatia, Magnes. carb., Natrum muriat.*

With DIARRHŒA:—*Natrum muriaticum.*

STINGING in the parts:—*Sepia.*

With yellow FACE:—1. *Natrum muriaticum.*
2. *China, Ferrum, Sepia.*

PALE:—1. *Pulsatilla.*
2. *Arsenicum, Sepia.*
3. *Graphites, Kreosotum, Natrum muriaticum.*

With weakness:—1. *Kreosotum.*
2. *Alumina, Baryta.*

With PAINS in SMALL of BACK:—1. *Magnesia muriatica.*
2. *Causticum, Kreosotum.*
3. *Baryta, Conium, Graphites, Kali, Nitrum.*

With voluptuous dreams:—*Petroleum.*

With TREMBLING:—*Alumina.*

ARTICLE X.

UTERINE CRAMPS, HYSTERALGIA.

SECTION 49.

SYMPTOMS, CAUSES, TREATMENT.—The pains which are known under the name of *uterine cramps*, or *hysteralgia*, are a real neuralgia of the uterus, and are both *idiopathic*, or existing independently of any organic affection of the uterus, and *symptomatic*, or depending upon some organic lesion of the womb. This neuralgia is generally characterized by intense, acute, lancinating or tearing pains, which are generally irregular, intermittent, recurring at more or less regular and well-marked intervals, and being principally seated in the hypogastrium, whence the pain radiates to the groins, external pudendum and anal region. Hysteralgia only occurs during the age when women menstruate, and attacks particularly nervous and irritable women, in whom it may be excited by any thing that has a tendency to exalt the sensitiveness of the uterus. Sometimes the disease accompanies the menstrual functions and, in such a case, manifest itself some time previous to the menses setting in. The best remedies for this affection are:

1. *Causticum, Cocculus, Conium, Ignatia, Magnesia muriaticum, Nux vomica.*

2. *Belladonna, Baryta, Chamomilla, Hyoscyamus, Natrum muriaticum, Platina, Sepia, Stannum.*

With the following particular indications:—

CAUSTICUM.—For *uterine cramps*, with pains in the hypogastrium, or in the stomach, chest or small of the back, obliging her to bend double; fulness, pressure in the abdomen as if it would burst; constant but ineffectual desire to raise wind; violent increase of the pain after taking the least nourishment, or after raising herself and tightening her clothes round the hypogastrium; relieved by external heat.

COCCULUS.—Painful pressure in the uterus, with pressure on the chest, restlessness, sighs, flatulence, fainting nausea, oppression and cramps of the chest; anxiety and starting of limbs; suppression of the menses, or leucorrhœa in their stead.

CONIUM.—*Uterine cramps with digging in the vulva*, distention of the abdomen and stitches extending to the right side of the chest; pinching and squeezing in the uterus.

IGNATIA.—*Uterine cramps* with cutting stitches, labor-pains; *compressive hysteralgia*, followed by puriform leucorrhœa, or accompanied by dyspnœa; relieved by external pressure or lying on the back.

MAGNESIA MURIATICA.—*Uterine cramps, with pains extending to the thighs* and *followed by leucorrhœa.*

NUX VOMICA.—*Contractive hysteralgia*, with digging and clutching pains, especially during the menses, with increase of the menstrual discharge and passage of coagula; painful pressure in the parts, especially in the morning in bed, or during a walk in the open air, with painful contraction in the hypogastrium.

DOSE.—Dissolve in globules or one or two drops of the attenuated preparation in ten table-spoonfuls of water, and give the patient a table-spoonful every half hour, or every hour or two hours until the pain is removed.

Also the following remedies:—

BELLADONNA, for:—Clutching pains in the hypogastrium, with pains in the small of the back and drawing pains down the thighs; heaviness and pressure on the parts; the pains are especially felt before the menses, with congestion of the head.

BRYONIA.—Uterine cramps, with pinching and uneasiness in the abdomen, as if the menses would make their appearance; burning pains in the uterus; pressure and fulness in the pit of the stomach.

CHAMOMILLA.—Uterine cramps, with pulling sensation down to the thighs; *pressure in the uterus* like labor-pains, with frequent urging to urinate.

HYOSCYAMUS.—*Uterine cramps*, with pains like labor-pains, especially before the menses, and with pulling in the loins and small of the back.

NATRUM MURIATICUM.—Uterine cramps, especially at the period of the menses, with burning, and cutting pains in the groins.

SABINA.—Lancinating *uterine cramps*, or pulling and cutting in the hypogastrium or groin, *as if the menses would make their appearance*, with pressure on the parts, groin and small of the back, and tenesmus at the anus.

SEPIA.—*Uterine pains*, like painful rigidity, or *pressure on the parts*, as if every thing would issue through the vulva, with cutting pains and jelly-like leucorrhœa.

STANNUM.—Uterine cramps, with pressure in the hypogastrium and uterus, as if the menses would make their appearance.

DOSE.—The same as page 145.

ARTICLE XI.

NYMPHOMANIA.

Section 50.

Symptoms.—Authors are exceedingly divided in opinion concerning the character of this affection, which consists in an excessive excitement of the sexual desire in females; some confound it entirely with *erotalgia* or *erotomania*, which is simply a platonic aberration of the mind, whereas nymphomania is a disease characterized by physical symptoms; some again do not look upon it as a disease, but only as an excessive development of a perfectly natural instinct; others again regard it simply as a surexcitation of the sexual organs. Our own opinion is, that nymphomania is a real disease, characterized by a violent desire for sexual union, which is manifested by improper expressions and signs, with or without physical excitement of the parts, but which is distinguished from *erotomania* by this, that, in the latter condition, the patient desires an absolute physical and spiritual union with the sole object of her love, without any expressed desire for the material act, which always remains subordinate to the higher desire; whereas a woman affected with nymphomania, desires sexual intercourse with any person indiscriminately. In erotomania the desire is of a spiritual, in nymphomania of a physical nature. Most authors who have treated of this disease, have distinguished three periods. In the first period, no external symptom reveals as yet the invasion of the disease, for the patients are still able to conceal the obscene ideas with which their imaginations are filled. Soon, however, relapsing into their amorous reveries in spite of all efforts to the contrary, the patients lose courage, seek solitary places, and finally abandon themselves to their unbridled fancies and desires, and sometimes even go so far as to gratify their passion by self-pollution. At this period we frequently observe a marked turgescence about the breasts and parts, with itching, tension, and a more or less copious leucorrhœa. In the second period, the patients abandon themselves without any restraint to their passions, and seize every opportunity of talking about amorous enjoyments; they lose all sense of modesty, inviting the men near them to have sexual intercourse with them; at the same time the patients try to inflame their desires by all sort of means, reading lascivious novels, conversation, voluptuous songs, stimulating diet, touch. In the third period the disease presents a truly sorrowful aspect of human misery; the female is totally insane; she invites the first man she sees to have intimacies with her; she throws herself upon him, exciting him by words, improper attitudes, and, if he resists, she becomes raving, and tears and strikes whatever is within her reach. The most timid girl becomes like a mad prostitute; modesty gives place to wild lust, and the horribly excited fancy frequently leads patients to self-abuse. At this period other symptoms generally manifest themselves, such as convulsive movements, or burning thirst, dry and burning mouth; discharge of a thick froth from the mouth; fetid breath; spasms of the throat, with hydrophobia, sleeplessness, restless sleep, with distressing, heavy and lascivious dreams. Sometimes the attacks are followed by a sort of prostration which it is of the utmost importance to arrest. Towards the close of the disease, the patients generally fall into a sort of slow fever, with colliquative diarrhœa and general consumption, and thus they die with all the symptoms of a most violent acute or chronic malady; sometimes they succumb even during a violent spasmodic paroxysm of the disease, although such an occurrence happens very rarely.

Section 51.

Causes, prognosis, treatment.—Nymphomania rarely ever breaks out before the age of pubescence, or after some critical period, although young girls as well as old women have, in isolated cases, been attacked with it. According to some authors, it is most frequently met with among women with strong muscles, rich and black hair, black, lively and large eyes, an expressive and animated countenance, well-formed, full and large breasts, round hips, a slender and straight waist, large mouth, red and thick lips, white, round and properly arranged teeth; in some cases, however, the disease has been met with among females of a totally different character. The disease has been observed in young widows of an ardent temperament, and who are suddenly deprived of the sexual pleasures which had been their delight; or it likewise attacks married women whom their feeble and sickly husbands could not satisfy. On the other hand, excessive sexual intercourse and onanism likewise lead to the disease. In other cases, nymphomania seems to arise from itching eruptions at the vulva, such as lichen, erythema, etc., in consequence of which the patients have to rub the parts all the time, by which means the sensitiveness of these organs is much increased; a similar effect appears to have resulted from the presence of ascarides in the rectum or anus. Sometimes the affection seems to be owing to organic diseases of the vagina, vulva, uterus or its appendages. Feather beds, sleeping too long in the morning, stimulating food or drink, coffee, liquor, chocolate; certain kinds of fish, truffles, cinnamon, vanilla, etc.; balls, theatres, novel-reading, a violent and unrequited passion, bad examples, and other influences that excite and inflame the imagination, may lead to the development of this horrible disorder. As regards *prognosis*, it is always favorable as long as the third stage has not yet set in. A good deal depends upon the treatment. Under old school treatment many cases have been pronounced incurable, which have yielded perfectly to homœopathic treatment. The best remedies for this disease, according to our provings and to positive clinical experience, are:

1. *Phosphorus*, *Platina*.
2. *Hyoscyamus*, *Stramonium*, *Veratrum*.
3. *Belladonna*, *Cantharis*, *Natrum muriaticum*, *Nux vomica*, *Pulsatilla*.
4. *China*, *Mercurius*, *Sulphur*, *Zincum*.
5. *Agnus*, *Majoran*.

Especially when the following conditions occur:

DURING CONFINEMENT:—1. *Platina*, *Belladonna*, *Pulsatilla*.
2. *Sulphur*, *Veratrum*, *Zincum*.

With physical WEAKNESS of the organs:
Agnus, *Calcar.*, *Conium*, *Graphites*, *Hyoscyamus*, *Lachesis*, *Moschus*, *Natrum mur.*, *Opium*, *Sepia*, *Stramonium*, *Sulphur*.

With LEUCORRHŒA:—1. *Calcarea*, *Mercurius*, *Pulsatilla*, *Sepia*.
2. *Carbo vegetabilis*, *China*, *Conium*, *Graphites*, *Natrum mur.*, *Nux vomica*, *Phosphorus*, *Sulphur*, *Zincum*.
3. *Agnus*, *Lachesis*, *Nitric acid*, *Silicea*.

With lascivious FUROR:—1. *Hyoscyamus*, *Stramonia*, *Veratrum*.
2. *Belladonna*, *Cantharis*, *Mercurius*, *Nux vomica*, *Phosphorus*, *Platina*, *Pulsatilla*, *Zincum*.

During PREGNANCY:—*Belladonna*, *Platina*, *Stramonium*, *Veratrum*, *Lachesis*, *Mercurius*, *Pulsatilla*.

With want of MODESTY:—1. *Hyoscyamus*, *Stramonium*, *Veratrum*.
2. *Belladonna*, *Nux vomica*, *Opium*, *Phosphorus*.

After ONANISM:—1. *Nux vomica*, *Sulphur*.
2. *Calcarea*, *Carbo vegetabilis*, *China*, *Mercurius*, *Natrum mur.*, *Phosphorus*, *Platina*, *Pulsatilla*.

With desire for ONANISM:—*Sulphur*.

With ITCHING at the vulva:—1. *Calcarea, Carbo vegetabilis, Conium, Natrum mur., Sepia, Silicea, Sulphur.*
2. *Lachesis, Mercurius, Nitric acid, Platina.*

At the time of the MENSES:—1. *Stramonium.*
2. *Hyoscyamus, Veratrum.*
3. *Platina, Pulsatilla, Sepia.*

With SPIRITUAL excitation without the physical:—
1. *Calcarea, Carbo vegetabilis, China, Phosphorus.*
2. *Cantharis, Graphites, Lachesis, Natrum mur., Pulsatilla, Sepia, Stramonium, Veratrum.*
3. *Conium, Ignatius, Majoran, Moschus, Nitric acid, Zincum.*

With EXCITEMENT of the parts, turgescence of the vulva, etc:
1. *Platina.*
2. *Cantharis, Natrum mur., Nux vomica, Phosphorus, Pulsatilla.*
3. *Graphites, Nitric acid., Opium, Silicea.*

ARTICLE XII.

CHLOROSIS, GREEN-SICKNESS.

SECTION 52.

SYMPTOMS AND COURSE.—Chlorosis, which seems to be a disease peculiar to females, although it has also been observed in males,* is characterized by discoloration and paleness of the skin, and more particularly of the face, habitual weakness, derangement of the digestive functions, embarrassed respiration, and frequently by the presence of amenorrhœa or dysmenorrhœa. The group of symptoms which is generally

* See Uzac, on Chlorosis in Males. Paris: 1853. In quarto.

present in this affection, is the following: yellowish or greenish paleness of the face, with bloatedness of the part, white lips, livid and swollen eyelids after sleeping; sad expression of the eyes and excessive whiteness of the conjunctiva; dryness, or dull leaden or earthy color of the skin; flabbiness of the flesh, œdema of the feet; diminished appetite, or loss of appetite, dyspepsia, desire for hearty food or for things which cannot be eaten, such as chalk, coal, etc.; constipation, nausea, vomiting; small and frequent pulse; palpitation of the heart; dyspnœa, especially when going up stairs or when ascending an eminence; spontaneous attacks of weariness even unto fainting; laziness, aversion to movement; desire to be alone; sadness, sighs, frequent weeping; menstrual irregularities or suppression; the menstrual discharge is scanty, pale and serous; aggravation of the symptoms at each menstrual period, with gastralgia, fainting, melancholy, foreboding, melancholy thoughts. If the disease continues, other symptoms develop themselves, such as headache at the occiput, painful distension of the abdomen, organic affections in various parts, hectic fever. Frequently the disease announces itself by sadness and indolence, followed by digestive derangements, discoloration of the skin, and all the other symptoms. In some cases the disease sets in with gastric derangement, or mucous inflammation of the stomach and bowels. At length incurable and fatal affections may develop themselves as consequences of this disease. Pathological anatomy has so far been unable to reveal any disorganizations that might be looked upon as peculiar to this malady, unless we may accept the statement of some authors that bodies have been found destitute of blood; for as to the other organic changes, such as serous effusions in the various cavities, pulmonary tubercles, organic lesions of the heart, liver, spleen, ovaries, etc., they do not belong to the chlorosis proper, but ought to be traced to affections that have developed themselves during the course of chlorosis, sometimes even in consequence of an improper management of the disease. Some authors regard chlorosis as a symptom of amenorrhœa, and not by any means as a disease by itself. It is true, in many cases, chlorosis only sets in after amenorrhœa has taken place; but there are also cases where chlorosis precedes the menstrual suppression, and where it exists without either amenorrhœa or dysmenorrhœa being present, so that it would seem as though chlorosis and amenorrhœa, so far from holding towards each other the relation of cause and effect, are, on the contrary, the effects of one and the same cause, which may perhaps be a deranged condition of the functions of digestion and reproduction.

Section 53.

Causes, diagnosis and prognosis.—According to some authors, the proximate cause of chlorosis is an inertia of the genital organs. This opinion will appear somewhat well founded, if we consider that chlorosis generally takes place at the period of pubescence, and if the menstrual functions are either delayed or otherwise irregular. It has, however, been met with in both widows and married women in consequence of excesses. Predisposing causes seem to be: a lymphatic temperament; a feeble constitution; the influence of a cold and damp dwelling or temperature; indigestible or not sufficiently nourishing food; abuse of watery, cold or warm beverages, (tea, coffee, decoctions, etc.;) warm baths; wines of bad quality, abuse of spirits; excessive sleeping or watching; sedentary habits, onanism, and other debilitating causes. As exciting causes we may likewise mention: disturbing emotions, ennui, imprisonment, unhappy or disappointed love, abstemiousness; accidental and prolonged menstrual suppression; debilitating, acute and chronic maladies. It is not always easy to distinguish between chlorosis and other affections where paleness is a prominent symptom. Such, for instance, as *anæmia*, which resembles chlorosis as far as the color of the skin is concerned; but the other symptoms and the causes which produce each malady, will enable us to distinguish one from the other. Whatever resemblance these two maladies may bear to each other, as far as the discoloration of the skin, of the conjunctiva, lips, mucous membrane of the mouth, and various other symptoms which both diseases have in common, are concerned, the derangement of the visceral functions is much more marked in chlorosis than in anæmia; moreover, we observe in chlorosis cerebral disturbances, melancholy, headache, pains in the stomach, and strange tastes which are entirely wanting in anæmia. It is much more easy to confound chlorosis with certain organic affections of the heart, so much more as dyspnœa, violent palpitation of the heart, various abnormal sounds, serous effusions, etc., are frequently present in chlorosis; what will enable us, however, to establish a correct diagnosis, is this, that, in chlorosis, all these signs are always irregular and changing; whereas, in organic diseases of the heart, they are more fixed and always permanent. We hardly need allude to the distinction between chlorosis and jaundice, since the color of the skin in these two diseases is not at all the same. As regards the other organic lesions which may occasion anæmia, such as: pulmonary tubercles, cancer, disorganizations of the stomach, etc., these diseases are so well marked, that they cannot well be mistaken for idiopathic anæmia; moreover, the paleness of the skin which exists in these diseases, is neither as universal nor as clear as in chlorosis. As far as *prognosis* is concerned, it depends upon the fact whether the disease is recent and uncomplicated or old and complicated. In the former case it is without any danger, and a cure is easily effected, if we but use a rational treatment. In the second case, the disease is always a serious, and often incurable malady, proportionate to the importance of the organic affections upon which it depends.

Section 54.

Treatment.—What we have said under Amenorrhœa concerning the necessity of a proper regime, is likewise and most emphatically applicable to the treatment of chlorosis, more particularly since these two classes of patients have tastes and desires entirely opposed to their health. The appetite is sometimes so depraved that things which are absolutely not fit to eat, are craved by such patients; exercise in the open air which is absolutely indispensable to the restoration of their health, and always does them a deal of good, is generally needed by such patients. Nevertheless the physician has to require of them that they take sufficient exercise, and he has to gradually bring them back to the use of nutritive beverages and solid food, without, however, opposing them in a rude and positive manner; for the strange fancies which these patients sometimes manifest for things which do not belong to the class of aliments, are natural indications rather than unmeaning caprices. As long as these patients do not exhibit a desire for things that are absolutely injurious either to the constitution or to the treatment, it is advisable to let them indulge their fancies, and so gradually prevail upon them, by gentle means and appropriate medical treatment, to resume a natural and rational diet. Any thing that has a tendency to excite the sexual organs, heating beverages and solid food, influences that work upon the imagination and excite the passions, novel-reading, dancing-parties, theatres, habits of indolence, etc., should be carefully removed from and avoided by the patient. A well-regulated physical and mental exercise, quiet, and a simple diet, are the best preventives and likewise indispensable to a successful treatment. As regards *treatment*, we are willing to admit with the other school, that iron is a very useful remedy, but not in the enormous doses in which it is prescribed by allœopathic physicians; for we are persuaded that the good effects of iron in this disease, do not result from its chemical, but from its dynamic action, and that if the desired result cannot be obtained by homœopathic doses, massive doses will be of no avail either. In homœopathic practice iron, however, is not the only remedy for chlorosis; we have other remedies which experience has shown to be, if not superior, at least equal to, iron in chlorosis; they are:

1. *Pulsatilla*, *Sulphur*, *Calcarea*, *Belladonna*, *Cocculus*, *Lycopodium*, *Nitri acid.*

2. *China*, *Conium*, *Helleborus*, *Kali*, *Natrum muriaticum*, *Nux vomica*, *Phosphorus*, *Platina*, *Plumbum*, *Sepia*, *Spigelia*.

3. *Arsenicum*, *Digitalis*, *Graphites*, *Mercurius*, *Phosphori acid.*, *Staphysagria*, *Valeriana*.

4. *Baryta*, *Carbo animalis*, *Carbo vegetabilis*, *Causticum*, *Ignatia*, *Oleander*, *Sabina*, *Sulphuris acidum*, *Zincum*.

With the following particular indications:—

BELLADONNA.—For frequent pressure on the genital organs, with or without leucorrhœa; jerking shocks in the vagina; heat in the vulva; fulness and pressure in the abdomen; scanty and painful menses, preceded by colic; weariness; anorexia; frequent paroxysms of anguish; numbness of the legs when sitting; lymphatic temperament with blue eyes and fair hair.

CALCAREA.—In many cases, after *Sulphur*, and particularly for the following symptoms; amenorrhœa, with congestive headache, vertigo, gastralgia with fulness in the hypochondria; weariness and heaviness in the body; *leucorrhœa*, anorexia, dyspnœa and frequent palpitation; nausea and vomiting; nervous prostration, with desire to be magnetized; frequent shuddering and chilliness; weary after the least effort; melancholy and inclined to weep; desire for wine and dainties, with aversion to flesh; obstinate constipation.

COCCULUS.—Particularly after abuse of coffee and chamomile-tea, or for frequent cramps in the bowels; suppressed or scanty and irregular menses; leucorrhœa; paralytic weakness; dyspnœa, cramps in the chest; sadness, uneasiness, anguish, sight; sensitiveness to the open air; whether cold or warm; frequent yawning; fainting nausea; gastralgia.

FERRUM.—In obstinate cases, when every other remedy seems to fail, especially when the following symptoms occur: complete suppression; *constant desire to lie or sit;* œdema of the face, hands and feet, *with bloat around the eyes;* weariness in the legs or after the least exercise in the open air; want of vital heat; uneasiness with throbbing in the epigastrium; gastralgia or vomiting after the least meal; dyspnœa as from contraction of the chest.

Lycopodium.—Especially after the favorable action of *Calcarea*, or for complete suppression, sensitiveness to the open air, vascular excitement or sensation as if the blood were colder and ceased to circulate; tendency of the limbs to go to sleep; lassitude with trembling; fainting turn; continual drowsiness; chilliness; melancholy, averse to company; falling off of the hair; desire for sweets; constipation; dryness of the vagina.

Nitri acidum.—Nourishment after *Calcarea*, especially suitable to girls with choleric temperament, brown or black hair or eyes, or when the following symptoms are present: hysteria, nervous prostration after the least pain; sadness, tendency to start, aversion to meat, desire for chalk, lime, clay; difficult digestion, with nausea, lassitude, drowsiness after eating; short and panting breathing; palpitation of the heart when going up stairs.

Pulsatilla.—Especially after abuse of Ferrum, or for suppression, *frequent leucorrhœa*, megrim, hysteric distress; buzzing in the ears, weariness and heaviness of the legs; dyspnœa, loss of breath after an exertion; *frequent palpitation of the heart;* cold hands and feet; pressure and heaviness in the abdomen; gastralgia, nausea, vomiting; chilliness and shivering, with yawning and stretching; œdema of the feet, melancholy mood, weeping, dread of dying; *marked desire for spirits or spicy things, stimulants;* gentle, timid disposition.

Sulphur.—In most cases, after *Pulsatilla*, or at the commencement of the treatment, for abdominal cramps, leucorrhœa, nervous debility, fainting, sensitiveness to the open air, tendency of the limbs to go to sleep; aversion to washing; constant drowsiness in the day-time; frequent shivering, coldness; melancholy, weeping mood, raw and burning eructations; difficult digestion, with pressure and fulness in the stomach; constipation, with hard stool; dyspnœa and sense of weight in the chest; frequent congestion of the chest.

Dose.—Of the appropriate remedy give five or six globules dry on the tongue, or one or two drops of the attenuated preparation on sugar or in a spoonful of water every morning or evening; or, after an improvement has set in, every two or three days.

ALSO:

CHINA.—For abdominal or pulmonary cramps, *leucorrhœa;* nocturnal, pressive headache; weakness, lassitude and heaviness of the legs; restless sleep, with anxious and fatiguing dreams; nervousness, with sensitiveness to noise; dyspepsia, pressive gastralgia especially after eating; hysteric ailments; watery, leucophlegmatic infiltration; distress in the limbs which feel as if broken; lowness of spirits and hypochondria; listless, apathetic; desire for dainties, wine, acids; frequent palpitation of the heart.

CONIUM.—Hysteric ailments; flabby and withered breasts; nervousness with involuntary weeping; anxiety, tendency to start; *leucorrhœa;* abdominal cramps with distention of the abdomen and stitches in the parts; hysteric cramps in the throat; aversion to bread; desire for acids; nausea after eating; palpitation of the heart after drinking.

KALI CARBONICUM.—Amenorrhœa, palpitation of the heart; œdema; fainting turns; aversion to open air; dry skin; desire for sweets; nausea, vomiting, constipation.

NATRUM MURIATICUM.—Hysteria, sadness, weeping; weakness of mind and body, aversion to movement; desire for bitter things, leucorrhœa, palpitation, irregular beating of the heart.

NUX VOMICA.—Menses not quite suppressed, but irregular, preceded by pains in the nape of the neck and back; nausea with fainting, especially in the morning; fatigue with aversion to movement; constipation, with frequent but ineffectual urging to go to stool; frequent urging to urinate, with tenesmus of the bladder; congestion of the head with pressive headache; irascible mood, or dedression of spirits.

PHOSPHORUS.—Scanty menses, preceded by leucorrhœa with weeping mood; frequent colic with pains in the small of the back and vomiting; weakness, nervous prostration and fainting turns; violent beating of the heart; dyspnœa, oppression; spitting of blood; hysteric symptoms.

PLATINA.—Uterine cramps, with pressure in the hypogastrium and on the parts; loss of appetite, constipation, vertigo; *deathly anguish, with dread of dying;* suspicious and proud disposition.

PLUMBUM.—Leucorrhœa; painful breasts; frequent cramps in the abdomen, paralytic weakness; constipation; hysteric spasms; flabby muscles; œdema; constant shivering; nausea and vomiting.

SEPIA.—Suppression of the menses; frequent leucorrhœa; hysteric or nervous headache; general weakness and disposition to perspire; frequent shiverings, alternating with heat; melancholy and weeping; catarrhal discharges from the nose, ears, bronchial passages, etc.; frequent colic and pains in the small of the back; tendency of the limbs to go to sleep; heaviness of the body, aversion to motion; sensitiveness to the open air; fainting spell; depression of spirits.

SPIGELIA.—Weariness after walking ever so little; yellowish margin around the eyes; sensitiveness of the pit of the stomach to the least contact; catarrhal, mucous discharges; œdema; dyspnœa; violent palpitation of the heart; irregular beating of the heart and abnormal sounds in the cardiac region.

DOSE.—The same as on page 164.

Also:

ARSENICUM.—For prostration that does not allow one to walk; frequent fainting turns; marked desire for acids, coffee or brandy; excessive desire for coit; corrosive leucorrhœa; nausea and vomiting.

DIGITALIS.—Weakness and frequent fainting turns; œdema; frequent drowsiness in the day-time; small, feeble, very *slow* pulse, accelerated by the least movement; frequent attacks of anguish, with weeping mood and dread of the future; marked desire for bitter food and sour drinks; nausea and vomiting in the morning; sense of weakness in the pit of the stomach, as if the patient would die; *audible palpitations of the heart*, with anguish and contraction in the chest.

GRAPHITES.—When the menses appear sometimes, but are

too pale, and do not last long enough; hysteric headache; frequent nausea; pains in the chest; abdominal cramps; hysteric spasms; mucous leucorrhœa and sterility; bronchial or nasal catarrh; œdema.

Mercurius.—Frequent leucorrhœa, œdema of the hands, feet and face; weakness with rush of blood after the least effort; irritable mood; sad, melancholy, contrary.

Phosphori acidum.—Leucorrhœa, with tympanitis of the womb; nervous prostration; constant drowsiness; sadness, with fear about one's health; marked desire for juicy and refreshing things; pressure at the stomach after eating.

Staphysagria.—Lassitude, as if the limbs were lame, especially after an effort; drowsiness in the day-time, with yawning and stretching; hypochondriac mood, sadness; fears about her health; frequent sweating; marked desire for wine and spirits; painful sensitiveness of the sexual organs.

Valeriana.—Chlorosis complicated with hysteria, with excessive nervousness.

Dose.—The same as on page 164.

Section 55.

Particular Indications.—Here follows a list of the principal indications regarding the use of the remedies which have been recommended for chlorosis. These indications refer both to the causes which induce chlorosis, and to the principal symptoms of this malady. We have arranged them in alphabetical order, as follows, referring the reader, for further details, to the article on Dysmenorrhœa, Sections 5–10.

Abdomen, pain in, colic:—1. *Belladonna*, *Nux vomica*, *Pulsatilla*.
2. *Arsenicum*, *Carbo vegetabilis*, *China*, *Cocculus*, *Ignatia*, *Lycopodium*, *Mercurius*, *Phosphorus*, *Sulphur*.
3. *Calcarea*, *Nitri acidum*, *Platina*.
4. *Causticum*, *Ferrum*, *Staphysagria*, *Zincum*.

Distended:—1. *Arsenicum*, *Belladonna*, *Calcarea*, *Carbo vegetabilis*, *China*, *Graphites*, *Mercurius*, *Phosphorus*, *Sepia*, *Sulphur*.

2. *Causticum*, *Conium*, *Digitalis*, *Lycopodium*.
3. *Kali*, *Natrum muriat.*, *Nux vomica*, *Pulsatilla*, *Valeriana*.
4. *Carbo animalis*, *Ferrum*, *Ignatia*, *Nitri acidum*, *Platina*, *Plumbum*, *Sabina*, *Spigelia*.

ABSTEMIOUSNESS, sexual, as a cause:—1. *Conium*.
2. *Calcarea*, *Cocculus*, *Sulphur*.
3. *Nux vomica*, *Phosphorus*, *Sepia*, *Staphysagria*.

APPETITE, gone:—1. *China*, *Nux vomica*, *Sepia*.
2. *Arsenicum*, *Belladonna*, *Cocculus*, *Conium*, *Ignatia*, *Lycopodium*, *Mercurius*, *Platina*, *Pulsatilla*, *Sulphur*.
3. *Digitalis*, *Ferrum*, *Nitri acidum*, *Sulphuris acid.*
4. *Carbo animalis*, *Carbo vegetabilis*, *Graphites*, *Kali*, *Plumbum*, *Sabina*, *Spigelia*.

BEVERAGES, SPIRITUOUS (cause):—1. *Nux vomica*.
2. *Arsenicum*, *Belladonna*, *Calcarea*, *China*, *Helleborus*, *Ignatia*, *Lycopodium*, *Pulsatilla*.
3. *Carbo vegetabilis*, *Cocculus*.
4. *Carbo animalis*, *Conium*, *Sulphur*, *Sulphuris acid.*

CEPHALALGIA:—1. *Belladonna*, *Calcarea*, *China*, *Ignatia*, *Mercurius*, *Nux vomica*, *Pulsatilla*, *Sepia*, *Sulphur*.
2. *Arsenicum*, *Carbo vegetabilis*, *Cocculus*, *Lycopodium*, *Platina*.
3. *Conium*, *Ferrum*, *Graphites*, *Kali*, *Phosphorus*.

COFFEE, ABUSE OF (cause):—1. *Causticum*, *Ignatia*, *Nux vomica*.
2. *Cocculus*, *Mercurius*, *Pulsatilla*, *Sulphur*.
3. *Belladonna*, *Carbo vegetabilis*, *Platina*, *Sepia*.
4. *Arsenicum*, *Nitri acidum*, *Sulphuris acidum*.

COLD and DAMPNESS (cause):—1. *Calcarea*.
2. *Mercurius*, *Sulphur*.
3. *Carbo animalis*, *Carbo vegetabilis*, *China*, *Ferrum*, *Nitri acidum*, *Pulsatilla*, *Staphysagria*, *Zincum*.
4. *Belladonna*, *Conium*, *Kali*, *Nux vomica*, *Phosphorus*, *Sepia*.

CONSTIPATION:—1. *Calcarea, Cocculus, Nux vomica, Plumbum, Sulphur.*

2. *Belladonna, Carbo vegetabilis, Conium, Graphites, Kali, Mercurius, Phosphorus, Platina, Sepia, Zincum.*

3. *Arsenicum, China, Natrum muriat., Pulsatilla, Sabina.*

4. *Carbo animalis, Digitalis, Ferrum, Ignatia, Spigelia.*

DAMPNESS, see Cold.

DESIRES, STRANGE, for

BITTER things:—*Digitalis, Natrum muriaticum.*

BRANDY:—1. *Arsenicum, Nux vomica, Sepia, Sulphur.*

2. *Spigelia, Staphysagria.*

3. *China, Pulsatilla.*

COFFEE:—*Arsenicum, China, Conium.*

COAL:—*Cicuta, Conium.*

CHALK, CLAY, etc.:—*Nitri acidum, Nux vomica.*

COOLING things:—1. *Cocculus, Pulsatilla.*

2. *Phosphorus, Valeriana.*

3. *Carbo animalis.*

HERRINGS:—*Nitri acidum.*

JUICY things:—*Phosphori acidum.*

PIQUANT things:—*Pulsatilla.*

SALT things:—1. *Calcarea, Conium.*

2. *Causticum, Nitri acidum.*

3. *Carbo vegetabilis, Phosphorus.*

SPIRITUOUS drinks:—1. *Calcarea, Staphysagria.*

2. *Arsenicum, Mercurius, Nux vomica, Pulsatilla, Sulphur.*

3. *China, Sepia, Spigelia.*

SOURCROUT:—*Carbo animalis, Chamomilla.*

SOUR things:—1. *Arsenicum, Phosphorus, Sulphur.*

2. *Digitalis, Ignatia, Kali, Sepia.*

3. *Carbo animalis, China, Conium, Sabina.*

Desire for SWEETS:—1. *China, Kali, Lycopodium.*

2. *Sulphur.*

3. *Calcarea, Carbo vegetabilis, Nux vomica.*

DYSPEPSIA, digestion difficult:—1. *Calcarea*, *China*, *Mercurius*, *Nux vomica*, *Pulsatilla*, *Sulphur*.
2. *Carbo vegetabilis*, *Natrum muriaticum*, *Sepia*.
3. *Arsenicum*, *Belladonna*, *Conium*, *Ferrum*, *Graphites*, *Ignatia*, *Kali*, *Lycopodium*, *Phosphorus*, *Staphysagria*.

DYSPNŒA, breathing oppressed:—1. *Arsenicum*, *Belladonna*, *Carbo vegetabilis*, *Ignatia*, *Nux vomica*, *Phosphorus*, *Pulsatilla*, *Sepia*, *Sulphur*.
2. *Calcarea*, *China*, *Cocculus*, *Kali*, *Lycopodium*, *Platina*, *Spigelia*, *Zincum*.
3. *Carbo animalis*, *Conium*, *Ferrum*, *Mercurius*, *Staphysagria*.
4. *Digitalis*, *Graphites*, *Nitri acidum*, *Phosphori acidum*, *Plumbum*, *Sabina*, *Sulphuris acid.*, *Valeriana*.

EXERCISE in the open air, aversion to:

As symptom:—1. *Calcarea*, *Cocculus*, *Kali*, *Nux vomica*.
2. *Belladonna*, *China*, *Conium*, *Ignatia*, *Sepia*, *Spigelia*, *Sulphur*, *Valeriana*.
3. *Arsenica*, *Carbo animalis*, *Mercurius*, *Nitri acidum*, *Plumbum*, *Staphysagria*.
4. *Carbo vegetabilis*, *Digitalis*, *Graphites*, *Phosphorus*, *Platina*, *Pulsatilla*, *Sabina*.

FACE, BLUEISH:—1. *Conium*, *Digitalis*.
2. *Arsenicum*, *Belladonna*, *Ignatia*.
3. *Lycopodium*, *Staphysagria*.
4. *Mercurius*, *Phosphorus*, *Pulsatilla*.

Round the eyes:—1. *Arsenicum*, *China*.
2. *Cocculus*, *Ignatia*, *Phosphori acid.*, *Staphysagria*.
3. *Ferrum*, *Nux vomica*, *Phosphorus*, *Sabina*, *Sepia*, *Sulphur*.
4. *Calcarea*, *Graphites*, *Kali*, *Mercurius*, *Spigelia*.

PALE:—1. *Arsenicum*, *China*, *Phosphori acid.*, *Sepia*, *Sulphur*.
2. *Cocculus*, *Conium*, *Ferrum*, *Kali*, *Lycopodium*, *Nux vomica*, *Phosphorus*, *Platina*, *Pulsatilla*, *Spigelia*.

3. *Belladonna*, *Calcarea*, *Carbo animalis*, *Digitalis*, *Helleborus*, *Ignatia*, *Nitri acidum*, *Plumbum*, *Sabina*, *Staphysagria*, *Zincum*.
4. *Carbo vegetabilis*, *Graphites*, *Mercurius*.

EARTHY:—1. *China*, *Ferrum*, *Mercurius*.
2. *Arsenicum*, *Ignatia*, *Nitri acidum*, *Nux vomica*, *Phosphorus*.
3. *Sepia*.
4. *Plumbum*, *Zincum*.

GREENISH:—1. *Arsenicum*, *Carbo vegetabilis*.

YELLOWISH:—1. *Conium*, *Ferrum*, *Nux vomica*, *Plumbum*, *Sepia*, *Sulphur*.
2. *Carbo vegetabilis*, *China*, *Digitalis*, *Mercurius*, *Nitri acidum*, *Phosphorus*.
3. *Arsenicum*, *Belladonna*, *Calcarea*, *Ignatia*, *Kali*, *Pulsatilla*, *Spigelia*.
4. *Causticum*, *Cocculus*, *Graphites*, *Helleborus*, *Natrum muriaticum*, *Sulphuris acid.*

Round the MOUTH:—1. *Sepia*.
2. *Nux vomica*.

The NOSE:—1. *Sepia*, *Nux vomica*.

At the temples:—*Causticum*.

Eyes:—1. *Nitri acidum*, *Spigelia*.
2. *Nux vomica*.

FAINTING, FREQUENT:—1. *China*, *Nux vomica*, *Sepia*.
2. *Arsenicum*, *Cocculus*, *Ferrum*, *Phosphorus*, *Spigelia*.
3. *Belladonna*, *Calcarea*, *Carbo vegetabilis*, *Ignatia*, *Kali*, *Mercurius*, *Plumbum*, *Pulsatilla*, *Sulphur*.
4. *Causticum*, *Conium*, *Graphites*, *Helleborus*, *Nitri acidum*, *Staphysagria*, *Valeriana*.

FLESH, FLABBY (symptom):—1. *Calcarea*, *Cocculus*.
2. *Conium*, *Mercurius*, *Sulphur*.
3. *China*, *Digitalis*, *Ferrum*, *Pulsatilla*.
4. *Graphites*, *Kali*, *Plumbum*, *Sulphuris acidum*.

HEART AFFECTED:—1. *Calcarea*, *Pulsatilla*, *Spigelia*, *Sulphur*.

2. *Lycopodium. Phosphorus, Sepia, Zincum.*
3. *Arsenicum, Belladonna, Carbo vegetabilis, China, Cocculus, Digitalis, Graphites, Kali, Mercurius, Nitri acidum, Nux vomica, Sabina.*
4. *Carbo animalis, Conium, Ferrum, Helleborus, Ignatia, Plumbum, Staphysagria, Valeriana.*

PALPITATION of:—1. *Calcarea, China, Mercurius, Phosphorus, Pulsatilla, Sepia, Spigelia, Sulphur.*
2. *Arsenicum, Belladonna, Carbo vegetabilis, Ignatia, Kali, Nitri acidum, Nux vomica, Zincum.*
3. *Carbo animalis, Cocculus, Digitalis, Ferrum, Graphites, Platina, Plumbum, Sabina, Sulphuris acid.*
4. *Conium, Staphysagria, Valeriana.*

INDOLENCE, aversion to motion:—1. *Arsenicum, Nux vomica.*
2. *Cocculus, Digitalis, Natrum muriaticum.*
3. *Belladonna, Mercurius, Phosphorus, Pulsatilla, Sepia, Zincum.*
4. *Calcarea, Carbo animalis, Carbo vegetabilis, China, Conium, Kali, Nitri acidum, Sulphur.*

INFILTRATIONS, œdematous:—1. *Arsenicum, China, Pulsatilla, Sulphur.*
2. *Belladonna, Lycopodium, Mercurius, Sabina.*
3. *Conium, Ferrum, Kali, Nitri acidum, Phosphorus, Plumbum, Sepia.*

IRON-PREPARATIONS, abuse of (cause):—1. *China, Pulsatilla.*
2. *Arsenicum, Belladonna, Mercurius.*

LEUCORRHŒA (symptom):—1. *Calcarea, Mercurius, Pulsatilla, Sepia.*
2. *Carbo vegetabilis, China, Cocculus, Conium, Ferrum, Graphites, Phosphorus, Sabina, Sulphur.*
3. *Arsenicum, Carbo animalis, Kali, Nitri acidum, Phosphori acid., Sulphuris acid.*
4. *Belladonna, Ignatia, Nux vomica, Platina, Plumbum, Zincum.*

LOVE, UNHAPPY (cause):—*Causticum, Ignatia, Kali, Nux vomica, Phosphori acid., Sepia, Staphysagria.*

NAUSEA:—1. *Nux vomica, Pulsatilla, Sulphur.*
2. *Arsenicum, Belladonna, Calcarea, Carbo vegetabilis, China, Cocculus, Conium, Digitalis, Kali, Mercurius, Nitri acidum, Phosphorus, Sepia.*
3. *Ignatia, Phosphori acid., Platina, Plumbum, Spigelia, Staphysagria.*
4. *Ferrum, Sabina, Zincum.*

ONANISM (cause):—1. *Calcarea, China, Conium, Nux vomica, Phosphori acid., Sepia, Staphysagria, Sulphur.*
2. *Carbo vegetabilis, Kali, Lycopodium, Mercurius, Phosphorus, Pulsatilla, Spigelia.*
3. *Arsenicum, Ferrum, Ignatia, Plumbum.*

SADNESS, melancholy:—1. *Cocculus, Ignatia.*
2. *Belladonna, Graphites, Lycopodium, Platina, Pulsatilla.*
3. *Calcarea, China, Conium, Nux vomica, Sepia, Staphysagria, Sulphur.*
4. *Carbo animalis, Causticum, Digitalis, Helleborus, Kali, Mercurius, Phosphorus, Phosphori acid., Spigelia.*

SIGHING, frequent:—1. *Belladonna, Ignatia, Nux vom.*
2. *China, Cocculus, Digitalis, Graphites, Kali, Mercurius, Nitri acidum, Plumbum, Pulsatilla, Sepia.*

SOLITUDE, desire of:—1. *Belladonna, Ignatia, China.*
2. *Carbo animalis, Conium, Digitalis, Graphites, Nux vomica, Sepia.*

WEEPING, frequent:—1. *Causticum, Platina, Pulsatilla, Sulphur.*
2. *Belladonna, Calcarea, Graphites, Ignatia, Natrum muriaticum, Sepia, Staphysagria.*
3. *Arsenicum, Carbo animalis, Carbo vegetabilis, China, Kali, Nitric acid, Nux vomica, Plumbum, Sulphuris acid.*
4. *Cocculus, Conium, Digitalis, Mercurius, Phosphorus, Zincum.*

ARTICLE XIII.

HYSTERIA.

SECTION 56.

REMARK:—We have spoken of this affection in detail somewhere else,* so that all we have to do here, is to point out the place where this article may be found by those who are unacquainted with our work on "Nervous Diseases." However, in order not to leave a gap in our series, we will here mention very briefly the principal remedies for this affection, referring the reader for the details to the work in question. These remedies are:

1. *Aurum*, *Conium*, *Ignatia*, *Moschus*, *Nux moschata*, *Nux vomica*, *Pulsatilla*, *Sulphur*.
2. *Asarum*, *Belladonna*, *Calcarea*, *Causticum*, *Cicuta*, *Cocculus*, *Magnesia muriatica*, *Natrum muriaticum*, *Nitric acid*, *Platina*, *Sepia*, *Silicea*, *Stramonium*, *Valeriana*, *Viola odorata*.
3. *Aconitum*, *Agaricus*, *Agnus*, *Bryonia*, *Chininum*, *Coffea*, *Hepar*, *Lachesis*, *Mercurius*, *Phosphorus*, *Plumbum*, *Stannum*, *Veratrum*, *Zincum*.
4. *Arsenicum*, *Cannabis*, *Chamomilla*, *Hyoscyamus*, *Opium*, *Phosphori acid.*, *Staphysagria*.
5. *Capsicum*, *Carbo vegetabilis*, *Cuprum*, *Digitalis*, *Dulcamara*, *Iodium*, *Ipecacuanha*, *Lycopodium*, *Rhus*, *Squilla*, *Sulphuris acid.*, *Tartarus*, *Thuja*.

With the following particular indications:

For GENERAL CONVULSIONS:—1. *Belladonna*, *Cicuta*, *Conium*, *Ipecacuanha*, *Moschus*, *Stramonium*, *Veratrum*.

* On the Homœopathic Treatment of Nervous and Menstrual Diseases, translated by Charles J. Hempel, M. D., and published by W. Radde, 332 Broadway, New York.

2. *Calcarea*, *Causticum*, *Conium*, *Cuprum*, *Platina*, *Sulphur*.

4. *Bryonia*, *Coffea*, *Opium*, *Pulsatilla*, *Secale*, *Sepia*.

For the LOCAL or partial symptoms in the moral sphere:—*Calcarea*, *Conium*, *Ignatia*, *Platina*, *Asa fœtida*, *Nux moschata*, *Nux vomica*, *Pulsatilla*, *Sepia*, *Sulphur*, *Silicea*.

HEADACHE: —*Aurum*, *Ignatia*, *Platina*, *Moschus*, *Sepia*, *Belladonna*, *Cocculus*, *Valeriana*, *Veratrum*, *Bryonia*, *Hepar*, *Nitri acidum*, *Phosphorus*.

THROAT:—*Belladonna*, *Ignatia*, *Nux vomica*, *Stramonium*, *Sulphur*, *Cocculus*, *Conium*, *Chamomilla*, *Nitri acidum*, *Pulsatilla*, *Sepia*.

STOMACH: —*Ignatia*, *Chamomilla*, *Cocculus*, *Nux vom.*

BOWELS:—*Ignatia*, *Cocculus*, *Ipecacuanha*, *Nux vomica*, *Moschus*, *Stannum*, *Valeriana*, *Arsenicum*, *Belladonna*, *Stramonium*, *Sulphur*, *Veratrum*.

URINARY organs:—*Asa fœtida*, *Pulsatilla*, *Sepia*, *Belladonna*, *Hepar*, *Nux vomica*, *Zincum*.

UTERUS:—*Cocculus*, *Ignatia*, *Cicuta*, *Conium*, *Nux vomica*, *Pulsatilla*, *Natrum muriaticum*, *Platina*, *Sepia*, *Stannum*, *Stramonium*, *Hyoscyamus*, *Phosphorus*.

LARYNX:—*Belladonna*, *Coffea*, *Cuprum*, *Moschata*, *Phosphorus*, *Natrum muriaticum*, *Platina*, *Hepar*, *Hyoscyamus*, *Pulsatilla*, *Sulphur*, *Veratrum*.

BRONCHIA:—*Belladonna*, *Ignatia*, *Moschus*, *Nux vomica*, *Phosphorus*, *Pulsatilla*, *Aconitum*, *Coffea*, *Cuprum*.

LUNGS:—*Ignatia*, *Moschus*, *Nux vomica*, *Aconitum*, *Belladonna*, *Coffea*, *Nux moschata*, *Pulsatilla*, *Stramonium*, *Aurum*, *Conium*, *Cuprum*, *Ipecacuanha*, *Phosphorus*, *Stannum*.

HEART :—*Aconitum*, *Pulsatilla*, *Chamomilla*, *Cocculus*, *Nux vomica*, *Veratrum*, *Arsenicum*, *Kali*, *Nitri acidum*.

However summary these few details may be, we trust that they will be found sufficient in every case where the different maladies treated of in this volume, are complicated with hysteric symptoms; as regards the treatment of hysteria in its fulness, we again refer the reader to our work on *Nervous Diseases*.

SECOND SECTION.

ORGANIC LESIONS OF THE UTERUS AND ITS APPENDAGES.

Section 57.

General Remark.—Organic affections of the uterus being infinitely more important than those of the remaining sexual organs, we shall first treat of each uterine affection in particular, leaving out only such details as belong exclusively to operative surgery, and we shall afterwards briefly and summarily advert to the treatment of the diseases affecting the remaining organs. In the present Section, we shall treat successively of 1st, the *displacement of the uterus;* 2d, of *endometritis;* 3d, of *metritis;* 4th, of *uterine dropsy;* 5th, of *physometry;* 6th, of *tumors, excrescences* and *foreign bodies in the uterus;* 7th, of *schirrous* and *cancer of the uterus;* 8th, of *noncancerous ulcerations;* 9th, of *gangrene of the uterus;* 10th, of *affections* of the *neck of the uterus;* 11th, of *ovaritis* and other organic lesions of the ovaries; 12th, of *vaginitis* and other affections of the vagina; 13th, of *vulvitis* and other affections of the vulva; 14th, of affections of the *breasts* and *nipples.* We shall only present the internal treatment to be pursued in these affections, and we shall leave out every thing that exclusively concerns the surgical treatment of these affections; at the same time we mean to show that a judicious homœopathic treatment is capable in many cases of superseding the employment of surgical means in organic affections of the sexual organs.

ARTICLE I.

DISPLACEMENTS AND DEVIATIONS OF THE UTERUS.

FALLING, HERNIA, OBLIQUITY AND INVERSION OF THIS ORGAN.

SECTION 58.

FALLING OF THE UTERUS.—By falling of the uterus we understand the displacement of the uterus downward, of which we generally distinguish three degrees; the first, called *relaxation of the uterus*, being simply a slight descension of the organ; the second, being a *falling* of the uterus to the fundus of the pelvis; and the third, consisting in an actual *protrusion* of the uterus outside of the vulva. The first degree is rarely accompanied by any ailments worthy the interference of art, and is very frequently present in the case of women who have had several children. Some practitioners only admit two degrees of this affection, 1st, an incomplete or partial descension of the uterus, and 2nd, an actual protrusion of the organ. In descending, the uterus carries along with it the superior portion of the vagina; the os tincæ either bears on the upper portion of the os cocyx or presents near the orifice of the vagina; the fundus of the womb is generally inclined laterally; the Fallopian tubes are almost in a vertical position, and the small intestines occupy the place of the womb. In complete prolapsus, the vagina is sometimes turned upon itself either partially or totally, forming the external surface of a tumor which, at its lower portion, exhibits the orifice of the uterus, and sometimes assumes the appearance of the skin. Enclosed in this species of sac, the fundus of the bladder and the anterior wall of the rectum are sometimes carried along with the womb. Sometimes the small intestines even descend into the upper part of the external tumor which has been known, in some instances, to go down to the knee. Prolapsus may take place both during and between the periods of pregnancy, or when the uterus is either in health or attacked with disease. The most frequent diseases of the uterus are: acute or chronic inflammation, schirrus or cancer, polypi and fibrous tumors. The organs which accompany the prolapsed uterus, have likewise been seen diseased, especially the bladder, where calculi have been discovered. The symptoms of falling at the first degree, are: pulling in the loins and groin; pains in the small of the back; sense of pressure in the rectum, and constriction of the anus, sensation as if something would issue from the vulva, dysuria and even retention of urine, inflammation and swelling of the uterus, leucorrhœa, pulling in the stomach and more or less considerable disgestive derangements. At the second stage all these symptoms become more marked; the urine which comes in contact with the surface of the tumor, frequently causes a violent inflammation and excoriation of the vaginal mucous membrane, followed by partial or total gangrenous sloughing. The predisposing causes seem to be a lymphatic constitution, chronic leucorrhœa, confinement, a large pelvis, emaciation, frequent constipation, and the presence of tumors bearing upon the uterus; it is more frequently met with in women who have had several children, although we likewise find it in unmarried females and even young girls. Exciting causes are: violent exertions, falling upon the nates or knees, violent shaking when riding in a carriage, long standing or walking, pressure upon the abdomen, pulling at the womb in consequence of large excrescences. As regards *diagnosis*, the disease is clearly revealed by an examination of the parts which exhibit a pear-shaped tumor with the larger portion upwards and the orifice of the womb downwards. This kind of prolapsus must not be confounded with falling of the vagina or elongation of the neck of the womb; in falling of the vagina the shape of the tumor differs from that of the prolapsed uterus, and the os tincæ is distinctly felt at the bottom of the cylindrical cavity which forms the arc of the tumor. As regards the elongated neck, its shape is less cylindrical than that of the womb, and if the finger be introduced in the uterine cavity, the os tincæ is found to be much nearer the vaginal orifice than ordinarily. As to *prognosis*, it depends entirely upon the nature of the causes and upon the duration of the disease, upon the condition of the parts and the constitutional volume of the patients; prolapsus depending upon malformation of the pelvis, is of course incurable; recent prolapsus, or such as results from some accidental cause, is cured the most easily; the diseased condition of the prolapsed parts aggravates the weakness and may portend the most distressing results, although patients have got well even after the sloughing of the gangrened womb. It is supposed by uninformed persons that pregnancy is favorable to the cure of prolapsus, but nothing is more ill-founded. In the fourth or fifth month the uterus indeed resumes its natural height, but after confinement the uterus prolapses again, and successive pregnancies make the weakness worse and worse. The *treatment* of this affection will be described hereafter, when the other organic lesions are treated of.

Section 59.

Hernia of the uterus and ovaries.—By *hernia of the uterus* or *hysterocele*, we understand the passage of this organ into the crural canal, which may take place both with the pregnated and unimpregnated uterus. If unimpregnated, the displaced uterus forms a hard tumor; the os tincæ is raised, turned towards the sacrum or enclosed in the hernial sac; the vagina is stretched, turned from above downwards, and curved forwards towards one or the other groin. During pregnancy hernia generally takes place in consequence of some violent effort; first we observe a rather small tumor in the hypogastrium or towards the groins, which increases gradually and soon reveals its true character by the movements of the fetus. This kind of hernia is occasioned by the weakness and relaxation of the uterine ligaments, contusion of the abdominal muscles, abscesses in the groin, etc.; generally it sets in in consequence of a violent effort. Recent hernia of this kind, of little extent, and without adhesions, can easily be reduced by moderate pressure to be made after the patient is first placed in a suitable position; but, if such hernia takes place during pregnancy, confinement is scarcely ever possible without an operation. Beside hernia of the womb, we sometimes, though very rarely, come across hernia of the ovary. Ovarian hernia may be crural, inguinal, ischiatic, umbilical, or even vaginal, according as the ovary becomes engaged in one or the other of these parts. Very young girls are more particularly subject to this disease, though no age is exempt from it. The most frequent predisposing causes seem to be, among full-grown persons: ascites, emaciation succeeding obesity, immoderate use of fat or oily substances, relaxing beverages, damp climates; among children, an insufficient development of the pelvis, the particular form and situation of the ovaries, etc. The exciting causes are the same as those which induce any other kind of hernia; among children they are, in particular, cries and badly-applied bandages. The accompanying symptoms are almost all of a purely local nature; there is no derangement of the digestive organs, no colic, no constipation or vomiting, no functional or material lesion of any other organ, or even of the uterus. As regards the tumor itself, the skin is not altered, it is circumscribed, has the volume and shape of a pigeon-egg, resisting, more or less uneven, and always the seat of a more or less acute pain, especially when pressed upon; the pain extending in the pelvis and towards the uterus. At the time of the menses, this tumor becomes considerably larger, and decreases again after the period. This hernia never disappears of itself, and it is always more or less difficult to effect reduction by taxis. It is generally difficult to diagnose this hernia; if reducible, it sometimes resembles epiplocele, except that, in this kind of hernia, the tumor is much less circumscribed, never painful to pressure, and the pulling pains are felt rather in the epigastrium than in the hypogastrium. If the hernia is not reducible, it might be confounded with a lymphatic ganglion; but such a tumor is likewise scarcely ever painful, and the gland is always moveable and scarcely ever isolated, nor is it exactly located opposite a hernial orifice; the most difficult cases are those where the hernia is complicated with hydatids or schirrous degenerations. In such cases a diagnosis may sometimes be facilitated by observing the influence which the movements of the neck of the uterus have upon the tumor, inasmuch as no trace of this influence exists in any of the other kinds of hernia with which ovarian hernia might be confounded. This hernia is never serious unless it becomes strangulated, in which case, as in the other kinds of hernia, gangrene is to be apprehended unless reduction is speedily effected.

Section 60.

Obliquity, anteversion and retroversion of the uterus.—By these terms we understand the various deviations of the uterus from the normal line; obliquity, properly speaking, being an accident peculiar to pregnancy, we shall revert to it when speaking of the accidents which may complicate utero-gestation; so that, in the present instance, we shall only treat of *anteversion* and *retroversion*. These names are applied to uterine displacements where the longitudinal axis of the uterus assumes an horizontal direction in the pelvis, in which case we term the displacement *anteversion* when the fundus of the uterus is turned forward, behind the os pubis, and *retroversion*, when the fundus of the uterus is directed toward the hollow of the sacrum. Either of these displacements may take place during and between the periods of pregnancy; *anteversion*, however, occurs more particularly when the uterus is empty, and *retroversion* during pregnancy. For this reason we shall likewise treat of retroversion when we come to speak of pregnancy, and shall here simply deal with anteversion. This defect is very much analogous to falling of the uterus, of which it is, so to say, only a variety. It is generally produced by the same causes, such as: relaxation of the ligaments of the uterus, excessive width of the pelvis combined with narrowness of the lower strait, a fall upon the feet, knees or nates; violent shaking when riding in a carriage, or similar concussions; the affection may also be owing to certain organic lesions, fibrous or other tumors in the anterior wall of the uterus, or tumors situated behind the body of this organ. Some look upon an engorgement of the anterior wall of the uterus as the only cause of the anteversion; but, according to recent observations, this engorgement which is indeed always present, is rather the effect than the cause of the anteversion. The symptoms of this affection are: sense of embarrassment and heaviness in the pelvis, especially at the extremity of the rectum, with more or less frequent tenesmus, frequent urging to urinate, pulling in the groin which sometimes extends to the thighs; pains in the small of the back, and aggravation of the pain by standing, walking or riding in a carriage. Sometimes the bowels are completely bound and the urine cannot be voided. Soon all these symptoms become complicated with symptoms of uterine inflammation, with pains in the pelvis and small of the back, leucorrhœa which is sometimes bloody, irregular menses which are at times too copious, at others too scanty, more or less fever having a remittent or continuous type, deranged digestion, emaciation and loss of strength, and in the event of continued inflammation, organic degenerations of the uterus. On the other hand, at the period of menostasis, all the symptoms of an anteversion sometimes disappear quite suddenly after the complete cessation of the menses and the loss of uterine vitality. The most certain diagnostic sign of this defect is derived from the touch. On inserting the finger into the vagina while the woman is standing erect, we soon meet a solid body engaged in the upper portion of the vagina, which being round in front and thinner behind, will soon be recognized as the displaced uterus, which can at once be restored to its natural position by hooking the os tincæ with the finger and bringing this part of the uterus forward. As regards *prognosis*, the difficulty is proportionate to the development of the organic affection and to the symptoms described above; sometimes anteversion becomes a cause of sterility. The *treatment* will be found described at the close of this article.

Section 61.

Inversion of the Uterus.—We understand by this defect, the complete turning of the uterus inside out, in the manner of a glove, stocking or hat, the internal becoming the external surface. We generally distinguish three degrees of this affection, namely: 1, *Simple depression*, where the fundus of the uterus is only a little depressed. 2, *Incomplete inversion*, when the fundus of the uterus has come down to the orifice, and has even penetrated into the vagina. 3, *Complete inversion*, when the uterus is completely turned inside out, and is suspended in the vagina, close to the vulva. These various degrees of inversion may take place after confinement, or at any other period entirely removed from this event. When occurring after confinement, a description of the treatment to be pursued will be furnished in the article devoted to the accidents and ailments incidental to confinement; here we have only to do with the other degrees. The symptoms which characterize this affection generally differ somewhat according as the inversion is more or less complete, or takes place suddenly or gradually, under circumstances which are more or less serious. Incomplete inversion sometimes announces itself simply by a more or less copious menorrhagia, or a simple leucorrhœic discharge when the accident occurs independently of parturition. Other symptoms gradually develop themselves, such as pullings and twitchings in the groin, pains in the small of the back, a sensation of distention and heaviness in the pelvis. If the inversion is not reduced in season, the inverted part in the vagina may become strangulated, and the fundus of the uterus may tear, whence inflammation, and subsequent gangrene, and lastly death, may result; or, if the inflammation should be less intense, a simple adhesion of such portions of the peritoneal coat of the uterus as are brought in contact with each other, may be the consequence. In complete inversion, all the above-mentioned symptoms become much more marked, with tearing pains, violent pullings, syncope, convulsions, and an hæmorrhage which may soon terminate fatally. Even if the patient's life is not destroyed by hæmorrhage or gangrene, the womb, hanging out of the vulva, irritated by the contact with urine, air and clothes, remains almost always in a permanent state of chronic inflammation, and becomes covered with more or less serious ulcerations. The causes of inversion, not induced by parturition, are most of them analogous to the traction and the pressure made on the uterus during parturition. For instance, inversion may be caused by extensive polypi, by uterine dropsies, by effusions of blood in the uterine cavity, which tends to thin the walls of this organ, to weaken its energies, and, by suddenly escaping from the uterine cavity, to drag the uterus after it. As regards the *diagnosis*, we become advised of a simple depression, and of an imcomplete inversion of the uterus, by the touch revealing the existing condition of the womb, and, in complete inversion, by the aspect and shape of the tumor within the vagina and outside of the vulva. Considering all that we have said here, and in Section 58, of falling of the womb, and of the shape and character of these tumors, it seems almost impossible to confound an inverted womb with any of the other tumors occurring in the vagina, or protruding from the vulva. The *prognosis* is always dubious, for the inversion may soon terminate fatally, unless repaired in season. The sooner the inversion takes place after confinement, the greater the danger; the further removed from the period of confinement, the less dangerous the accident becomes. Reduction immediately after inversion is not so very difficult; the longer reduction is delayed, the more difficult it becomes. Some authors speak of old cases of inversion, that became reduced spontaneously in consequence of some sudden concussion of the female body. If inversion is caused by a polypus, the womb resumes of itself its original position, after the removal of the weight that drew it down.

SECTION 62.

TREATMENT OF ALL DISPLACEMENTS.—In order to avoid frequent repetitions, we have condensed the treatment of the various forms of displacements into one paragraph. Our business is not to point out the surgical means that it may be necessary to resort to in these affections, but to show the internal treatment, which will sometimes enable us to do without surgical operations, or, at any rate, which will wonderfully facilitate the use of instruments. Thanks to Hahnemann, these internal means are furnished by homœopathy. A few globules of the proper remedy will sometimes do more for the patient, in such affections, than all the appliances of surgery. Of course, the necessary external means should not be neglected, for no cure can be affected without them. Whatever may be the nature of the displacement, the patient should always be placed on her back, in a horizontal position, and, as a general rule, should be kept in this position until health is totally restored. In recent and complicated cases of inflammation, strangulation, gangrene or hæmorrhage, some remedy which will facilitate the reduction should at once be administered, particularly *Nux vomica*, *Sepia*, *Ignatia*, or one of the remedies mentioned below; after which the patient should be left undisturbed by work or mental excitement. In most cases, such treatment may be sufficient to effect a reduction without any surgical means. Even in severe cases of inflammation, hæmorrhage or strangulation, a well chosen remedy, corresponding to all the symptoms of the case, will be found sufficient to effect a cure, without the interference of the surgeon. If the displacement is of long standing, and the patient has to attend to her business, it will not always be found possible to effect a cure without well applied bandages, provided they are adapted to the case before us, and constructed by an intelligent maker; for a badly made or improperly applied bandage may do as much harm as a well made and properly applied bandage may do good. The principal remedies which are to be administered internally, in the various displacements, are:

1. *Belladonna, Ignatia, Mercurius, Nux vomica, Sepia, Sulphur.*
2. *Ferrum, Kreosotum, Stannum.*
3. *Aconitum, Aurum, Cocculus, Colocynthis, Lycopodium, Natrum muriat., Nitri acidum.*
4. *Cantharides, Dulcamara, Graphites, Nux moschata, Silicea, Thuja, Veratrum.*

For FALLING of the womb:—1. *Nux vomica, Platina, Thuja.*
2. *Belladonna, Sepia.*
3. *Aurum, Calcarea, Kreosotum, Mercurius.*
4. *Ferrum, Nux moschata, Stannum.*

Of the vagina:—1. *Mercurius, Sepia.*
2. *Ferrum, Ammonium.*
3. *Belladonna, Nux vomica.*
4. *Aurum, Calcarea, Ferrum, Nux moschata.*

For HERNIA of the womb:—1. *Nux vomica, Sulphur.*
2. *Aurum, Cocculus, Silicea, Veratrum.*
3. *Chamomilla, Colocynthis, Nitri acidum, Opium, Phosphorus, Rhus, Staphysagria.*
4. *Aconitum, Carbo animalis, China, Pulsatilla, Thuja, Zincum.*

For ANTEVERSION:—1. *Nux vomica, Platina.*
2. *Belladonna, Sepia.*
3. *Aurum, Calcarea, Ferrum, Mercurius, Vux vom., Stannum.*

For INVERSION:—1. *Belladonna, Nux vomica.*
2. *Calcarea, Mercurius, Stannum.*
3. *Aurum, Ferrum, Nux moschata.*

For STRANGULATION of the parts:—1. *Aconitum, Sulphur.*
2. *Lachesis, Opium.*
3. *Arsenicum, Vux vomica, Belladonna, Veratrum.*

For GANGRENE:—1. *Arsenicum, Belladonna.*
2. *Cantharides, Kreosotum, Lachesis, Sulphur.*

For HÆMORRHAGE:—1. *Belladonna, Ferrum, Mercurius, Nux vomica, Sepia, Sulphur.*
2. *Aconitum, Calcarea, China, Lycopodium, Nitri acidum.*
3. *Phosphorus, Zincum.*

For INFLAMMATION:—1. *Aconitum, Belladonna, Mercurius, Nux vomica, Sepia, Sulphur, Sulphuris acidum.*

For LEUCORRHŒA:—1. *Belladonna, Mercurius, Sepia, Sulphur.*
2. *Ferrum, Kreosotum, Nux vomica, Stannum.*
3. *Cocculus, Nitri acidum.*

DOSE.—For chronic cases give three or four globules, or one or two drops of the attenuated preparation on sugar or in a spoonful of water every morning and evening, and in acute cases dissolve this dose in ten tablespoonfuls of water, and give a tablespoonful every five minutes, or every half hour, hour, or two and three hours, according to the gravity and intensity of the case.

ARTICLE II.

ENDOMETRITIS, OR SUPERFICIAL METRITIS.

SECTION 63.

GENERAL OBSERVATION.—We understand by endometritis, or superficial metritis, an inflammation of the uterine lining membrane. Some authors have confounded it with metritis or parenchymatous inflammation of this organ; but the ancients have always described it as a separate malady under the name of blennorrhagia of the uterus or uterine catarrh. This inflammation may either be acute or chronic, each of which presents symptoms which it may be well to distinguish. In the following paragraphs we shall treat, 1st, of acute *endometritis* or *blennorrhagia* of the uterus, and 2nd, of chronic endometritis or *uterine catarrh*, giving the symtomatology, etiology and diagnosis of each disease. As regards the treatment of these two affections, it has so many points of contact that we shall unite in one paragraph all we have to say on the subject. The treatment will be indicated after the pathology of these two affections.

SECTION 64.

BLENNORRHAGIA, OR ACUTE SUPERFICIAL METRITIS.—This affection is a superficial phlegmasia of the internal lining membrane of the uterus, and is characterised by acute, inflammatory leucorrhœa. The irritation may either be confined to the uterus, or may be accompanied with inflammation of the vaginal mucous membrane. At first the symptoms with which the disease sets in, are: a more or less marked febrile movement, with malaise, spontaneous lassitude, headache, though these symptoms only exist in the severer forms of this inflammation, but are almost always absent in the lighter ones. These precursory symptoms generally last from four to six days, at the termination of which period a heavy pain is generally experienced above the pubes extending to the loins, perinæum, groin and thighs, with heat, itching and smarting at the genital organs, difficult, painful and smarting micturition. In many cases the inflammation invades the external parts; they become sensitive, moist, red and swollen; at the same time the mouth of the uterus becomes more open, softer, moister, warmer and more painful than usual. The catarrhal discharge generally sets in as soon as the uterus begins to show signs of sensitiveness; at first it is serous and bloody, but it soon becomes thick, yellowish or greenish, ropy, fluid or purulent; after drying up, it leaves yellow or greenish stains on the linen, and stiffens it as if it had been starched; afterwards the discharge sometimes becomes whiter, milky and mixed with transparent pieces of thick mucus. If this change in the discharge sets in, the inflammatory condition is almost entirely dispersed, which may take place at the end of thirty-six or forty days or even sooner, when the discharge becomes chronic, or reappears again at the time of the menses, after sexual excesses, overeating or drinking, or even without any apparent cause. As a general rule, the more acute the inflammation, the thicker and darker the discharge. The discharge always has an alkaline reaction, whereas vaginal secretions always react like acids. Examined by the microscope, the discharge looks homogeneous, thick, containing globules resembling those that float in pus or healthy mucus. As regards the course of this affection, we may distinguish four periods. The first period sets in with a rather slight itching at the vulva, in the interior of the vagina and sometimes in the uterus, with sense of heat in the uterus, pains in the small of the back and in the back, increase of the sexual desire and frequent urging to urinate. In the second period, which sets in about the third or fourth day, a serous discharge takes place which is at first scanty, but soon becomes more profuse, assumes a greenish or yellowish, rather dark appearance, and is accompanied with increased burning at urination. In the third period, which generally commences about the ninth day, the inflammation becomes less intense, is still very copious, thickens, becomes more and more whitish, and then decreases, with diminution of the flow of urine. In the fourth period, when the disease inclines to become chronic, the discharge disappears and reappears again repeatedly, and frequently without any known cause. The causes of this affection are frequently the same as those that give rise to vaginitis; in many cases the uterine blennorrhagia is nothing more than a development of a pre-existing vaginal irritation. Most frequently this phlegmasia becomes developed at the menstrual periods, especially when the normal menstrual discharge is either insufficient or remains entirely absent. Another cause of this disease are long and painful confinements, miscarriages, the presence of polypi or hydatids in the uterus, engorgements, indurations or other organic lesions of this organ, and more particularly sexual abuses, onanism, irritating injections and any other irritating causes. As regards DIAGNOSIS; an inflammatory catarrhal discharge can easily be distinguished from a simple and mild leucorrhœa; it will likewise be an easy matter to distinguish between acute blennorrhagia and a parenchymatous inflammation of the uterus, inasmuch as there is scarcely any or very little discharge in the latter disease, and the body of the uterus is moreover enlarged, which is not the case in uterine catarrh; as regards symptomatic discharges of the uterus, such as take place in cancer, engorgements, etc., all doubts will likewise be removed by the touch or by an exploration of the parts. The greatest difficulty will be found in distinguishing this discharge from syphilis; in such a case all absence of other syphilitic signs, and a history of the case, will enable us to decide. The PROGNOSIS of acute blennorrhagia is never serious; when not complicated, in healthy and otherwise well formed women, it generally terminates in resolution. In vicious, lymphatic, scrofulous or herpetic constitutions, or when other disorganizations of the uterus are present, or when the exciting cause continues to operate, the disease inclines more than any other to pass into the chronic form, and becomes exceedingly obstinate even under treatment.

Section 65.

Uterine catarrh or superficial chronic metritis.—In most cases, or perhaps in all cases, this affection is only the consequence of an acute blenorrhagia of the uterus, so that even where it appears to be a primary disease, it may always be supposed that it has been preceded by an acute stage which has passed over without having been observed. The symptoms by which this affection manifests itself, are: dull pains in the hypogastrium aggravated by pressure, with pulling in the loins, groin, thighs, frequent urging to urinate and painful urination. These pains are accompanied by a leucorrhœal discharge of a dirty-white or yellowish color, more or less consistent, having a sickening and insipid smell, an alkaline reaction and being more or less profuse. If proceeding from the neck of the uterus, it is more abundant and more tenacious than that which is secreted from the body of the uterus. In most cases the disease is accompanied by digestive derangements, bulimia alternating with anorexia, pains in the stomach, nausea, vomiting of ropy mucus in the morning. These symptoms, especially the discharge, become generally worse immediately before or after the menses, under the influence of a stimulating diet, or in consequence of sexual excesses, onanism, etc. In some women, this affection increases the sexual desire; in others, this desire is diminished, and even gives place to positive repugnance.—Chronic catarrh of the uterus being the result of an acute blennorrhagia which had probably passed unnoticed, the exciting or predisposing causes of catarrh are the same as those of acute blennorrhagia. The diagnosis is obtained by the touch and by an exploration of the affected parts; the mucous membrane of the neck is generally red and inflamed and at the uterine orifice we discover traces of the matter that is discharged from the vagina; the orifice is open and the parts composing it are soft and swollen.—The PROGNOSIS is not serious except where a continuance of this affection has given rise to uterine disorganizations; sometimes the disease terminates spontaneously in resolution; in other cases it disappears and gives rise to some other affection; still more frequently it continues for years unless it is removed by rational and truly efficacious treatment.

SECTION 66.

TREATMENT.—The best means for acute as well as chronic blennorrhagia, are:

1. *Alumina, Calcarea, Kreosotum, Mercurius, Pulsatilla, Sepia.*
2. *Ammonium, Bovista, Carbo vegetabilis, China, Cocculus, Ferrum, Graphites, Lycopodium, Phosphorus, Sabina, Silicea, Sulphur.*
3. *Arsenicum, Borax, Cantharides, Carbo animalis, Iodium, Kali, Magnesia carbonica, Mezereum, Natrum, Natrum muriatica, Nitri acidum, Phosphori acidum, Platina, Stannum, Veratrum, Sulphuris acidum.*
4. *Belladonna, Coffea, Lachesis, Nux vomica, Zincum.*

With the following particular indications:

In the FIRST PERIOD:—1. *Pulsatilla, Mercurius, Sepia, Kreosotum.*
2. *China, Cocculus, Ferrum, Phosphorus, Platina, Sabina.*

In the SECOND PERIOD:—1. *Mercurius, Pulsatilla, Sabina, Sepia.*
2. *Alumina, Calcarea, China, Cocculus, Kreosotum, Lycopodium, Natrum, Nitri acidum.*

In CHRONIC catarrh, or in the third or fourth period of acute blennorrhagia:—1. *Alumina, Calcarea, Mercurius, Pulsatilla, Sepia.*

2. *Ammonium, Carbo vegetabilis, China, Cocculus, Ferrum, Graphites, Lycopodium, Phosphorus, Sabina, Silicea, Sulphur.*

And particularly:

For sexual APPETITE increased:—1. *Belladonna, Platina, Veratrum.*

2. *China, Coffea.*

3. *Arsenicum, Cantharis, Kreosotum, Lachesis, Nux vomica, Sulphuris acidum, Zincum.*

ABDOMEN PAINFUL:—1. *Belladonna, Carbo vegetabilis, Lycopodium, Magnesia muriat.*

2. *Causticum, Conium, Drosera, Ignatia, Pulsatilla, Sepia, Silicea, Sulphur, Zincum.*

3. *Alumina, Ammonium muriat., Belladonna, Graphites, Kali, Mercurius, Natrum, Natrum muriat.*

Desire, SEXUAL, less:—*Belladonna, Kali, Natrum muriat.*

DISCHARGE, ACRID:—1. *Alumina, Ferrum, Mercurius, Phosphorus.*

2. *Arsenicum, Bovista, Carbo vegetabilis, Conium, Iodium, Sepia, Silicea.*

3. *Ammonium, Chamomilla, Ignatia, Kreosotum, Lycopodium, Pulsatilla, Ruta, Sulphur, Sulphuris acidum.*

4. *Antimonium, Calcarea, Cannabis, Cantharis, Carbo animalis, China, Hepar, Kali, Magnesia carbonica, Magnesia muriatica, Mezereum, Nitri acidum, Phosphori acidum, Thuja.*

BLOODY:—*China, Cocculus.*

2. *Kreosotum, Nitri acidum.*

3. *Arsenicum, Lycopodium, Sepia, Silicea, Sulphuris acidum.*

4. *Alumina, Antimonium, Cantharis, Carbo veget., Conium, Magnesia muriatica.*

BROWN:—*Nitri acidum.*

BURNING:—1. *Calcarea, Pulsatilla.*

2. *Conium, Kreosotum.*

3. *Ammonium, Cantharis, Carbo animalis, Kali, Sulphuris acidum.*
4. *Arsenicum, Borax.*

CORROSIVE, see ACRID.

FETID:—1. *Kreosotum, Sabina.*
2. *Natrum.*
3. *China, Nitri acidum, Nux vomica, Sepia.*

GREENISH:—1. *Sepia.*
2. *Bovista, Mercurius.*
3. *Carbo vegetabilis, Pulsatilla.*

ITCHING:—1. *Calcarea.*
2. *Alumina, Kreosotum, Mercurius.*
3. *Sabina, Sepia.*
4. *Arsenicum, China, Ferrum, Kali, Phosphori acid.*

MILKY:—1. *Calcarea, Pulsatilla.*
2. *Ammonium, Silicea.*
3. *Carbo vegetabilis, Ferrum, Sulphur.*
4. *Conium, Graphites, Kreosotum, Lycopodium, Phosphorus, Sabina, Sepia, Sulphuris acidum.*

PURULENT:—1. *Cocculus, Mercurius, Sabina.*
2. *China, Kreosotum, Sepia.*
3. *Calcarea, Ignatia.*

THICK:—1. *Pulsatilla.*
2. *Sabina.*
3. *Arsenicum, Carbo vegetabilis, Natrum, Natrum muriatica, Zincum.*
4. *Ambra, Bovista, Sepia.*

VISCID:—1. *Borax, Stramonium.*
2. *Bovista, Sabina.*
3. *Aconitum, Phosphorus, Phosphori acidum.*

WATERY, serous:—1. *Graphites.*
2. *Ammonium, Pulsatilla, Sepia.*
3. *Antimonium, Carbo animalis, Carbo vegetabilis, Chamomilla, China, Kreosotum, Magnesia carbon., Magnesia muriat., Mercurius, Nitrum, Silicea, Sulphur.*

YELLOWISH :—1. *Sepia.*

2. *Kreosotum, Lycopodium, Sabina.*

3. *Aconitum, Carbo animalis, Carbo vegetabilis, Chamomilla, Nux vomica.*

4. *Alumina, Arsenicum, Bovista, Kali, Phosphori acidum, Sulphur.*

MENSES SUPPRESSED :—1. *Conium, Graphites, Kali, Pulsatilla, Silicea, Sulphur.*

2. *Aconitum, Calcarea, Chamomilla, Cocculus, Ferrum, Phosphorus, Sepia.*

3. *Arsenicum, China, Lachesis, Magnesia carbonica, Mercurius, Nitri acidum, Platina, Sabina, Zincum.*

TOO SCANTY :—1. *Ammonium, Conium, Graphites, Kali, Pulsatilla, Sulphur.*

2. *Alumina, Cocculus, Lachesis, Lycopodium, Mercurius, Phosphorus, Silicea.*

3. *Aconitum, Ferrum, Sabina, Sepia.*

PAINS in SMALL of back :—1. *Magnesia muriatica.*

2. *Baryta, Conium, Graphites, Kali, Kreosotum.*

VAGINA AFFECTED :—1. *Calcarea, Kali, Sepia.*

2. *Belladonna, Cantharis, China, Kreosotum, Ferrum, Lycopodium, Mercurius, Nux vomica, Pulsatilla, Thuja.*

3. *Arsenicum, Carbo vegetabilis, Cocculus, Conium, Graphites, Natrum muriaticum, Nitri acidum, Phosphorus, Platina, Sabina.*

4. *Borax, Carbo animalis, Magnesia muriatica, Natrum, Silicea, Sulphuris acidum, Zincum.*

VULVA affected, LABIA swollen :—1. *Sepia.*

2. *Carbo vegetabilis, Mercurius, Nux vomica.*

3. *Aconitum, Belladonna, Calcarea, Conium, Natrum muriat., Nitri acidum, Silicea, Sulphur, Thuja.*

4. *Ammonium, Graphites, Kali, Kreosotum, Nitri acidum, Pulsatilla.*

WOMB, PAINFULNESS of :—1. *Belladonna, Conium, Nux vomica, Platina, Pulsatilla, Sepia, Sulphur.*

2. *Chamomilla, Cocculus, Graphites, Kreosotum, Magnesia carbon., Magnesia muriat., Sabina.*
3. *Carbo animalis, China, Ferrum, Kali, Natrum muriaticum.*

WORSE *before* the menses :—1. *Calcarea, Lachesis.*
2. *Baryta, Carbo vegetabilis, China, Phosphorus.*
3. *Kreosotum, Pulsatilla.*
4. *Alumina, Graphites, Ruta, Sepia, Sulphur, Zincum.*

During the menses :—1. *Alumina.*
2. *China, Cocculus, Graphites, Lachesis, Pulsatilla, Zincum.*

Following the menses :—1. *Alumina.*
2. *Pulsatilla, Ruta, Sabina.*
3. *Cocculus, Kreosotum, Mercurius, Nitri acidum, Silicea, Sulphur.*
4. *Bovista, Graphites, Magnesia carbonica, Phosphori acidum.*

For further information concerning the use of the abovementioned drugs, see the articles on *dysmenorrhœa* and *leucorrhœa.*

DOSE.—In acute cases dissolve six globules, or one or two drops of the liquid attenuation in ten table-spoonfuls of water, and give the patient a table-spoonful of this solution every two hours; in chronic cases give a few globules every night before retiring, dry on the tongue or dissolved in a spoonful of water.

ARTICLE III.

TRUE OR PARENCHYMATOUS METRITIS.

Section 67.

General Observations.—After long and serious reflections we have been induced to reserve the name of *metritis* for an inflammation of the tissue of the uterus; for whatever opinions modern authors may express on the subject, in the so-called *superficial metritis,* it is only the mucous lining that is inflamed; but just as palpable a mistake it would be to designate by the term carditis an inflammation of the external or internal membrane of the heart, which would constitute either *pericarditis* or *endocarditis*, just as false it would be to call metritis an inflammation of the lining membrane of this organ. By metritis we understand an inflammation of the uterine substance itself. But, in order to avoid all confusion resulting from the fact that our learned professors have ranged all kinds of uterine inflammation under the name of *metritis,* we will designate an inflammation of the uterine tissue by the adjective *tune* or *parenchymatous metritis*. The acute form of this disease generally occurs only during confinement; the chronic form is frequently met with in the unimpregnated uterus, in which case the neck of the uterus is most frequently the seat of the disease. Hence result tolerably characteristic differences between the acute and chronic forms of metritis, which we will describe in the following paragraphs in this order; 1st, *acute* metritis; 2d, *chronic* metritis, to be followed by the *treatment* of both of these affections.

Section 68.

Acute Metritis.—The symptoms of this affection differ

according as the neck alone, or the neck and body of the uterus are affected. An acute inflammation of the neck of the uterus generally sets in after the first embrace or in consequence of severe labor. In the former case the neck is a little swollen, warm and very sensitive to contact; in the latter case, the pain deep in the vagina is more or less acute; there is a discharge of blood or of bloody mucus, and an examination shows that the neck is swollen and sometimes covered with cracks having more or less depth. Febrile symptoms are generally absent, and the affection is without danger; in most cases a cure takes place without the interference of art, although this acute form sometimes passes into the chronic stage. When the whole body of the uterus becomes inflamed, other symptoms develop themselves beside those which we have described above. General metritis commences most frequently with a more or less acute pain in the hypogastrium; if the peritoneum should be involved, this pain is felt in all the parts of the abdomen. It is a continuous, fixed pain, aggravated by pressure, cough, deep inspirations. At the same time a sense of heaviness, heat and tension is felt in the hypogastrium. An examination shows that the neck is soft, swollen, painful to contact and warmer than the vagina. Sometimes the uterus forms a round tumor above the pubes which, being deep-seated, is more easily discovered by the touch than by sight. Frequently a species of tenesmus of the rectum and dysuria with painful urination supervenes. The loins, the groins and the thighs are equally affected by pains consisting for the most part in painful twitchings and pullings. Most patients complain moreover of headache, especially in the frontal region, with vanishing of sight and hearing, vomiting, partial sweat, pains in the small of the back, lassitude, fainting turns, profound changes in the features, pale face, etc. Fever is not wanting; it consists in a violent chill which lasts a long time, and is followed by heat with a torpid character. The pulse is hurried, the skin dry and warm, the urine red. In fatal cases we have afterwards meteorism, singultus, delirium, coldness of the extremities and discharge of fetid matter from the vagina. Sometimes the affection involves the neighboring organs, the peritoneum, ovaries, fallopian tubes, etc., which may happen even in the mildest cases. As to the CAUSES of this disease, it is rarely ever noticed before the age of pubescence, and after the critical period; it occurs quite frequently during confinement, but rarely during pregnancy. *Exciting causes* are: serious wounds, compression, ligatures, cauterizations, commotions of the uterus in consequence of too much vehemence during intercourse, sudden suppression of the menses, vaginal injections, mechanical or external irritations, tetter at the parts, ascarides in the anus or vagina, violent straining at stool, etc. The DIAGNOSIS of acute metritis is sometimes rather obscure; but an attentive exploration of the sexual parts may help us establish it, especially when the inflammation is confined to the neck; but if both the uterus and the peritoneum are invaded, metritis can readily be diagnosed; for, in simple peritonitis, the symptoms of metritis are always absent; whence we may infer that, whenever the symptoms of peritonitis and metritis co-exist, the inflammation was originally a case of genuine metritis. As regards the COURSE and TERMINATION of acute metritis, it may terminate in death even on the third or second day after the disease had set in, but which generally happens within seven days, or within two, three or four weeks after the invasion of the disease. Sometimes the inflammation terminates in gangrene, in consequence of which the dead uterus has been known to become detached from the body, expelled through the vagina, and the patient nevertheless to survive such a terrible accident. Metritis however does not always terminate fatally or lead to disastrous results. Cases which happen between the periods of pregnancy, and which do not involve the peritoneum or the whole womb, generally terminate happily, within a few weeks, or after three or four days, especially under homœopathic treatment. Metritis setting in during pregnancy, often leads to the destruction of the fetus and even to the death of the mother. Among the consequences of acute metritis, we have to note an obstruction of the Fallopian tubes as occurring quite frequently, in consequence of which sterility of course result. The PROGNOSIS of course depends upon the extent of the inflammation, upon its intensity and upon existing complications. Inflammations occurring during pregnancy or immediately after confinement, are always more dangerous than those which occur at other periods.

SECTION 69.

CHRONIC METRITIS.—This affection occurs much more frequently than acute metritis. It may set in in consequence of an acute inflammation or as a primary disease, and may either affect the whole of the uterus or the neck only. The primary disease seems to be principally owing to sexual excesses, to onanism, the use of pessaries, or to some herpetic or rheumatic metastasis; often it sets in without any apparent cause; it occurs most frequently between the twentieth and the fortieth year. The characteristic SYMPTOMS of this disease are: dull and heavy pain in the hypogastrium, extending to the loins, groin, thighs and sometimes to the breasts, the pain being aggravated by long standing, walking or by sexual excesses; sometimes the pain is accompanied by a discharge of opaque, milky, inodorous mucus from the vagina, and sometimes by hæmorrhages with paleness of the face, weakness, emaciation. With some exceptions most women preserve their volume, good looks and even strength. The os tincæ appears more elongated than in its normal state; the neck is very soft, its surface is smooth and the orifice generally closed; touch always causes a more or less acute pain, or aggravates the pain generally experienced by the patient. When the disease is confined to the neck, the womb preserves its mobility and ordinary weight; but when the body of the uterus is involved, this organ always seems heavier when attempted to be raised by the finger introduced into the vagina, and it is less moveable on examining the hypogastrium, or on introducing the finger in the rectum, we sometimes discover a round tumor in the region of the womb, which is easily recognised as the uterus by the various movements imparted to it by the exploring finger. The menstrual discharge is generally painful and difficult, though not necessarily suppressed.—This affection generally runs a slow COURSE; it may continue for years without any noticeable change in the symptoms or without any local changes; often the disease may terminate favorably, in which case the swelling of the womb diminishes gradually and the symptoms which the patient experienced disappear, or become reduced to some obscure and not very embarrassing sensations in the hypogastrium; in some cases the trouble remains unchanged for an indefinite period. It is a mistake to suppose that cancerous ulcerations and degenerations can result from chronic metritis; this is about as true as it is that tubercular phthisis can result from some neglected catarrh of the lungs. Cancerous and schirrous degenerations are idiopathic affections resulting from pre-existing germs in the diseased organ; this germ may indeed be developed but cannot be created by succeeding or continuous inflammations or catarrhs; on the contrary, its presence is very frequently the only *pathological cause* of these repeated catarrhal inflammations. Uterine catarrh is readily DIAGNOSED; it cannot well be confounded with cancer or polypus of the womb, both of which diseases are characterized by symptoms which are wanting in catarrh. In cancer the affected part is hard, uneven, and the seat of lancinating pains; there is a reddish discharge, frequent flooding, and the face of the patient has the straw-colored complexion which we observe in all cancerous diseases. In a case of polypus, if it has not yet grown outside of the uterine orifice, the neck will be found open, and the expulsive pains which frequently accompany the repeated hæmorrhages, may at least lead us to suspect the presence of polypus. The *prognosis* of chronic uteritis may be inferred from what we have said of the course of the disease; if no cancerous diathesis or polypi are present, the affection is not as serious as one would suppose; simple cases yield more or less promptly to homœopathic treatment.

Section 70.

Treatment.—The principal remedies for acute or chronic parenchymatous metritis are:

1. *Pulsatilla*, *Sepia*, *Belladonna*, *Chamomilla*, *Kali*, *Platina*, *Sabina*.
2. *Bryonia*, *Carbo animalis*, *Conium*, *Crocus*, *Ferrum*, *Graphites*, *Kreosotum*, *Mercurius*, *Nux vomica*, *Opium*, *Rhus*, *Secale*, *Sulphur*.
3. *Aconitum*, *Arnica*, *Calcarea*, *China*, *Cocculus*, *Coffea*, *Colocynthis*, *Hyoscyamus*, *Ignatia*, *Ipecacuanha*, *Magnesia muriatica*, *Natrum*, *Natrum muriaticum*, *Phosphoric acid*, *Thuja*.
4. *Arsenicum*, *Cantharis*, *Lachesis*, *Lycopodium*, *Magnesia carb.*, *Phosphorus*, *Stramonium*, *Sulphuris acid.*, *Veratrum*, *Zincum*.

With the following particular indications:

For acute metritis:—1. *Mercurius*, *Belladonna*.
2. *Aconitum*, *Chamomilla*, *Coffea*, *Nux vomica*.
3. *Bryonia*, *Cantharis*, *China*, *Cocculus Ignatia*, *Lachesis*, *Platina*, *Pulsatilla*, *Rhus*, *Sabina*, *Secale*, *Sepia*.
4. *Arnica*, *Arsenicum*, *Cocculus*, *Crocus*, *Ferrum*, *Hyoscyamus*, *Stramonium*, *Sulphur*, *Veratrum*.

For chronic metritis:—1. *Belladonna*, *Calcarea*, *China*, *Cocculus*, *Conium*, *Kali*, *Kreosotum*, *Nux vomica*, *Platina*, *Pulsatilla*, *Sabina*, *Secale*, *Sepia*.
2. *Bryonia*, *Ferrum*, *Graphites*, *Lycopodium*, *Magnesia carbonica*, *Magnesia muriatica*, *Natrum*, *Natrum muriaticum*, *Phosphorus*, *Zincum*.

And with these complications:

With gangrene:—1. *Sabina*, *Secale*.
2. *Arsenicum*, *Belladonna*, *Lachesis*, *Silicea*.
3. *Aconitum*, *Conium*, *Mercurius*, *Plumbum*, *Sulphur*, *Sulphuris acid.*

Hiccough:—1. *Nux vomica*.
2. *Ammonium muriaticum Hyoscyamus*, *Ignatia*.
3. *Belladonna*, *Pulsatilla*, *Veratrum*.

4. *Aconitum*, *Cocculus*, *Lycopodium*, *Magnesia muriaticum*, *Mercurius*, *Natrum*, *Staphysagria*, *Stramonium*, *Sulphur*.

LEUCORRHŒA:—1. *Calcarea*, *Kreosotum*, *Mercurius*, *Pulsatilla*, *Sepia*.

2. *Ammonium*, *Carbo vegetabilis*, *China*, *Cocculus*, *Conium*, *Ferrum*, *Graphites*, *Lycopodium*, *Phosphorus*, *Sabina*, *Sepia*, *Sulphur*.

3. *Arsenicum*, *Cantharis*, *Carbo animalis*, *Chamomilla*, *Magnesia carbonica*, *Natrum muriaticum*, *Phosphori acid.*, *Sulphuris acidum*.

Complications with frequent METRORRHAGIA:—1. *Belladonna*, *Calcarea*, *China*, *Ferrum*, *Nux vomica*, *Sabina*.

2. *Bryonia*, *Chamomilla*, *Crocus*, *Lycopodium*, *Mercurius*, *Nitri acidum*, *Phosphorus*, *Pulsatilla*, *Secale*, *Sepia*, *Stramonium*, *Sulphur*.

3. *Aconitum*, *Cantharis*, *Coffea*, *Platina*, *Silicea*, *Sulphuris acidum*.

MENSES SUPPRESSED:—1. *Conium*, *Graphites*, *Kali*, *Lycopodium*, *Pulsatilla*, *Sulphur*.

2. *Aconitum*, *Calcarea*, *Chamomilla*, *Cocculus*, *Ferrum*, *Phosphorus*, *Sepia*, *Staphysagria*.

3. *Arsenicum*, *Bryonia*, *Colocynthis*, *Cocculus*, *Crocus*, *Ignatia*, *Mercurius*, *Stramonium*, *Veratrum*.

PAINFUL:—1. *Belladonna*, *Bryonia*, *Chamomilla*, *Nux vomica*, *Platina*, *Pulsatilla*, *Secale*, *Sepia*, *Sulphur*.

3. *Calcarea*, *Cocculus*, *Coffea*, *Graphites*, *Ignatia*, *Phosphorus*, *Veratrum*.

3. *Ammonium*, *Carbo vegetabilis*, *Kreosotum*, *Lachesis*, *Magnesia muriaticum*, *Mercurius*, *Zincum*.

OVARITIS:—1. *Cantharis*, *Staphysagria*, *Thuja*.

2. *Carbo animalis*, *China*, *Conium*, *Lachesis*, *Lycopodium*, *Secale*, *Sepia*, *Zincum*.

3. *Aconitum*, *Carbo vegetabilis*, *Colocynthis*, *Graphites*, *Ignatia*, *Mercurius*, *Nitri acidum*, *Nux vomica*, *Sulphur*.

PERITONITIS:—1. *Aconitum*, *Belladonna*, *Bryonia*, *Hyoscyamus*, *Nux vomica*.

2. *Chamomilla*, *Coffea*, *Colocynthis*, *Rhus*, *Sulphur*.

3. *Colocynthis*, *Mercurius*, *Pulsatilla*, *Veratrum*.

POLYPUS, probable in persons who had been so affected before:—1. *Calcarea*, *Conium*, *Phosphorus*, *Staphysagria*.

2. *Lycopodium*, *Mercurius*, *Silicia*, *Thuja*.

3. *Belladonna*, *Graphites*, *Hepar*, *Mezereum*, *Natrum muriaticum*, *Nitri acidum*, *Phosphori acid.*, *Sulphur.*, *Sulphuric acid.*

4. *Ambra*, *Pulsatilla*.

Schirrus or cancer, in persons with this diathesis:—

1. *Graphites*, *Kreosotum*.

2. *Carbo animalis*.

3. *Arsenicum*, *Belladonna*, *China*, *Clematia*, *Mercurius*, *Sepia*, *Silicea*, *Sulphur*.

4. *Calcarea*, *Lachesis*, *Phosphorus*, *Sabina*, *Staphysagria*, *Thuja*.

VOMITING, frequent:—1. *Nux vomica*.

2. *Conium*, *Ipecacuanha*, *Pulsatilla*.

3. *Arsenicum*, *Ferrum*, *Natrum muriaticum*, *Sepia*.

4. *Aconitum*, *Kreosotum*, *Lachesis*, *Magnesia muriatica*, *Phosphorus*, *Veratrum*.

And when the affection breaks out:

After CONFINEMENT:—1. *Nux vomica*.

2. *Aconitum*, *Belladonna*, *Bryonia*, *Chamomilla*, *Coffea*, *Colocynthis*, *Rhus*.

3. *Arnica*, *Arsenicum*, *Hyoscyamus*, *Ipecacuanha*, *Lachesis*, *Mercurius*, *Platina*, *Pulsatilla*, *Secale*, *Stramonium*, *Veratrum*.

Retrogressed ERUPTIONS:—1. *Bryonia*, *Graphitis*, *Ipecacuanha*, *Phosphori acid*.

2. *Belladonna*, *Chamomilla*, *Lycopodium*, *Natrum Pulsatilla*, *Rhus*, *Sepia*, *Staphysagria*.

3. *Aconitum*, *Alumina*, *Ambra*, *Arsenicum*, *Carbo vegetabilis*, *Causticum*, *Dulcamara*, *Hepar*, *Kali*, *Lachesis*, *Mercurius*, *Phosphorus*, *Silicea*, *Stramonium*, *Thuja*, *Veratrum*.

EXCESSES, sexual, or after onanism :—1. *Nux vomica*, *Sepia*.

2. *Calcarea*, *Phosphori acid.*, *Staphysagria*.
3. *Carbo vegetabilis*, *China*, *Conium*, *Kali*, *Mercurius*, *Phosphorus*, *Pulsatilla*, *Silicea*.
4. *Arsenicum*, *Ferrum*, *Ignatia*, *Lycopodium*, *Natrum muriaticum*, *Sulphur*.

IRRITATION, by pessaries, etc. :—1. *Arnica*, *Conium*, *Hepar*, *Nux vomica*, *Pulsatilla*, *Rhus*, *Sulphuris acidum*.

2. *Chamomilla*, *Lachesis*, *Phosphorus*, *Ruta*, *Staphysagria*, *Sulphur*.
3. *Bryonia*, *Calcarea*, *China*, *Hyoscyamus*, *Kali*, *Kreosotum*, *Lycopodium*, *Mercurius*, *Natrum*, *Natrum muriaticum*, *Nitri acidum*, *Platina*, *Secale*.

RHEUMATISM, metastatic :—1. *Aconitum*, *Belladonna*, *Bryonia*, *Chamomilla*, *Mercurius*, *Nux vomica*, *Phosphorus*, *Pulsatilla*, *Rhus*.

2. *Arsenicum*, *Carbo vegetabilis*, *China*, *Ferrum*, *Ignatia*, *Lachesis*, *Lycopodium*, *Sepia*, *Sulphur*, *Thuja*, *Veratrum*.
3. *Cantharis*, *Colocynthis*, *Kreosotum*, *Mezereum*, *Nitri acidum*.

SECTION 71.

SYMPTOMATIC DETAILS.—In all cases of metritis, no matter of what kind, we may administer the following remedies when indicated by the symptoms :

ACONITUM.—For acute metritis, at the commencement of the treatment, especially if the disease was caused by fright during confinement or menstruation, or for the following symptoms : *inflammatory fever with dry and burning heat*, *violent thirst with desire for cold drinks, red and warm face, short, oppressed breathing and sighing;* distention of the abdomen, with sensitiveness to contact and cutting pains through the whole abdomen.

BELLADONNA.—Often after *Aconitum*, especially when the abdomen is distended, with lancinating, digging pains, or violent cramp-colic, *as if part of the intestines were seized with nails; painful pressure on the genital organs as if every thing would issue through the parts;* sensitiveness of the abdomen to contact; shivering in some parts, with heat in others; *heat about the head and eyes, with redness of the face;* pressive headache, with throbbing of the carotids; spasmodic dysphagia; sleeplessness, with uneasiness and tossing of the limbs; sopor, *furious delirium;* suppression of the menses, or metrorrhagia with discharge of foul blood; lancing pain in the hips, permitting neither contact nor motion; pains in the small of the back as if the sacrum were broken.

BRYONIA.—Distention of the abdomen and excessive sensitiveness to the least contact or motion; *constipation;* lancinating pains in the abdomen aggravated by pressure; violent fever, with burning heat through the whole body; burning thirst for cold beverages; irascible mood, with apprehensions, dread of the future and uneasiness about her condition.

CARBO ANIMALIS.—In some cases of chronic metritis, for: painful pressure in the loins, groins and thighs, with ineffectual urging to raise wind; shivering and gaping; lassitude which scarcely permits her to remain up; distention of the abdomen; leucorrhœa which tinges the linen yellow; lassitude in the thighs.

CHAMOMILLA.—In acute metritis when caused by severe disappointment, fit of anger, during the catamenia or after confinement, with discharge of a black blood, mixed with coagulated blood; distention and sensitiveness of the abdomen to contact; colic like labor-pains; heat all over, with red face and thirst; nocturnal exacerbation, followed by sweat; restlessness; *impatience, nervousness.*

COFFEA.—In acute metritis, for nervousness, with sensitiveness to contact, or metritis is caused by excessive joy that had induced menstrual suppression.

Colocynthis.—Sometimes after Chamomilla, in acute metritis resulting from suppression of the menses or lochia in consequence of a violent indignation, or for: delirium alternating with sopor; heat about the head, red face, glistening eyes; dry heat; hard, full and hurried pulse; cutting in the bowels as with knives, with shiverings, tearing pains along the thighs; crampy colic as if the bowels were clutched, or were squeezed between stones.

Conium.—In chronic metritis, with or without ovaritis or peritonitis, especially for the following symptoms: distended abdomen, with digging above the pubes, and stitches extending to the side of the chest; clutching, squeezing in the womb; painful pressure downwards, with pulling in the thighs; suppressed or scanty menses; paralytic weakness in the small of the back; bloody or milky leucorrhœa; vomiting, hiccough; excessive sensitiveness of the abdomen to the least contact.

Crocus.—For profuse flooding, with discharge of a *viscid blood mixed with black coagula;* heaviness and pressure in the groin and hypogastrium, as if the menses would make their appearance; violent stitches as with knives in the sexual organs, extending into the abdomen; movements in the bowels as from a fœtus.

Ferrum.—In chronic metritis, with great pain during an embrace; colic like labor-pains; suppressed or scanty menses; lancinating headache; milky and corrosive leucorrhœa.

Graphites.—In chronic metritis, with or without ovaritis, especially for painful pressure on the parts, especially after long standing; eruptions, fetters, excoriations or ulcerations at the vulva; pains in the small of the back not permitting her to move; weariness in the hypogastrium, with dulness in the head; eructations and nausea, with lassitude; sense of heat at the hypogastrium; leucorrhœa; suppressed or scanty menses.

Kali carbonicum.—In chronic metritis, especially for aversion to sexual intercourse or else excessive irritation of the sexual instinct; painfulness of the parts during intercourse, with tearing and stitches in the womb; erythema and excoriations at the vulva; menses suppressed or scanty; menstrual blood corrosive and fetid; abdominal cutting pains or pressure in the hypogastrium as if everything would issue below; frequent eructations and vomiting.

KREOSOTUM.—In chronic metritis, with stitches through the vagina and uterus like electric shocks; sore pain at the neck of the uterus during intercourse, especially in the morning; indurations at the neck, increased sexual desire; leucorrhœa which stains the linen grey; swelling of the pudendum; violent cramp-pains in the groin; violent pressure downwards like labor-pains; nausea, vomiting.

LYCOPODIUM.—In chronic metritis, with tearing stitches in the parts; burning pain during and after intercourse; pulling and pressure in the groin, as if the menses would appear; *dryness of the vagina;* pressure from within outwards, above the pubes, when stooping; frequent passage of wind from the vagina; *suppressed menses;* heaviness of the legs; melancholy, sadness, lowness of spirits, peevishness.

MERCURIUS.—In acute metritis, especially when the pains in the womb are lancinating, boring or pressing; slight fever, not much heat, but shivering and frequent sweating.

NUX VOMICA.—In most cases of acute metritis, with or without peritonitis, when the fever is not very high, or after the fever had abated under the use of Aconite or Belladonna; also in many cases of chronic metritis, more particularly for the following symptoms: pressive pains in the hypogastrium, aggravated by pressure and contact; violent pains in the small of the back; swelling of the uterine orifice, with pains as if bruised, and stitches in the lower abdomen; heaviness and burning in the hypogastrium and in the parts; suppressed menses, or else too profuse, with violent pains in the small of the back, dysuria and burning urine; tearing or cramp-pains in the thighs and legs, with numbness of these parts; pulsative or pressive headache, with vertigo, blur before the eyes, buzzing in the ears and fainting turn; constipation or hard stool; in the morning the symptoms are worse.

Opium.—sometimes in acute metritis, with meteorism, hiccough, delirium, cold extremities, discharge of fetid matter, or else violent pains like labor-pains, with spasmodic contraction of the abdomen.

Platina.—In acute metritis, especially after confinement, with increased sexual desire, voluptuous tingling in the womb and external pudendum; painful pressure at the hypogastrium and on the parts, with shuddering and coldness; hardness of the womb; profuse discharge of a thick and black blood; sensitiveness of the parts; headache, restlessness and weeping.

Pulsatilla.—For *pulling, tension and contraction in the hypogastrium,* as *if the menses would make their appearance, with desire to vomit;* cutting pain in the uterine orifice; shiverings with yawning and stretching; weight in the hypogastrium as from a stone; pressure at the rectum, with tenesmus; *colic and vomiting,* also with discharge of mucus from the vagina; pressure at the sacrum and hypogastrium, with numbness of the limbs; pale face; semi-lateral headache; scanty or suppressed menses.

Rhus toxicodendron.—In acute metritis, especially after confinement, or after a sudden suppression of the menses, or if cerebral or typhoid symptoms become developed from the commencement of the disease, or if the symptoms are made worse by the least disappointment; *pulling in the hypogastrium,* as if labor would set in; excoriation-pain in the vagina when touching it.

Sabina.—In acute or chronic metritis, especially after miscarriage or confinement, with increased sexual desire; contractive pain in the uterus; pressive heaviness in the hypogastrium, as if the menses would make their appearance; violent stitches at the bottom of the vagina; *metrorrhagia, with discharge of coagula;* inflamed urine, with painful urination; discharge of a mucous liquid from the vagina.

Secale Cornutum.—Often in the most acute cases of metritis, with tendency to gangrene or putrescence; metritis caused by suppression of the lochia or menses; distention of the uterus; metrorrhagia, with tingling in the legs, debility, and discharge of a thin and black blood.

SEPIA.—In chronic metritis, especially for the following symptoms:—Painful rigidity in the hypogastrium and uterine region; *choking pressure downwards*, as if everything would pass through the vagina, with abdominal cutting pain and jelly-like leucorrhœa; hardness of the neck of the womb; falling of the uterus; *itching, erythematous redness* and *excoriations at the vulva;* suppressed or scanty menses; stitches in the womb, with distention and heaviness; nausea and vomiting.

SULPHUR.—When the other remedies, which have been named for acute and chronic metritis, have proved fruitless, especially for the following symptoms:—Excoriation-pain at the bottom of the vagina, during an embrace; suppressed or scanty menses; flooding between the periods, almost every day; violent pains in the hypogastrium, with heat, shivering and epileptiform convulsions; violent colic and pains in the small of the back, with distention of the abdomen; uterine cramp-pains; itching, inflammation, swelling and excoriation of the labia.

For further details concerning the use of the other remedies, see *Dysmenorrhœa*, Sections 5–10, and *Amenorrhœa*, Sections 23–32.

DOSE.—In acute cases, dissolve six globules, or one or two drops of the liquid attenuation, in ten table-spoonfuls of water, and give a table-spoonful every two or three hours. In chronic cases, give this dose twice a day, morning and evening.

ARTICLE IV.

HYDROMETRA, OR UTERINE DROPSY.

SECTION 72.

SYMPTOMS.—Most authors distinguish three kinds of hydrometra or dropsy of the uterus, namely: 1, *uterine ascites*, where the liquid is contained within the cavity of the uterus; 2, *hydatids* in the womb; and 3, *hydrometra of pregnant women*, which developes itself during pregnancy. Having to treat of the two last named varieties in the articles on *Foreign bodies in the womb*, and *Ailments during pregnancy*, we have here only to treat of the first form, *ascites*. The symptoms of this disease differ according as the disease is *persistent* or *periodical*, that is to say, according as the fluid contained in the womb remains there until the patient either gets better or dies, or according as it escapes at certain intervals from the uterine orifice. In the former case, the patient complains of pains in the lumbar region and in the hypogastrium, progressive swelling of the abdomen, menstrual suppression; sometimes swelling of the breasts, and discharge from the breasts of a certain quantity of milky lymph, so that the symptoms are often mistaken for those of pregnancy. This condition may last one, two or more months, and even years. The swelling of the abdomen increases from below upwards, and the accumulation of the secreted fluid gives rise to a round, circumscribed, soft, fluctuating, more or less voluminous tumor, yielding a dull sound to percussion. This dropsy may terminate in the spontaneous discharge of the fluid, in consequence of a contusion, fall, hurried motion, effort when coughing, sneezing, or in consequence of any other concussion of the body. In this case, uterine pains soon set in, the uterine orifice becomes dilated, and the fluid either escapes gradually or all at once, after which the cure is sometimes completed. In other cases, the fluid in the uterine cavity sometimes distends the womb to a certain extent, and occasions a sort of swelling of the abdomen; but from time to time, and more particularly at the period of the menses, or in consequence of some concussion, sometimes, without any appreciable cause, the neck of the uterus becomes dilated, so that the fluid which is enclosed in the uterine cavity is able to pass out, which does not prevent, however, the collection of another quantity of serum, that is expelled again, in its turn, after a certain period. This variety is termed, by some authors, periodical ascites of the womb, and is distinguished from the former variety by this, that, in the former variety, the secretion of the fluid *ceases* after its expulsion; whereas, in the periodical variety, the secretion continues after the expulsion. In either of these two varieties, it is only the external symptoms that are either permanent or variable; whereas, the pathological condition—namely, the abnormal secretion,—remains the same in either case. In either variety the abnormal secretion remains permanent until the definite cessation of the disease by a radical cure, or by death. Whenever a considerable quantity of fluid is secreted in the uterine cavity, or whenever this secretion is accompanied by other organic lesions of the womb, the patient experiences pains, a sense of heaviness in the loins, groins, and in the hypogastrium, with difficulty of urinating or going to stool, infiltration of the eyelids and straw-colored complexion.

Section 73.

Causes, diagnosis, prognosis, and treatment.—Hydrometra never sets in before the menstrual functions have commenced, or after they have entirely ceased. It is almost always the result of a tubercular, schirrous or hydatic degeneration of the walls of the uterus, but it may also exist independently of these alterations. Sometimes it sets in, in consequence of blows in the hypogastric region, or of a miscarriage, suppression of leucorrhœa or of the lochia, or it may be induced by any other cause that may induce inflammation of the uterine mucous membrane. As regards DIAGNOSIS, hydrometra might be most readily confounded with pregnancy; but the absence of all the real signs of pregnancy, such as the movements of the fœtus, the sounds of the fœtal heart, etc., will soon clear all doubt regarding it. As regards dropsies of the nervous cysts, of the Fallopian tubes or of the ovaries, they can scarcely be mistaken for dropsy of the womb; for in all these affections the womb remains unaltered, and the swelling is located on the right or left of the median line. Sometimes the accumulation of the menstrual blood, in amenorrhœa, may occasion a more or less considerable swelling of the abdomen; but, such a swelling corresponds more particularly to the menstrual period, increasing at such a period and decreasing again afterwards. Finally, in *physometra* the abdominal swelling sometimes reaches a considerable volume, but there is always resonnance in such a tumor, and an absence of fluctuation; these two characteristic signs are wanting in hydrometra. The PROGNOSIS is not very unfavorable unless there are deep-seated organic alterations of the uterus, and when the affection only depends upon chronic inflammation, a polypus, mucous concretions or spasmodic closing of the neck of the uterus; but, if the disease is occasioned by cancerous or schirrous degenerations, or by any other disorganizations of the uterus, it becomes exceedingly serious. The TREATMENT should be determined with reference to the cause of the disease, although the following remedies will be found generally sufficient:

1. *Arsenicum*, *Belladonna*, *China*, *Helleborus*, *Mercurius*, *Sulphur*.
2. *Bryonia*, *Calcarea*, *Conium*, *Ferrum*, *Iodium*, *Kali*, *Lachesis*, *Lycopodium*, *Pulsatilla*, *Ruta*, *Sabina*, *Sepia*.

3. *Aconitum*, *Ambra*, *Arnica*, *Cantharis*, *Dulcamara*, *Hyoscyamus*, *Nux vomica*, *Opium*, *Plumbum*, *Secale*, *Veratrum*.
4. *Ammonium*, *Antimonium*, *Aurum*, *Carbo vegetabilis*, *Cocculus*, *Hepar*, *Ignatia*, *Ledum*, *Nitri acid.*, *Phosphorus*, *Phosphoric acid*, *Silicea*, *Stannum*, *Stramonium*.

And in particular:

After a MISCARRIAGE:—1. *Belladonna*, *Sabina*, *Secale*, *Sepia*.
2. *Bryonia*, *Calcarea*, *China*, *Ferrum*, *Kali*, *Pulsatilla*, *Sulphur*.
3. *Arnica*, *Cantharides*, *Hyoscyamus*, *Lycopodium*, *Nitri acid.*, *Nux vomica*, *Phosphorus*, *Rhus*, *Silicea*.

BLOWS on the hypogastrium:—1. *Arnica*, *Conium*, *Pulsatilla*, *Rhus*.
2. *Bryonia*, *Iodium*, *Lachesis*, *Phosphorus*, *Ruta*, *Sulphur*.
3. *Calcarea*, *Cantharides*, *Carbo vegetabilis*, *Dulcamara*, *Kali*, *Lycopodium*, *Mercurius*, *Nitri acid.*, *Nux vomica*, *Silicea* *Veratrum*.

With hydatids:—1. *Cantharides*, *Mercurius*.

INFLAMMATION of the mucous lining (endometritis):—
1. *Mercurius*, *Pulsatilla*, *Sepia*.
2. *Ammonia*, *Calcarea*, *China*, *Conium*, *Ferrum*, *Lycopodium*, *Sabina*, *Sulphur*.
3. *Arsenicum*, *Cantharides*, *Kali*, *Nitri acid.*, *Phosphorus*, *Veratrum*.

Suppressed LEUCORRHŒA:—1. *Bryonia*, *China*, *Nux vomica*, *Pulsatilla*, *Sulphur*.
2. *Aconitum*, *Ammoniacum*, *Arsenicum*, *Belladonna*, *Lachesis*.
3. *Calcarea*, *Carbo vegetabilis*, *Conium*, *Nitri acid.*, *Phosphorus*, *Sepia*.

SUPPRESSION OF LOCHIA:—1. *Belladonna*, *Nux vomica*, *Pulsatilla*, *Secale*.
2. *Hyoscyamus* *Veratrum*.

POLYPI:—1. *Calcarea, Conium, Phosphorus, Staphysagria.*

2. *Lycopodium, Mercurius, Silicea, Thuya.*

3. *Belladonna, Graphites, Hepar, Mezereum, Nitric acid, Phosphori acid., Pulsatilla, Sulphur.*

SUPPRESSED MENSES:—1. *Conium, Kali, Lycopodium, Pulsatilla, Sulphur.*

2. *Ammonium, Dulcamara, Ferrum, Graphites, Hyoscyamus, Ignatia, Lachesis, Mercurius, Phosphorus, Sepia, Silicea, Veratrum.*

SCHIRROUS or CANCEROUS affections:—1. *Graphites, Kreosotum.*

2. *Arsenicum, Belladonna, Carbo animalis, China, Mercurius, Sepia, Sulphur.*

3. *Calcarea, Lachesis, Phosphorus, Sabina.*

For further details concerning the use of these remedies see *Dysmenorrhœa, Amenorrhœa, Leucorrhœa, Endometritis* and METRITIS.

DOSE.—Dissolve six globules, or one or two drops of the liquid attenuation in ten tablespoonfuls of water, and give the patient a tablespoonful of this solution every three or four hours, or even more frequently in urgent cases.

ARTICLE V.

PHYSOMETRA, TYMPANITIS OF THE WOMB.

SECTION 74.

SYMPTOMS, CAUSES AND TREATMENT.—This affection consists in a distension of the uterus, caused by gas which accumulates in the cavity of the uterus without being able to escape from it. The distended uterus forms a round, more or less extensive tumor in the hypogastric region, according as more or less gas is accumulated. If this affection sets in immediately after confinement, the swelling may sometimes attain to a size equal to that before confinement, and other symptoms may develop themselves with it, such as coma, turgescence of the face and head, loss of consciousness, and other cerebral symptoms. If the distension of the uterus is at all considerable, there is an embarrassment and tension about the hypogastrium; the uterine pains extend to the loins, groin and thighs, and even to the epigastrium; in many cases the menses cease. Sometimes a little fever is present, with evening exacerbations; shivering, thirst, loss of appetite, scanty and difficult stool, frequent urging to vomit, dyspnœa, laziness, aversion to physical exercise, swelling of the breasts and discharge of a milky fluid from the nipples. All these symptoms disappear after the escape of the gas through the vagina, which takes place at irregular periods and sometimes with a loud explosion. As regards the CAUSES of this affection, it is most frequently owing to the decomposition of coagula or of the placenta after confinement, or even of the dead fœtus in the uterus. In some cases, however, gas accumulates within the uterine cavity, to such an extent that the abdomen acquires the same dimensions as during pregnancy. The DIAGNOSIS of physometra is readily obtained; the elasticity of the tumor and its resonance when percussed, will remove all doubt as soon as we have become satisfied that the womb and not the intestines are the seat of the affection. The PROGNOSIS is not serious; the disease is not dangerous in itself, and only becomes so when it results from the putrefaction of a fœtus, of the placenta, or from the presence of some other primary trouble. As regards TREATMENT, if the expulsion of the gas should be prevented by some mechanical cause, this should be of course removed; for which purpose the finger is generally the best instrument. If medicines are required, the following are the best remedies:

1. *Phosphori acid.*
2. *Belladonna, China, Cocculus, Hyoscyamus, Lycopodium, Magnesia carb., Nux moschata, Sepia.*
3. *Carbo vegetabilis, Chamomilla, Graphites, Ignatia, Kali, Nux vomica, Phosphorus, Pulsatilla, Staphysagria, Veratrum.*
4. *Arnica, Calcarea, Colocynthis, Conium, Nitri acid., Platina, Plumbum, Sulphur.*

DOSE.—One or two drops of the liquid attenuation, or six globules dry on the tongue, morning and evening.

ARTICLE VI.

FOREIGN BODIES IN THE WOMB.

MOLES, HYDATIDS, SANGUINEOUS CONCRETIONS, MEMBRANEOUS FORMATIONS, POLYPI AND OTHER EXCRESCENCES.

SECTION 75.

MOLES.—We unite in this article all the foreign bodies which are found in the uterus, and which may require some peculiar treatment. As regards *moles*, authors are not at all agreed about the definition and meaning of this term. According to ancient authors, a mole is a shapeless and inert mass of flesh caused in the womb, in consequence of an imperfect conception. Afterwards all sorts of confused ideas were attached to this term, until modern authors finally agreed to admit three kinds of moles: 1st, *the fleshy mole*, resulting from false conception; 2d, the *hydatic mole*, being a heap of hydatids; and 3d, the *sanguineous mole*, which is a sanguineous concretion in the womb. We shall here treat only of the mole resulting from false conception, and defer a description of the other kinds to the next two paragraphs. The fleshy mole seems sometimes to be an hypertrophied placenta, containing within its cavity a fœtus which often continues to grow even after all life is extinguished. These fleshy moles always result from false conception, and should not be confounded with the fibrous concretions which are sometimes found even among unmarried girls, and of which we shall treat by and by when speaking of polypi. These masses of hypertrophied placenta frequently exist in the womb simultaneously with a fœtus, although in most cases the development of the fœtus is not only interfered with, but the fœtus is destroyed. Sometimes the placental hypertrophy only commences after the expulsion of the fœtus in consequence of some cause. As regards DIAGNOSIS, it is exceedingly difficult to establish it correctly. At the onset the swelling may be confounded with pregnancy. Even after the contents of the womb are changed, the signs of pregnancy still continue; only the movements of the fœtus are not perceived, and the development of the womb does not continue its regular course; everything seems to point to the presence of a foreign body in the uterus; but it is impossible to tell whether it is an hypertrophied placenta or a slowly-formed coagulum in the uterine cavity. Even after the body has protruded through the uterine orifice, the uncertainty is not always removed by an ocular inspection of the body. The expulsion of these bodies always takes place by means of contractile efforts on the part of the uterus, with pains and phenomena similar to those of confinement, and resembling a case of miscarriage after the death of the fœtus. In most cases, it is preceded and accompanied by a more or less profuse uterine hæmorrhage, which is often very rebellious to old school treatment, especially when the uterus is not entirely freed from the presence of the foreign body. As regards TREATMENT, the best means to favor the expulsion of the womb, are:

1. *Pulsatilla*, *Secale* or *Cantharis*.
2. *Calcarea*, *Silicea*.
3. *Belladonna*, *Kali*, *Opium*, *Platina*.
4. *Chamomilla*, *Cocculus*, *Nux vomica*, *Sabina*, *Sepia*.
5. *Arnica*, *Carbo veget.*, *Graphites*, *Ignatia*, *Magnesia muriat.*, *Natrum*, *Natrum muriaticum*, *Nux moschata*, *Ruta*, *Sulphur*.

And for UTERINE HÆMORRHAGE:

1. *Belladonna*, *Platina*, *Sabina*.
2. *China*, *Ferrum*.
3. *Arnica*, *Chamomilla*, *Crocus*.
4. *Bryonia*, *Hyoscyamus*, *Ipecacuanha*.

DOSE.—The same as at the end of Section 74, and if

hæmorrhage or other acute symptoms occur, mix one or two drops of the liquid attenuation in ten tablespoonfuls of water, and give the patient a spoonful every few minutes or every hour or few hours, according as the symptoms are more or less acute or dangerous.

For other details see *Metrorrhagia*, *Pregnancy* and *Confinement*.

Section 76.

Hydatids.—Like moles, hydatids are rather a disease of the fœtus than of the womb. They are a sort of hollow moles, caused by changes of the ovum. These formations may become exceedingly numerous, and have been known to exceed several thousand; fecund women are generally the most subject to such alterations. Such hydatids sometimes induce all the signs of true pregnancy: increase of the volume of the abdomen, menstrual suppression, frequent nausea, sadness without any apparent motive. This condition may last from one to twelve and even fifteen months. During the expulsion of the hydatids, acute uterine pains, like labor-pains, are experienced, and copious hæmorrhages frequently set in, which are followed by great weakness, and are accompanied by the expulsion of hydatids through the vagina. These masses are often lobular on the outside, granular like a full-grown placenta, and the lining membranes in the interior of these formations, often contain quantities of these vesicles which we term hydatids, from the size of an almond to that of a little grain of sand. Sometimes even the remnants or origin of the umbilical cord, or some other appendage of the ovum, is distinctly recognized in one or the other group of these vesicles. Beside these hydatids or hollow moles, there are others formed by small vesiclar acephalocysts, but differing from the preceding variety less than might be supposed. These vesicular hydatids, the animal nature of which is contested by some authors, exist under two distinct forms. Sometimes they are attached to several partial stems, which are ingrafted upon one larger common pedicle, thus constituting a variety known as grape-shaped moles. Sometimes these vesicles, in the cavity which contains them, are free from the vascular pedicles through which those of the preceding species receive their nourishment. Either species may give rise to false pregnancy, known under the name of *hydatid dropsy*. These moles induce an alternate occurrence of small, red and watery losses, commencing in most women from the second month, and continuing at longer or shorter intervals until the period of parturition, which generally takes place from the second to the tenth month. Their expulsion is very apt to take place when they are isolated, and it may be followed by all the symptoms setting in after confinement, such lochia, milk fever, and even metro-peritonitis. The CAUSES of this affection are not much known; some authors think, however, that an excessive use of vegetable and unwholesome food, and living in a damp and unwholesome dwelling may cause the disease. Like the hollow moles, hydatids may take place in married women, and like the former, seem a disease of the first product of gestation, though some authors pretend to have seen them likewise in unmarried women, whose purity could not be suspected. As regards the TREATMENT of this disease, the following remedies may be used to combat it:

1. *Calcarea*, *Sulphur*, *Silicea*, *Mercurius*.
2. *Aconite*, *Arsenicum*, *China*, *Ferrum*, *Graphites*.
3. *Belladonna*, *Hyoscyamus*, *Kali*, *Lycopodium*, *Sabina*, *Sepia*.

DOSE.—The same as at the end of the preceding paragraph.

SECTION 77.

SANGUINEOUS AND LYMPHATIC CONCRETIONS.—Beside the moles of which we have treated, there are other bodies of a widely different nature, but which are often confounded with moles. These are the sanguineous and lymphatic concretions formed in the womb. The sanguineous concretions are a species of coagula, which might be compared to the polypous concretions in the heart and larger vessels, although the coagula in the womb are generally more consistent and show some signs of organization; often they are surrounded by a fibrinous layer of a greyish-white color which envelops them like a membrane and increases this organized appearance; but in dissecting them carefully, this appearance disappears, and no cavity with smooth walls is found in their interior, as is the case with fleshy moles. These concretions may acquire a considerable volume, and may exist in the womb together with a large mass of liquid or coagulated blood. The formation of these coagula takes place most frequently in women who menstruate profusely and are subject to uterine hæmorrhages; they are likewise met with pretty frequently in women who were recently confined and whose lochia do not flow regularly; even young unmarried females are attacked by such disorders. When such concretions take place, the menses cease; afterwards, after a lapse of from one to two or three months, an hæmorrhage takes place which increases little by little, with labor-pains; the foreign body is expelled and the hæmorrhage diminishes gradually, undergoing the same changes as the lochial discharge. In other cases the expulsion does not take place so promptly, and the hæmorrhage may last longer and be followed by all the consequences of a serious flooding. The foreign body may also become decomposed, giving rise to a sanious and putrid discharge, the absorption of which into the organism sometimes increases the gravity of the case. Lymphatic concretions are membraneous bodies of integumentous consistence and a dirty-white color, resembling the membranes in croup. They are formed in the uterine cavity and are afterwards expelled, either shaped as a sac, or as a bursa, the external surface of which is studded with filaments, and the internal surface is smooth and moistened with a serous liquid; they form patches of various shapes, some of them having even been shaped exactly like the neck of the womb. Sometimes these patches are expelled together with menstrual blood. These formations seem to arise from a certain degree of inflammation or exuding irritation of the uterine mucous membrane; they affect more particularly women whose menses flow scantily and induce pain. In most cases these formations are accidental, and never occur again; sometimes they are reproduced at longer or shorter intervals. Their presence in, and expulsion from the womb, are generally accompained by the same symptoms as sanguineous concretions. The best remedies for these two kinds of concretions are:

1. *Nitri acid., Phosphori acid., Strontiana.*
2. *Bryonia, Carbo animalis, Kreosotum, Nux vomica, Secale, Sepia.*

For LYMPHATIC concretions:—1. *Suphuris acid.*

2. *Ammonium, Borax, Bromine, Iodium, Nux vomica, Spongia, Sulphur.*
3. *Alumina, China, Hepar, Nitric acid.*
4. *Arsenica, Euphorbium, Kreosotum, Lachesis Tart.*

For further details concerning the use of the remedies, see *Dysmenorrhœa, Amenorrhœa, Metrorrhagia, Confinement, Pregnancy,* etc.

DOSE.—The same as at the close of the last paragraph.

SECTION 78.

UTERINE POLYPUS.—Such polypi are fleshy, spongy, fibrous and other excrescences developing themselves in the sub-mucous cellular tissue of the womb. We distingush five varieties, namely:

1st. VESICULAR POLYPI—Composed of a soft, homogeneous tissue, and containing a liquid which is discharged when the polypus is torn.

2d. SARCOMATOUS OR FLESHY POLYPI.—Almost the same as fibrous bodies in the womb, except that the polypi grow out on the side of the uterine mucous membrane, whereas the fibrous bodies grow out of the peritoneal surface.

3d. CARTILAGINOUS, OSSEOUS AND STONY polypi,—Which are simply successive transformations of the former.

4th. SPONGY, FUNGOUS polypi.—Soft, red, looking like

tomatoes, frequently of a livid color, bleeding a good deal, sometimes like hæmorrhage, with tendency to change to cancer or to reappear.

5th. GRANULAR polypi.—Not very large, developed along the surface in the shape of whitish, grayish, or rose-colored granules with very thin pedicles, resembling cauliflowers or syphilitic vegetations for which some authors really take them.

All these polypi, some of which appear even in a mixed form, may occupy the most diversified portions of the womb, and differ vastly as regards insertion, shape, volume and duration. By growing thinner and longer either in the body or stem, or by inverting the fundus of the womb, the uterine polypi may even descend into the neck of the womb, and pass even into the vagina. All these polypi may grow without causing any sense of embarrassment in the sexual organs; whereas, at other times, their appearance may be preceded for a long period by a whitish, yellowish or greenish, purulent or puriform leucorrhœa, or by hæmorrhages or reddish discharges. In this case, such symptoms are accompanied by a sense of embarrassment, weight and pain in the hypogastrium, when walking; hysteric symptoms, such as heat in the face, sensation of a ball ascending to the throat, chest or abdomen, etc. All these symptoms may be caused by the smallest polypus, the presence of which may render walking or riding in a carriage exceedingly painful, or even impossible, cause great sensitiveness during sexual intercourse, disturb sleep, digestion and the other principal functions. If remaining enclosed within the uterine cavity, the uterus may become dilated to such an extent that it may simulate pregnancy; it presses upon the rectum and bladder, causing frequent urgings to evacuate these parts, colic pains in the small of the back, pullings in the groin, swelling of the feet, legs, thighs, and varices on the legs. At last all these symptoms grow worse, the limbs become dropsical, ascites sets in, and a hectic fever terminates the sufferings of the patient by death. In some cases all these symptoms remain stationary; but sooner or later, in consequence of some favorable cause, the polypus escapes from the womb, and protrudes at the vulva where it becomes irritated, inflamed, and then ulcerates in consequence of the friction of the clothes and the contact of the urine, until finally hectic fever sets is, and the patient dies likewise. At other times the polypi become transformed into encephaloid cancers, before issuing from the womb, they suppurate and ulcerate, with ichorous, bloody and very fetid discharges, which generally cause a number of very serious accidents. In other cases the polypi become gangrenous, with all the symptoms which characterise this affection. As regards the DIAGNOSIS of polypi, it is exceedingly obscure as long as these excrescences remain enclosed in the uterus, and the neck remains closed; but what may distinguish them from pregnancy with which they might be confounded, is the absence of the characteristic signs of pregnancy, and the slower development of the uterine symptoms. Prolapsus or inversion of the womb cannot be mistaken for polypus, if the parts are carefully examined, more particularly if the womb should be found to have remained in its place. The PROGNOSIS depends upon the age, shape, seat and nature of these excrescences. At first they are not very serious, unless debilitating hœmorrhages should set in. Polypi enclosed in the uterine cavity, are more serious than those that have protruded; but the most to be dreaded are such as have degenerated into cancerous or gangrenous tumors. As regards TREATMENT, neither ligature nor excision need ever be resorted to under proper homœopathic treatment; well chosen homœopathic remedies always secure the expulsion of polypi without instruments being resorted to. We would recommend the use of a single dose, which should be allowed to act for three or four weeks. No polypus comes off before the end of the seventh or eighth week, and, if we give the remedy every day or several times a week, the organism becomes used to the drug long before the polypus has been touched by the medical action to the foundation; or else, so many accessory symptoms set in that we are obliged to abandon the use of the remedy before it has had time to act. We have cured several polypi with two globules of *Calcerea* 30, which we allowed to act for ten weeks without repeating it. The best remedies to bring about the expulsion of polypi, are: .

1. *Calcarea.*
2. *Conium*, *Phosphorus*, *Staphysagria.*
3. *Aurum*, *Hepar*, *Lycopodium*, *Mercurius*, *Mezereum*, *Sepia*, *Silicea*, *Thuja.*
4. *Belladonna*, *Graphites*, *Natrum muriat.*, *Nitri acidum*, *Phosphori acid.*, *Sulphuris acid.*

And in particular for FLESHY polypi:—1. *Calcarea.*

2. *Staphysagria*, *Thuja.*
3. *Lycopodium*, *Mercurius*, *Nitri acid.*, *Phosphorus.*

For FUNGOUS polypi:—1. *Calcarea.*

2. *Lycopodium. Mercurius*, *Nitri acidum*, *Staphysagria*, *Thuja.*
4. *Phosphorus*, *Sepia*, *Silicea*, *Sulphur.*

For GRANULAR polypi: — 1. *Nitri acidum*, *Staphysagria*. *Thuja.*

2. *Calcarea*, *Lycopodium.*

For frequent HÆMORRHAGES:—1. *Calcarea.*

2. *Belladonna*, *Lycopodium*, *Mercurius*, *Nitri acid.*, *Phosphorus*, *Pulsatilla*, *Sepia*, *Sulphur.*
3. *Silicea*, *Sulphuris acid.*

SECTION 79.

CALCULI, OR FIBROUS BODIES OF THE WOMB.—These bodies are in structure analogous to the fibrous tissue; they are more or less globular, and are seated in the tissue of the uterus. These tumors may either grow out from the external surface of the womb on the side of the peritoneum, or from the internal mucous membrane. In this latter case, these tumors form the *fibrous polypi*, of which we made mention in the former paragraph. As a general rule, they may be seated either in the fibrous tissue of the uterus, or between this tissue and the peritoneal covering, or between this tissue and the mucous membrane. The *volume* of these bodies differs considerably. Some are no bigger than a little pea; others are of the size of a hazelnut, a chestnut, or a hen's egg; others again are bigger than a fist; some even have been known to weigh thirty pounds. When they are very numerous, they disfigure the body of the uterus completely, and if they attain to the size of a man's head, they dilate the uterine cavity in every direction. The structure of these tumors is likewise exceedingly varied: some are like *fleshy* bodies, others *fibro-cartilaginous*, others *osseous*. It may be that these differences simply denote the various periods of development which these tumors have to pass through before they reach their full growth. When *fleshy*, these tumors are so much paler the denser they are, and when they are soft, like muscular substance, they are red; when cut into, it is seen that they are formed of bundles of muscular fibres, which are interlaced here and there in an inextricable manner. Sometimes portions of the same fibrous body are still red and pretty soft, while other portions have already become whitish, gray, and much harder. These denser portions are the first to assume a fibro-cartilaginous consistence, and, if ossification sets in, it is here that the process of ossification first commences in a number of points, whence it spreads until the whole tumor has become ossified, after which it is hard and heavy. It frequently occurs that fibrous bodies, in the various stages, are found in the same uterus, or bodies, portions of which are still fleshy while other portions are already ossified. They do not seem to grow before the age of thirty years, and unmarried women seem more subject to them than married females. Moreover, the more children a woman has had, the less is she liable to such tumors. As a general rule, they are found quite frequently; on five women who are examined after death, one generally is found to have had one or more of such tumors in the womb. When these tumors are seated in the uterine tissue, and project towards the abdominal cavity, they are sometimes seen near the os tincæ, occupying the body of the uterus or the thickness of the neck. In the former case they are easily recognized by the touch; but this is not so easy when they are seated within the tissue of the uterus. Bodies which are seated near the peritoneal surface remain sometimes unknown for a long time, especially if they are small and pedunculated; but after they have acquired a considerable volume, they may be known by an external examination of the hypogastrium. As regards tumors with pedicles and projecting on the side of the uterine cavity, we refer the reader to what has been said in the preceding paragraph about *fleshy polypi*, which are nothing else than fibrous bodies with pedicles. The PROGNOSIS is not very serious in itself, but in some cases these tumors may act like foreign bodies, and induce all sorts of serious ailments, and even death. They may interfere with the menses, cause leucorrhœa, hæmorrhages, obstruct the development of the fetus, compress the rectum and bladder. For the TREATMENT, see the remedies for fibrous polypi mentioned in the preceding paragraph.

ARTICLE VII.

SCHIRRUS AND CANCER OF THE WOMB.*

SECTION 80.

DEFINITION AND VARIETIES OF CANCER.—Most authors now understand by cancer of the uterus, every affection which, *at the same time as it changes the tissue of the uterus, naturally tends to spread all around, and to destroy itself by ulceration in the centre.* Latterly, these ulcerations have been a good deal divided and subdivided, though some of them seem only different conditions of one and the same changes. Be this as it may, here are the different varieties admitted by modern authors.

1. SCHIRROUS or TUBEROUS cancer, consisting in a general or partial indurated swelling of the uterus, with change of tissue that is not susceptible of reduction, and must necessarily extend and ulcerate, unless we succeed in removing the affection of the tissues. To this variety belongs the *creeping cancer* of Duparcque, which sometimes commences in the vagina, with elongated, uneven, indurated and irregular elevations, not very extensive at first, and gradually spreading from a limited point over the whole vagina, with tendency to invade the neck of the uterus, and to change to a cancerous ulcer.

2. FUNGOUS cancer, FUNGUS HÆMATODES, or HYPERSARCOSIC cancer, being a swelling that spreads like a mushroom

* For a complete study of this subject, we refer the reader to "*Traité Pratique des Maladies Cancéreuses et des affections curables confonderes avec le cancer,*" by Dr. H. Zebert, Paris, 1851; and to a discussion in the Academy of Medicine (Bulletin of the Academy, Paris, 1854, Vol. xx.)

over the surface of the neck, of lobular or granular appearance, in some cases soft, and in others hard and firm ; of a brownish or violet color ; secreting a reddish, serous, puriform or ropy fluid ; discharging a black blood, in some cases continually ; termination in sphacelus or cancerous ulceration.

3d. BLOODY cancer, or cancerous engorgement of the womb, characterised by violet-colored, but uniform swelling of a portion of the uterus, and especially of the neck, where this variety is often seated without spreading any further; remarkable softness of the tissue, increasing in proportion as the tumor is nearer the uterine orifice; marked crepitating noise when compressing the tumor ; incessant discharge of a black and granulated blood, mixed with more or less extensive coagula ; oozing out of a milky, whitish fluid, which becomes afterwards mixed with a cerebriform matter, and with fetid substances; marked tendency to spread towards the body of the uterus.

4th. CEREBRIFORM OR ENCEPHALOID cancer, MEDULLARY cancer, characterised by the presence of this substance with which the tumor is either infiltrated, or which is found agglomerated in the cancerous engorgements; fetid, puriform or purulent discharge; discharge of putrid flocks; uneven surface of the ulcer ; the degeneration of the tissue is sometimes limited to the environs of the ulcer, sometimes it spreads over the whole womb ; a white liquid of the consistence of cream may be squeezed out of the tumor.

5th. ULCERATED, OPEN OF CONFIRMED cancer, or the cancer of the ancients properly speaking, being *schirrous*, *fungous*, *sanguineous* or *medullary* engorgements transformed into a corroding or spreading ulcer. This cancer may likewise be a primary ulcer. In such a case it generally commences at the neck of the uterus, in the shape of a superficial ulcer, (the *superficial* cancer of some authors) upon a basis of inconsiderable elevation, but very hard, with an irregularly circumscribed, unevenly granulated surface, the whole having a grayish color. In the cases where the cancerous ulceration forms only the last stage of preceding changes, the ulcer destroys successively the engorged parts; but where the cancerous affection commences with ulceration, the sore parts become indurated, the ulceration spreading more and more, and changing to an open ulcer, in proportion as the hardness keeps spreading.

As regards the *lardaceous* cancer of some authors, it only seems to form a variety of the *schirrous* cancer which becomes soft and ulcerated.

Cancers composed of a mixture of various tissues, do not constitute a separate variety: there may be ever so many modifications of this kind arising from peculiar combinations of the above-mentioned forms.

Section 81.

Symptoms and diagnosis of cancer.—The first invasion of the disease is often over-looked by the physician and the patient who scarcely thinks of the ailments she had experienced for a long time already. An examination of the parts would show considerable disease even at this period. The first symptoms generally are: menstrual irregularities, a temporary increase of the menstrual flow, leuchorrhœa, which is either continual or lasts only for a short time, white or yellowish, sometimes changing to a reddish color after intercourse or after any other local irritation; sense of weight at the hypogastrium, with pressure on the rectum, or the urinary organs; stool and emission of urine sometimes more painful, and always more or less difficult; disagreeble sensation during intercourse; occasional transitory shooting stitches, especially at the period of the menses, or after physical or moral excitement; transitory pullings in the loins or groin; hysterical ailments; hæmorrhoidal distress; alternate distension and caving in of the abdomen, etc. Sometimes we discover even at this period, slight swellings or indurations of the womb, occupying rather the neck than the body of the womb, with a sort of irregularity in the shape of the neck. These symptoms may remain unchanged for a long time; but as soon as cancer has openly set in, the neck and even the body of the uterus, and likewise the lips of the os tincæ are swollen, hard, knotty, lobed, and more or less red, but smooth and not sore, covered with a bloody mucus or with pure blood, painful to pressure, and sometimes accompanied with engorgement of the ovaries. In some cases there is only a single clearly circumscribed tumor, the seat and extent of which may be discovered by an examination through the rectum; in most cases there are several tumors, or even if the entire uterus should be invaded, a group of several rounded inequalities at the surface. These tumors might sometimes be confounded with fibrous bodies, if the other signs that accompany the cancer, did not render such a mistake impossible. As soon as the cancer has broken out, the pains, which until recently had been transitory, become permanent, with acute lancinating pains like needles or knives thrust through the part; the loss of blood becomes more frequent and sometimes habitual, and a fetid serous or bloody leucorrhœa sets in, which becomes fouler the more the ulceration progresses, being sometimes mixed up with small flocks of putrid matter, of a brownish color, and frequently having an excessively pungent odor, or also with little coägula of blackish blood. If the menses have continued so far, they often increase to a flooding; in women, where they have stopped, they act as if they would reappear; others discharge constantly a profuse watery liquid without smell, or having an insipid, sickening odor; stiffening the linen somewhat, and leaving grayish stains after dying; at the menstrual period this liquid becomes rose-colored. This serous discharge generally indicates that the ulceration has either commenced or is imminent. Pain now succeeds pain; loins, small of the back, hypogastrium, iliac region, even the nates down to the thighs become the seat of contusive tearing, or distensive pains, sometimes mingled with smarting pains or acute stitches in the neck of the uterus, and sometimes preventing sleep to such a degree that the patients dare not give themselves up to it. In spite of these sufferings, the cerebral functions remain frequently intact even until the moment of death. What is most remarkable is, that these cancers do not always prevent conception; women affected with enormous cancers, have been known to go their full term and to give birth to children who, however, did not survive; in most cases the children were putrified. As regards constitutional symptoms, uterine cancer seems to influence the general well-being less than other cancers; as long as it remains at the first stage, and is confined to a single point in the uterus, the constitution does not suffer, and the appetite remains unimpaired. Cases have been known where the patients retained a certain freshness and rotundity even after the cancer had progressed quite considerably. Other women, on the contrary, experience an intolerable malaise from the commencement of the disease. The appetite is gone, they become melancholy, are attacked with pains in various parts of the body, sudden and transitory swellings, and they become so restless that they cannot remain an instant in the same position. Fever generally does not set in until the cancer has arrived at its last stage; it is a hectic fever with several exacerbations every day. When the third stage is reached, a general constitutional derangement sets in. The process of nutrition becomes slower; the skin assumes a pale, yellowish, earthy color, sometimes with bluish streaks over the face; a general emaciation sets in, a flabbiness and thinness of all the tissues; the flesh becomes soft, the muscles lose their tone; the appetite is entirely gone; the bowels are completely bound, the stools are brown and hard; the horrible pains which the patients experience, and the loss of sleep, exhaust the remainder of their strength, and they gradually go into decline and perish.

Section 82.

Causes, course and terminations.—The etiology of cancer of the womb is not near so well known as is generally supposed. It is true, as has been asserted by some authors, that physical as well as vital derangements of the uterus, may be more or less instrumental in ushering in this disease;

but how often do not such causes exist without resulting in cancer, and, on the other hand, how often do not cancerous affections develop themselves without any appreciable cause? Where a cancerous germ exists, physical or moral commotions of the system may contribute to develop it; but a germ must pre exist in order that a cancerous disease may become developed, and such a germ cannot be created by any of the above-mentioned causes. In our judgment, the true cause of cancer, is a *cancerous diathesis* which, if once existing, may afterwards be developed by all sorts of moral or physical influences that have a tendency to irritate the uterus. Cancer may happen at any period of life, from the age of twenty to the most advanced old age. It occurs most frequently between the ages of forty and fifty, less frequently between thirty and forty, and least frequently before twenty-five and after seventy. The critical age is generally the period when cancer develops itself more openly and rapidly; but the first origin of this affection generally dates much farther back. According to some authors celibacy, or sexual excesses, onanism, frequent miscarriages, or uterine hæmorrhages, repeated menstrual irregularities, or even syphilis, are some of the exciting causes of cancer. It is very probable, that frequent or chronic uterine inflammations or discharges may develop a cancerous germ, in which case everything that tends to foster or create such diseases, may be looked upon as capable of producing cancer. This disease runs a very uncertain course, and its duration is inversely proportionate to its intensity. Generally it lasts from twelve to eighteen months. It may terminate fatally in five or six months, or after five or six years. Some patients, especially such as have suffered agonizing distress, die without having lost any of their stoutness; others die of peritonitis, a violent hæmorrhage; chronic fever, or in consequence of convulsions caused by the intense pain. If the disease continues uninterruptedly, the symptoms get worse and worse; the appetite is lost; frequent vomitings of bile and mucus set in; the patient is troubled with rumbling in the bowels, eructations, violent flatulent colic, obstinate constipation or excessive diarrhœa; afterwards aphthæ break out in the mouth; the patients become emaciated even so as to resemble skeletons; in other patients, the lower limbs become infiltrated; sometimes the whole body looks somewhat bloated, the strength gets lost, the patients are scarcely able to remain up for a few hours, and the ulcerative process gets worse and worse until death takes place. After death, the organs adjoining the uterus, are generally found intact, especially if only a part of the organ has been affected; but if the uterus had grown much larger, the fatty tissue near the neck sometimes becomes more voluminous, denser, and covered with little ulcers and foul and fungous vegetations. Sometimes the disease extends to the rectum and bladder, portions of which become schirrous, and are even destroyed by cancerous ulceration. The vagina may also become involved in the general affection, and even the peritoneum may become the seat of a chronic inflammation with effusion of an ichorous pus. As regards the more distant organs, scarcely any other derangements are discovered in them than are found in persons who have died with any other deep-seated diseases of the viscera accompanied by general marasmus.

Section 83.

Diagnosis and prognosis.—Although from our description of the disease, it might seem easy to infer its existence whereas the disease is really present, yet there is probably no disease that has been as frequently misapprehended where it was really present, or as frequently supposed to be present where it really did not exist. A chronic but uncomplicated inflammation of the uterus may be mistaken for cancer; so may certain forms of leucorrhœa, various other uterine degenerations, simple ulcerations and other affections, unless we take great care to direct our attention to the totality of the morbid phenomena.

In *chronic metritis* we likewise find the volume of the uterus enlarged, or at any rate of some of its parts, sometimes with intolerable pains, heaviness at the bottom of the vagina, pains in the small of the back, and painful pullings in the loins and hypogastrium; but these pains generally manifest themselves only when pressure is made upon the uterus, the inflamed and swollen portion of which remains soft, the neck remaining either smooth and even, or at most exhibiting only some small indurations about two lines deep. *Simple ulcerations* are distinguished from cancer by the manner in which they commence, by the matter which they secrete, by the absence of all schirrous characteristics in the parts where the ulcers are seated, and by the course which they pursue in their development. *Fibrous bodies* are sometimes more difficult to distinguish; but whatever may be the character of the swelling to which these tumors give rise, and however hard these tumors may be, they always remain indolent, and frequently project from the neck of the uterus, or from the uterine orifice, where they can be readily found out by the touch. As regards *polypi*, it is more difficult to diagnose them correctly, especially when they originate in a pure degeneration of the uterine substance, or when they are contained in the uterine cavity, where they often determine hæmorrhages, discharges of various kinds, and sometimes even ulcerations of the os tincæ, which may simulate a cancerous ulcer. However, the smoother, softer condition of the os tincæ, the more or less marked opening of the uterine orifice, and the absence of all induration, may lead us to establish our diagnosis even before the polypus had passed out of the neck of the womb, or before the orifice of the neck should have become sufficiently dilated to enable us to recognise the polypus by the touch. As regards the *discharges*, we have to pay particular attention to them, in order not to fall under the most serious mistakes. A most profuse and malignant leucorrhœa may exist without there being any trace of cancer, and there may even be prickings in the womb and vagina, profuse menstruation, an uneven surface in the orifice of the womb, and other symptoms resembling those of cancer. In such cases the true condition of the parts is frequently not recognized, except after long and patient observations; however, the fetid and ichorous discharges of cancer do not generally set in until the disease has advanced so far, that it is no longer possible to mistake it for something else, after an examination by the touch; so that, in spite of the apparently malignant nature of the discharge, we may always be sure not to have a cancer before us as long as none of the disorders characteristic of cancer, are recognized by the touch.

The PROGNOSIS of cancer is always highly dubious under any treatment; the more inveterate and extensive the cancerous ulceration, the less hope there is of a cure. Schirrous cancers seem to be the most difficult to cure, no matter at what stage of their growth, whereas fungous and medullary cancers seem often more than any other variety, disposed to yield to a rational treatment. It seems as though all the cases of cancers that have been set down as cured, could not possibly imply an error of diagnosis. It seems to us that a cure may be possible, although it must always be extremely difficult.

SECTION 84.

TREATMENT.—Homœopathy repudiates all cauterizations and external applications to cancerous sores, because all these ordinary means to which surgeons have been in the habit of resorting, are more injurious than useful. On the other hand, we have no positive remedies for this disease, especially when it has reached the last stage; nevertheless partial relief has been obtained in slightly, and even sometimes in desperate cases, by the use of some well chosen remedy. The best remedies which analogy and experience seem to point to as most adapted to uterine cancer, are:

1. *Graphites*, *Kreosotum*, *Sepia*.
2. *Arsenicum*, *Silicea*, *Sulphur*, *Mercurius*.
3. *Aurum*, *Belladonna*, *Carbo animalis*, *China*, *Lachesis*, *Lycopodium*, *Mercurius*.
4. *Cicuta*, *Cocculus*, *Conium*, *Dulcamara*, *Iodium*, *Magnesia*, *Mercurius*, *Nitri acid.*, *Staphysagria*, *Thuja*.

5. *Calcarea, Carbo veget., Phosphorus, Rhus, Sabina.*

And particularly:—

For SCHIRROUS cancer, before ulceration:—1. *Carbo animalis, Sepia.*

2. *Aurum, Belladonna, China, Staphysagria.*

3. *Calcarea, Carbo veget., Clematis, Cocculus, Conium, Lycopodium, Phosphorus, Rhus.*

For FUNGOUS cancer:—1. *Graphites.*

2. *Arsenicum, Carbo animalis, Kreosotum, Lycopodium, Sepia, Staphysagria, Thuja, Belladonna, Carbo veget., Lachesis, Mercurius, Nitri acidum, Phosphorus, Sabina, Silicea, Sulphur.*

3. *Aurum, Calcarea, Cocculus, Conium.*

For BLOODY cancer:—1. *Belladonna, Carbo animalis, China, Graphites, Kreosotum, Sepia.*

2. *Aurum, Carbo veget., Lachesis, Mercurius, Silicea, Sulphur.*

3. *Arsenicum, Cicuta, Cocculus, Conium, Phosphorus, Sabina.*

4. *Calcarea, Dulcamara, Iodium, Lycopodium, Magnesia muriat., Nitri acid., Staphysagria, Thuja,*

For MEDULLARY cancer:—1. *Belladonna, Phosphorus, Silicea, Sulphur.*

2. *Arsenicum, Carbo animalis, China, Graphites, Kreosotum, Mercurius, Sepia.*

3. *Aurum, Cicuta, Clematis, Cocculus, Conium, Dulcamara, Iodium, Magnesia muriat., Nitri acidum, Staphysagria, Thuja.*

4. *Calcarea, Carbo veget., Rhus, Sabina.*

For ULCERATIVE cancer:—*Graphites, Kreosotum.*

2. *Arsenicum, Belladonna, Carbo animalis, China, Lycopodium, Mercurius, Sepia, Silicea.*

3. *Aurum. Calcarea, Carbo veget., Lachesis, Phosphorus, Sabina, Staphysagria, Thuja.*

4. *Cicuta, Cocculus, Conium, Dulcamara, Iodium, Magnesia muriat., Nitri acidum, Rhus tox.*

With the following particular indications :

ARSENICUM.—For open cancer, with burning and agonizing pains, secretion of fetid, brownish or blackish ichor.

AURUM.—At the onset, when the indurations are still of a schirrous nature, with falling of the womb and pressure on the fundus of the bladder.

BELLADONNA.—For frequent hæmorrhages from the womb, painful pressure on the parts, violent pains in the small of the back and nervous excitement.

CARBO ANIMALIS.—For *schirrous* cancer, with pressive pains in the loins, groins and thighs, with distention of the abdomen, flatulence, frequent eructations and desire to vomit.

CHINA.—Sometimes at the commencement of the affection, when the indurations first commence, with ichorous leucorrhœa, dysmenorrhœa, etc.

CLEMATIS.—Sometimes for softened schirrus, with corrosive leucorrhœa and lancinating pains.

CONIUM.—For *intolerable lancinating* pains, with frequent nausea, vomiting, odd fancies for various things to eat, and other symptoms similar to such as occur during pregnancy.

GRAPHITES.—A powerful remedy in open cancer, especially for *warmth and painfulness of the vagina*, engorgement of lymphatic vessels and mucous follicles, hardness of the neck of the womb, which is swollen covered with fungous excrescences; heaviness of the abdomen, with exacerbation of the pains and fainting when standing; retarded and painful menses, with discharge of black, coagulated and fetid blood; stitches through the thighs and hypogastrium like electric shocks; *burning pains, constipation*, earthy complexion, sadness and restlessness.

KREOSOTUM.—For swelling of the labia, with *itching in the vagina;* stitches through the thighs, like electric jerks; dark, coagulated menstrual discharges, followed by an ichorous and corrosive discharge; painful pressure on the parts.

LACHESIS.—Sometimes after Kreosotum, at the critical age, for frequent hæmorrhages; stitches as with knives, sickly and distressed looks.

Lycopodium. — For open cancer with tearing stitches, burning pains in the vagina after intercourse; *warmth* and *dryness of the vagina,* bloody leucorrhœa.

Mercurius bromatus.—For itching, erythematous redness and swelling of the labia, with inflammatory egorgement of the vagina; serous, purulent and greenish leucorrhœa.

Sepia.—For soft schirrus, with painful pressure downwards, burning heat in the parts, eructions on the inside of the labia, soreness and redness of the vulva; lancinating jerks from the fundus of the vagina to the umbilicus; frequent bloody discharges between the periods, especially after intercourse; putrid leucorrhœa.

Silicea.—For open cancer, with bloody discharges from the vagina, especially after the menses, or fetid, brownish purulent, ichorous leucorrhœa.

Sulphur.—In most cases at the onset, especially in open cancer, with violent, burning pain in the vagina; painful soreness during intercourse; constant bloody discharges or else foul, corrosive, ichorous leucorrhœa.

For further details see *Dysmenorrhœa*, *Metrorrhagia*, *Leucorrhœa*, *Metritis*, *Endometritis*, *etc.*

Dose.—One or two drops of the liquid attenuation on sugar or in a little water, or six globules dry on the tongue, morning and evening.

ARTICLE VIII.

SIMPLE ULCERATIONS OF THE WOMB.

Section 85.

Symptoms.—Superficial erosions. — Simple and non-cancerous ulcerations of the uterus scarcely affect any other part than the neck, so that it would seem as though we ought not to have mentioned them until we treat of the diseases of the neck of the womb. But inasmuch as these ulcerations have often been confounded with cancer, we have deemed it advisable to give them a place immediately after the chapter on cancerous ulcerations. Simple ulcerations are of various kinds; some are quite *superficial*, consisting of single *erosions;* others, being more penetrating, form true ulcers without however becoming malignant. Moreover, several authors distinguished *herpetic*, *scrofulous* and *scorbutic* ulcerations, not to mention *syphilitic* ulcers, which may likewise invade the neck of the uterus. In this paragraph we will first treat of simple erosions, in the following paragraphs we will treat of other ulcerations, mentioning their symptoms, causes and diagnosis; in the last paragraph of this article will be found a description of the treatment. *Superficial erosions* are commonly seated at the lower extremity of the neck, at the os tincæ, most frequently on the posterior lip. The most simple of these ulcerations constitute red patches which are sometimes so superficial that they cannot even be recognised by the touch, unless the area or edges of the ulcer should be slightly raised and the existence of the erosion should be revealed by this tumefaction of the affected part. In most cases the neck is swollen, and a tenacious, transparent or whitish mucus is discharged from the orifice; sometimes the mucus is like pus or resembles an old catarrhal discharge from the nose and generally hides the os tincæ over which it is spread. Sometimes these erosions exist for a long time without the patient being aware of it; some only complain of a little embarrassment and pain in the pelvis, accompanied by a very slight leucorrhœal discharge assuming a slightly reddish or bloody color after intercourse which is scarcely ever painful. Other patients experience a sense of burning heat, a painful itching at the bottom of the vagina, pretty acute pains in the small of the back, and sometimes intolerable pains during intercourse; and a profuse discharge of white mucus takes place from the vagina being mixed with a good deal of blood after coit. The CAUSES of these erosions are very often sexual excesses, be it in consequence of the excitement which they cause in the organ, or of the friction which the sexual act may cause in the os tincæ. Other causes are: frequent and deep seated digestive derangements, or a general sinking of health. In other women such erosions seem to be caused by the pressure or friction which the neck of the uterus exercises against the walls of the vagina, in cases of deviation of the uterus from the normal line; sometimes they owe their existence to an acrid and corrosive leucorrhœa, to a gonorrhœal discharge, to acute or chronic inflammatory catarrh of the uterus or vagina. As regards the COURSE of such erosions, they have often been known to induce fungous or varicose tumors, especially in cases where these erosions showed a tendency to bleed profusely; a circumstance which, in some cases, may render the PROGNOSIS much more dubious than it may seem. In other cases, such erosions have been succeeded or accompanied by ovarian engorgements. The TREATMENT will be given in the last paragraph of this article.

SECTION. 86

DEEP-SEATED ULCERATIONS. — These ulcerations which sometimes penetrate the substance of the uterine neck to considerable depth, are almost always seated on the inside of the os tincæ, most frequently on the posterior lip; but very often they develop themselves in the fissures occasioned in the neck by parturition. In some cases they ascend pretty high up in the neck, and even extend into the body of the uterus. If these ulcerations are divided by cracks and marked by little tubercular elevations, they may assume the appearance of cancerous ulcerations. Leucorrhœa is not necessarily present; but they give rise to frequent hæmorrhages or an almost continual bloody discharge; the general health is not often affected by them. If no proper treatment is pursued, the disease may continue for months. Some authors think that these ulcerations may degenerate into cancer; this is a mistake, for simple ulcers always terminate in cicatrization, and if cancer becomes developed in the end it is because a cancerous germ existed from the commencement. As regards CAUSES, these ulcers seem for the most part to result from an inflammation of the vagina or from an acute or chronic uterine catarrh, during the course of which they become frequently developed, with simultaneous engorgement of the uterus or its neck. The same causes which produce chronic metritis or vaginitis, may likewise cause these ulcerations, especially if the catarrhal discharge should have become suppressed without the inflammatory condition of the womb or its neck having disappeared. The DIAGNOSIS is not very difficult except when the ulcer is deep-seated, bleeding and of a fungous character, which might lead one to confound it with cancer. We may guard against such an error by remembering that in cancer, the tissue of the neck is either much softer or much harder, bleeds more readily and is more livid than in veinal ulcerations; moreover the lancinations are more frequent and more marked, and the secretions are fouler and have a more unhealthy look. A simple ulcer is moreover much more easily controlled and cured than an ulcer having a cancerous character. For the TREATMENT we refer the reader to the last paragraph of this article.

SECTION 87.

HERPETIC, SCORBUTIC, SCROFULOUS and SYPHILITIC ULCERATIONS.—We have not much to offer concerning these different varieties of ulcerations, which are of the same nature, when attacking the neck of the uterus, as when breaking out on the skin, or on any portion of the lining membrane in other cavities. Herpetic ulcers generally arise from some preexisting herpetic eruption on the neck of the uterus. These eruptions consist most frequently in red tips, or in transparent vesicles on the neck, which is more or less swollen, and which secrete a more or less copious quantity of mucus. In most cases these eruptions are accompanied by an herpetic eruption on the skin; and if this eruption disappears, it will be generally found that leucorrhœa breaks out after it, or that an existing leucorrhœa becomes more profuse. Frequently the neck is more swollen, more puffed, and looks more angry than it does in simple erosions. *Scrofulous* ulcerations are characterised by a tuberculous matter which they secrete, and these tubercles sometimes form roughnesses that may give rise to the suspicion of a cancer having developed itself. The destruction caused by these ulcers, may be quite extensive, involving even the whole neck of the uterus, even down to the lower portion of the vagina; they generally follow the course of hot or cold abscesses, forming tumors where fluctuation is felt, as in softened cancer, or in a suppurating gland. In almost all cases, these ulcerations are complicated with engorgements of the body of the uterus, whence the tubercular process may spread onward, inflaming the peritoneum and causing effusions in the peritoneal cavities. These scrofulous ulcerations are so rare, that scarcely one is found in a hundred. As regards the so-called *scorbutic* ulcerations, it is more than probable that they are mercurial ulcerations arising from the abuse of mercury, when given for syphilis, similar to the ulcers which are frequently seen at the prepuce and scrotum, after the use of excessive doses of mercury, although the regular doctors deny that mercury has anything to do with such sores, which they attribute to some other morbid diathesis. As regards *syphilitic ulcers*, it is an established fact, that chancre may break out on the neck of the uterus. Some authors relate cases of chancre contracted by intercourse with women who were supposed to be affected with uterine cancer; if we consider the uncertainty which prevailed in the diagnosis of cancer at the time when these cases took place, we need not make a great effort of the imagination in order to believe that these pretended cases of uterine cancer were cases of true chancre. As a general rule, it is very difficult to establish a sure diagnosis of these syphilitic ulcerations, unless we choose to resort to the inoculation of the syphilitic virus on some other part of the body, in consequence of which the sufferings and dangers of the patient would be increased. Nevertheless, however difficult it may be to diagnose simple syphilitic erosions, there are cases of fully developed chancre, which cannot be mistaken for any other kind of ulcer.

Section 88.

Treatment of non-cancerous ulcerations of the womb.—In the treatment of these ulcers, which should be exclusively internal, all external applications should be avoided, as was likewise recommended for cancer, and the remedies should be selected in conformity with the symptoms furnished by the aspect and nature of the ulcers, and by the constitutional symptoms of the patient. The main remedies for such ulcerations, are:

1. *Nitri acidum*, *Thuja*.
2. *Arsenicum*, *Belladonna*, *China*, *Cicuta*, *Cocculus*, *Mercurius*, *Pulsatilla*, *Sepia*, *Silicea*, *Sulphur*.
3. *Calcarea*, *Carbo vegetabilis*, *Conium*, *Nitri acidum*, *Phosphorus*, *Phosphori acidum*, *Staphysagria*.
3. *Aurum*, *Carb. animalis*, *Causticum*, *Chomomilla*, *Graphites*, *Kreosotum*, *Mercurius*, *Petroleum*, *Ruta*, *Sabina*, *Secale*.

4. *Antimonium*, *Argentum nitricum*, *Clematis*, *Hepar*, *Kali*, *Muriatis acidum*, *Nux vomica*, *Petroleum*.

And in particular:

For superficial EROSIONS:—1. *Arsenicum*, *Lachesis*.

2. *Carbo vegetabilis*, *Lycopodium*, *Mercurius*, *Nitri acidum*, *Phosphorus*, *Pulsatilla*, *Secale*, *Silicea*, *Sulphur*, *Thuja*.
3. *Ammonium*, *Belladonna*, *Causticum*, *China*, *Kreosotum*, *Petroleum*, *Phosphori acidum*, *Sepia*.

For deep-seated ULCERATIONS:—1. *Belladonna*, *Calcarea*, *Nitri acidum*, *Pulsatilla*, *Silicea*.

2. *Aurum*, *Conium*, *Graphites*, *Kreosotum*, *Lycopodium*, *Mercurius*, *Sulphur*.
3. *Antimonium*, *Asafœtida*, *Carbo vegetabilis*, *Hepar*, *Lachesis*, *Muriatic acidum*, *Petroleum*, *Phosphori acidum*, *Rhus*, *Ruta*, *Sepia*.
4. *Causticum*, *Clematis*, *Kreosotum*, *Natrum muriat.*, *Phosphorus*, *Sabina*, *Staphysagria*, *Thuja*.

For HERPETIC ulcerations:—*Calcarea*, *Graphites*, *Lycopodium*, *Mercurius*, *Sepia*, *Silicea*, *Sulphur*.

2. *Arsenicum*, *Clematis*, *Conium*, *Dulcamara*, *Rhus*, *Staphysagria*, *Zincum*.
3. *Belladonna*, *Cicuta*. *Cocculus*, *Hepar*, *Magnesia*, *carbonica*, *Natrum muriat.*, *Petroleum*, *Pulsatilla*, *Thuja*, *Veratrum*.

For SCORBUTIC ulcerations:—1. *Arsenicum*, *Carbo animalis*, *Carbo vegetabilis*, *Lachesis*, *Mercurius*, *Staphysagria*, *Sulphur*.

2. *Ammonium*, *Ammonium muriat.*, *Clematis*, *Conium*, *Hepar*, *Phosphorus*, *Pulsatilla*, *Sepia*, *Silicea*, *Thuja*.
3. *Alumina*, *Ambrosia*, *Causticum*, *Iodium*, *Kreosòtum*, *Natrum muriat.*, *Nitri acidun*, *Nux vomica*, *Ruta*.

4. *Belladonna, Calcarea, Cantharis, China, Graphites, Lycopodium, Phosphori acidum, Sabina, Zincum.*

For SCROFULOUS ulcerations :—1. *Arsenicum, Belladonna, Calcarea, Carbo vegetabilis, Lycopodium, Silicea, Sulphur.*

2. *Aurum, Graphites, Hepar, Lachesis, Phosphorus.*
3. *Carbo animalis, Clematis, Conium, Dulcamara, Iodium, Mercurius, Nitri acidum, Phosphori acid., Sepia, Thuja.*
4. *Alumina, Ammonium, Cantharis, Kali, Kreosotum, Mezereum, Pulsatilla, Sulphuris acidum.*

For SYPHILITIC ulcerations:—1. *Mercurius.*

2. *Nitri acidum, Thuja.*
3. *Aurum, Carbo vegetabilis, Kali, Iodium, Lachesis. Nux juglans.*
4. *Carbo animalis, Clematis, Lycopodium, Phosphorus, Phosphori acidum, Sepia, Staphysagria.*

For further details see the articles: *Leucorrhœa, Endometritis, Metritis, Metrorrhagia,* and *Dysmenorrhœa;* the symptoms by which these affections are characterized, frequently accompany the above described ulcerations, which can often only be cured by attending to the complaint of which the ulcers are mere symptoms. This remark applies more particularly to *uterine catarrh,* which is often the fundamental cause of the ulcerated condition of the neck of the womb.

DOSE.—Give one or two drops of the liquid attenuation, or six globules dry on the tongue, morning and evening.

ARTICLE IX.

GANGRENE AND PUTRESCENCE OF THE WOMB.

Section 89.

Symptoms and treatment.—Gangrene or putrefaction of the uterus, is a disease which sometimes supervenes as one of the frightful terminations of acute metritis, and particularly of malignant epidemic puerperal metritis. According to Boer, it first attacks the neck of the uterus, whence it extends to the more remote parts; the uterus increases in volume; its walls become thickened and spongy; the tissue of the organ becomes soft and friable between the fingers, looking sometimes like decayed fruit, either pale or dark-colored and blackish; the internal surface is generally softer than the other parts, sometimes ulcerated and covered with a layer of viscid, putrid, blackish and fetid substance; often we find beneath this layer the tissue of the uterus altered to the depth of 2, 3, and even 6 lines. During the patient's life-time it is often very difficult to recognise this affection, especially, when the entire surface of the uterus has not been invaded, or when it only exists here and there, and occasions a few scattered eschars. However, inasmnch as the affection always commences at the neck, and its presence is at all suspected, we may recognize it by the touch. It is only in the most serious cases, where the whole surface of the uterus is invaded, that the disease will develop all its characteristic symptoms; in such a case, the pains in the hypogastrium which existed until then, disappear; a brownish liquid of a fetid odor, is discharged from the vulva: a diarrhœa of a cadaverous smell sets in, and a cold and clammy sweat breaks out either over the whole body or only on some parts; the pulse becomes frequent, small and intermittent; the features are deeply altered, the extremities become colder, and the patient sinks into syncope or a prolonged coma, with or without delirium. If the disease is not arrested by proper treatment, death almost always sets in a few days after these dangerous symptoms have made their appearance. This affection is almost always occasioned by a violent metritis, or it sets in in consequence of tedious and difficult labor. However, it may likewise set in in women who went through their confinement without any untoward symptoms. We likewise meet with it in epidemic puerperal fever; but nothing has yet occurred that might lead us to assert that this disease is contagious.

The TREATMENT of this disease is always very difficult, even in homœopathy, although we do sometimes obtain some success. The principal remedy is undoubtedly SECALE CORNUTUM, which may be tried even in the most unpromising cases; not, however, in large doses, such as are recommended by Hartmann, but, on the contrary, in the 30th to the 200th potency, six globules in half a tumblerful of water, of which the patient may take a teaspoonful every hour. Next to Secale, we may try *Arsenicum* and *Kreosotum*, also *Carbo vegetabilis*, which may be useful as long as the organic reaction has not entirely ceased. Experience will teach us whether *Phosphorus*, *Carbo vegetabilis*, *Nitri acidum*, *Sabina*, *Squilla*, *Belladonna*, may effect any good in this disease.

ARTICLE X.

DISEASES OF THE NECK OF THE UTERUS.

SECTION 90.

INFLAMMATIONS.—Inflammations of the neck of the womb are induced by the same causes as those of metritis generally. We distinguish three forms of such inflammations, namely: 1st, *acute;* 2d, *chronic;* 3d, *granular.*—The two former may, like metritis, affect only the mucous membrane, (*catarrhal* inflammation,) or the parenchyma, (*parenchymatous* inflammation.) The catarrhal form is scarcely ever present without uterine catarrh, of which it is only an extension; parenchymatous inflammation, on the contrary, is very often limited to the neck of the uterus, or even to one of the lips of the os tincæ, which is, in such a case, harder, longer, thicker and redder than its fellow. Either variety inclines to pass from the acute to the chronic stage, and the parenchymatous form is very apt to develope ulceration. In *granular* inflammation, we find the os tincæ surrounded by small vegetations, generally of the size of a millet-seed, whitish, soft, pretty numerous, and secreting from their interstices the blood which exudes, after contact, sexual intercourse or pressure at stool. At other times the granulations are hard, of the size of peas, and pediculated. In many cases this inflammation seems idiopathic, consequent upon menstruation, fatigue, long standing, constipation, and such like causes. It is also present in induration of the neck of the womb, fibrous tumors of the womb, herpes, or syphilis. If entirely idiopathic, the inflammation is not dangerous; but if complicated with other affections, the prognosis is more doubtful.

As regards TREATMENT, the *catarrhal* variety is treated exactly like *Endometritis*, described in Sections 63—66.

The principal remedies for *parenchymatous* inflammation of the neck, are: *China, Belladonna, Sepia, Platina, Natrum, Thuja, Nitri acidum, Mercurius, Conium, Kreosotum, Graphites.*

For idiopathic *granular* inflammation, we give, *Nitri acidum, Thuja, Staphysagria.* If of a *syphilitic* character, *Cinnabaris, Nitri acidum, Thuja, Mercurius, Lycopodium.* If accompanying indurations or fibrous tumors of the womb, see these affections and their treatment, Sections 78, 79.

DOSE.—One or two drops of the liquid attenuation in ten tablespoonfuls of water, a tablespoonful every three or four hours.

SECTION 91.

NEURALGIAS, REDNESSES, ENGORGEMENTS, ERUPTIONS, ULCERS AND CANCERS OF THE NECK OF THE WOMB.—Having mentioned ulcerations and cancer of the womb, in Sections 80—88, and the other derangements which we have just named, resembling a good deal those which have been treated in the preceding paragraph, we have but little to say concerning the affections which form the subject of this paragraph.

Neuralgia of the neck of the womb exists often independently of any other lesion of this organ or of the body of the uterus; the patients complain of pains that are seated high up in the vagina, without any alteration being perceptible even after the most minute investigation. Contact is always painful, and sexual intercourse often produces such an agonizing distress, that the patients would rather bear any other torture. The best remedies for this condition are:

1. *China.*
2. *Kali, Ferrum, Causticum, Natrum muriaticum, Kreosotum, Sepia, Belladonna.*

The *rednesses* of the neck of the womb consist in red or rose-colored patches on or near the neck, breaking out at the time of, or after the menses, or in consequence of sexual excitement. They are likewise seen on the posterior lip of the neck, in women who flood copiously, and where they seem induced by the contact of the secreted fluid. Other of these efflorescences resemble herpes, and are often accompanied by a simple engorgement of the neck. According to some practitioners, all such efflorescences manifest a predisposition to ulcerations, and old-school physicians at once advise to cauterize the parts. We do not look upon these efflorescences as any thing serious, and, if they coexist with engorgements of the neck, we have to treat them altogether and not the spots alone.

Engorgements of the neck of the womb may either be *simple* or *complicated.* They are termed complicated when they are united to inflammations, ulcerations, degenerations, or any other organic lesions of the womb or neck of the uterus. If existing without any of these affections, they are termed *simple.* In this instance we have only to do with simple engorgements; the other kinds will be found mentioned in the chapters where the affections to which those engorgements are united, are treated of. Generally we distinguish three kinds of simple engorgements: *congestive, hard* and *œdematous.* The congestive engorgement most frequently extends over the whole neck and may vary from a simple catarrh to a state of turgescence, where the accumulated blood imparts to the tissue of the neck the appearance of an engorged spleen. The neck is in such a case softened, larger and darker-colored, with sense of heaviness in the pelvis, pullings in the groin, and generally copious menstruation, sometimes amounting to hæmorrhage. The *hard* engorgement can hardly be distinguished from schirrus, and may easily degenerate into cancer; like schirrus, it exists with or without roughnesses. The *œdematous* engorgement is rarely ever found except after confinement, and seems to be induced by the violent treatment which the neck of the womb has to suffer. As regards TREATMENT, the congestive engorgement yields very generally to *Belladonna* or *Platina,* beside which we may have to employ *Sepia, Mercurius,*

Ammonium, *Conium*, *China*, *Crocus*, *Sabina*, *Sulphur*. The best remedies for the *hard* or *indurated* engorgement, which it is much more difficult to disperse, are: *Belladonna*, *Sepia*, *Carbo animalis*, *Aurum*, *China*, *Magnesia muriatica*, *Angustura*, *Staphysagria*, *Clematis*, *Conium*, *Cocculus*. For *œdematous* engorgements, we recommend: *Arnica*, *China*, *Lycopodium*, *Sepia*.

As regards the ERUPTIONS on the neck of the womb, some authors speak of *phlyctænæ* and *herpetic efflorescences*, which, according to their statement, degenerate in ulcers. We have not had an opportunity of treating such affections. However, the reader may consult the article *Ulcerations*, Sections 85—88, and our previous remarks in this paragraph, about efflorescences or rednesses of the neck of the womb.

ARTICLE XI.

OVARITIS AND OTHER AFFECTIONS OF THE OVARIES.

SECTION 92.

OVARITIS.—Ovaritis, like any other inflammation, may either be acute or chronic. Acute ovaritis is most generally caused by pregnancy and confinement; but it may likewise result from retrocession of gonorrhœa, in which case we term it *blennorrhagic ovaritis.* The acute ovaritis, which is consequent upon pregnancy or confinement, is frequently a sort of latent disease, characterized by a violent fever, which continues for several days, without causing any derangement in the secretion of milk or the lochial discharge; no local symptom, exploration of the abdomen, touch, etc., indicate the presence of the organic disorder; but all at once the patient becomes delirious, comatose and death ensues. In other cases the local affection is revealed by a sense of heaviness in the groins and small of the back, the lochial discharge becomes less; other symptoms set in, such as: hysteric ailments, nausea, mucus on the stomach, vomiting, convulsions even; the emission of urine and the passage of stool become painful. The pain sometimes extends down to the thigh on the affected side, which becomes stiff and numb; the pain is increased by suddenly raising herself when lying down, or by bearing-down at stool. At the same time we discover on one, and sometimes on both sides of the uterus a tumor, which is more or less painful when pressed upon, and where sometimes a throbbing or fluctuation is perceived. In the *first stage* of the disease, the ovary is a little harder than generally, but scarcely any larger; in the *second stage* its volume becomes double and even quadruple that of the natural size, sometimes larger than a hen's-egg; the organ becomes rounded, soft, friable or infiltrated with serum; in the *third stage* the serum is changed to pus, which is either infiltrated in the tissue or deposited in mass in the interior and softened organ; in the *fourth stage*, the whole or part of the ovary becomes soft or even completely dissolved. Arrived at this point, the ovarian abscess generally breaks and the contents become scattered in the peritoneal cavity, or in the bladder or rectum; at other times they pass off by the vagina, or the abscess burrows onwards to the crural arch or presents itself at the inguinal ring. The affection may likewise terminate in *softening* of the ovary, or, according to some authors, in *gangrene.* A frequent termination of the disease is *induration* of the ovary. In any event, ovaritis is always a dangerous disease; it may terminate fatally in three or four days; suppuration generally sets in about the fifteenth day, and resolution, if it take place at all, between the eighth or twelfth day, or even sooner, if a rational treatment be pursued. Resolution is undoubtedly the most fortunate result; but even if an *abscess* should already have formed, help is sometimes possible. Beside pregnancy and confinement, other causes of this disease are: traumatic lesions, blows on the hypogastrium, vehement exercise of the sexual act, onanism, menstrual suppressions, drugs used to effect miscarriage, etc.

Chronic ovaritis scarcely differs from the acute form, except that it is slower. Sometimes it follows acute inflammation; but it may likewise develop itself imperceptibly and terminate in softening, induration or other degenerations of the ovary. As long as suppuration has not set in, it is difficult to recognise the disease, and we may barely suspect its presence, when a sensitive and painful, but not stinging tumor forms in the ovarian region, which becomes from time to time the seat of a new inflammation. If suppuration sets in, the affection sometimes assumes the form of ovarian dropsy; we discover in the tumors a partial fluctuation, with hardness in various points; or in other words, the hardness is less uniform, but likewise less evident than in *ovarian dropsy*, with pains and sensitiveness from the commencement of the formation of the tumor, whereas in ovarian dropsy, the tumor forms and fluctuation is perceived before the pain is felt. We have already stated that the most frequent terminations of this inflammation are softening, induration and other degenerations of the ovary. Prostitutes and young girls addicted to secret vices, seem principally exposed to this disease; often, however, it originates in moral causes, which render the cure very difficult.

Gonorrhœal ovaritis corresponds in women to the gonorrhœal orchitis of men; it is a metastasis of the inflammatory process of the urethral mucous membrane of the ovary, where it develops itself as an acute disease.

The principal remedies for *acute* and *chronic* ovaritis are:

1. *Belladonna.*
2. *Mercurius*, *Lachesis.*
3. *Conium*, *Platina.*
4. *Sabina*, *Dulcamara*, *China.*
5. *Staphysagria*, *Ambra*, *Antimonium*, *Arsenicum*, *Aconitum*, *Cantharis.*

In *acute* ovaritis *Aconite* will be found very serviceable as long as the fever is high; but inasmuch as *Aconite* has not any specific effect upon the ovary, we had better not stop to trouble ourselves about the fever, but at once give *Belladonna*, which may be alternated every three hours with *Mercurius*, if the pain is very violent. *Mercurius* is an excellent remedy, if suppuration may be apprehended; if it should have set in already, *Lachesis* is the best remedy. In a case of acute ovaritis supervening during chronic inflammation of this organ, and where the face had already become hippocratic and the pulse filiform, *Conium* brought about a cure. In some cases where the pain is excessive, and the sexual system is very much excited, *Cantharis* will be found highly useful.

In chronic ovaritis, besides the remedies named, we may derive benefit from *Platina*, *Lachesis*, *Staphysagria*, *Sabina*, *Bryonia*, *Rhus*, *Arsenicum*, *Colocynthis*, *Ignatia*, *China*, *Nux vomica*, *Phosphori acid.*, and other remedies have likewise been recommended for ovaritis. But these remedies have no specific relation to the ovaries, and can only be used as intercurrent remedies for accidental symptoms, for instance: *Ignatia*, *Staphysagria*, *Phosphori acid.*, where the affection is fed by moral causes, disappointments, grief, etc.; *Staphysagria*, *Phosphori acid.*, *China*, when it is caused by onanism; *Bryonia*, *Arsenicum*, *Rhus* and other remedies, when the peculiar character of the pain indicates these drugs.

Blennorrhagic ovaritis generally yields to the remedies that were specifically required by the original disease, such as *Mercurius*, *Aurum*, *Nitri acid.*, *Thuja*, *Pulsatilla*.

Section 93.

Dropsy of the ovaries.—At the commencement nothing seems more obscure than this affection, which consists in the formation of a sac or cyst containing a liquid. The only sign that betokens its existence, is a tumor, the growth of which gradually impedes the functions of the adjoining organs; but this tumor may exist for a long time without any pain, menstrual irregularities, or other changes in the condition of the patient. It is only after a period, when the abdomen becomes very much distended, that dyspnœa, a sense of weight and gastric derangements set in. The size of the tumor may vary from that of a hen's egg to a tumor of six feet and more in circumference. At first it is seated in the region of the ovary, but afterwards it may descend into the inferior portions of the pelvis or occupy the middle of the abdominal cavity. The liquid it encloses, is of different kinds, sometimes transparent or colorless, at other times milky or purulent, gelatinous, lemon or coffee-colored, or like honey, vinous sediment, tallow, oil, etc. If developed to a certain degree, ovarian dropsy may easily be confounded with ascites; the diagnosis is aided by the fact that the ovarian tumor is always round, irregular and not level at the upper surface, and that the bowels and the stomach are situated above the tumor; percussion yields a much duller sound than in ascites; finally, the commencement of the trouble in one side, its primitive limits, the undiminished quantity of the urine, the preservation of the general health, the absence of the horizontal level when the patient sits down, and the natural shape of the sides when she is lying on her back; the tympanitic sound of the bowels on the sides of the tumor, where the dulness of sound seems circumscribed by curvilinear outlines, are so many signs which distinguish in a positive manner ovarian dropsy from ascites. Moreover the tumor is always moveable, and if the patients turn suddenly from one side to the other, they experience a sensation as if a round and cold body were falling from side to side. Internal exploration shows the uterus more or less pushed to the opposite side. The *cause* of this disease, and the influences that lead to it, are almost unknown; according to some authors the disease scarcely ever sets in before the age of forty or fifty, and married women are more subject to it than unmarried; we have seen cases of ovarian dropsy at twenty and at thirty years, and in young girls of acknowledged purity. Ovarian dropsy, though sometimes incurable, is not very serious; it develops itself slowly, and the general health does not suffer much. Such tumors have existed for thirty and more years in some cases, and yet the patients lived up to eighty and even more years. According to most authors, the average duration of the disease from the commencement to its fatal issue, is from six to twelve years; death taking place either in consequence of the compression of the thoracic organs, or of the rupture of the tumor and effusion into the peritoneal cavity, which almost always causes sudden and malignant peritonitis.

As regards TREATMENT, the old-school looks upon this disease as incurable, and rebelling against all possible remedies. Allœopathic practioners resort to puncture, incision, and extirpation as their only means of cure. So far homœopathy has not been much more successful in the treatment of this malady; there are cases, however, where *Arsenicum*, *Lycopodium*, *Sepia*, *Iodium*, and *Platina*, seem to have affected an improvement, and these remedies might, perhaps, effect a cure if used in time:—*Mercurius*, *Phosphori acid.*, *Graphites*, *China*, *Staphysagria*, *Thuja*, have also been recommended.

Section 94.

Various other affections of the ovaries: hydatids, cysts, calculi, fibrous bodies, tubercles, cancer, hernia.—All we do is to mention these affections, the treatment of which is the same as that which has been recommended for similar diseases of the womb. In order not to leave any gap in our work, we will mention some remedies that seem to us to deserve particular attention when these diseases affect ovaries:

For Hydatids:—*Cantharis*, *Mercurius*.

Fibrous bodies:—*Calcarea*, *Platina*, *Staphysagria*, *Thuja*.

Ovarian cancer:—*Graphites*, *Arsenicum*, *Kreosotum*,

Hernia:—*Nux vom.*, *Silicea*, *Conium*, *Magnesia muriat.*, *Cocculus*, *Sulphur*, *Sulphuris acidum*.

ARTICLE XII.

VAGINITIS AND OTHER DISEASES OF THE VAGINA.

SECTION 95.

VAGINITIS.—This inflammation is likewise either *acute* or *chronic*. Both forms only affect the mucous membrane of the vagina to which they remain confined during the whole course of the disease, and are characterised by more or less copious blennorrhœa or leucorrhœa, with swelling and more or less marked heat of the vaginal mucous membrane. *Acute* vaginitis, generally commences with itching and painful tension extending from the vulva through the vagina, and which, together with the heat and swelling, increases for the first five or six days. The walls of the vagina close in upon each other, and are very painful when a finger is introduced; the emission of urine is more painful and frequent; there is a sense of weight on the anus, and the pains are worse during stool; walking is impeded, especially if the inflammation extends as far as the vulva. The intensity of the pains varies according to circumstances, from a simple malaise to intense agony, without these pains being at all proportionate to the perceptible signs of the inflammation. At the onset, the mucous membrane is generally drier than in the normal condition; but soon a quantity of serous fluid of a light color is secreted and discharged by the vulva. Gradually this fluid becomes creamy, yellowish or greenish, sometimes bloody; its quantity varies, from a hardly perceptible discharge to a flow equal to the catamenial discharge. In all cases of *simple* vaginitis, this discharge is almost transparent, with round globules floating in it, such as are found in pus and mucus;

but, if vaginitis is caused by impure coit, the discharge contains moreover small animalculæ. The mucous lining is generally more or less intensely and more or less uniformly red, with or without puffiness of the affected portions. In a few rare cases, the inflammation penetrates to the subjacent tissues, becoming *phlegmonous*, with acute and continuous pains, febrile motions and other accessory symptoms such as headache, weight in the stomach, nausea, vomiting, etc.; even abscesses may form in the substance of the vaginal walls, which may break either at the perinæum or at the labia majora. The course of acute vaginitis varies; generally the acute symptoms decrease after eight or ten days, after which the discharge becomes less copious, and finally ceases altogether, provided the inflammation does not become chronic. In most cases *chronic* vaginitis which differs from acute vaginitis only in the intensity of its symptoms and its slower course, is only a sequel of the *acute* form, although it may, however, be a chronic inflammation from the first, with all the signs of such a form.

According to the condition of the mucous membrane, both the *acute* and *chronic* variety may assume a good many modifications. We distinguish in this respect:—

1. *Erysipelatous* and *erythematous vaginitis*, where there is scarcely any discharge, but where the vagina exhibits intensely-red, painful, more or less extensive patches, somewhat raised and causing a sense of pain and smarting.

2. *Papulous vaginitis*, where the vagina and the neck of the womb are covered with papulæ or follicles that are more or less developed, and present themselves in the shape of small spots of the size of a pin's head, or in the shape of granulations that resemble fleshy granulations, and may form real vegetations.

3. *Vesicular vaginitis*, caused by a spreading of the eczema from the vulva to the vagina and which may produce a true herpes phlyctenoides in the deep-seated parts of the vagina, and on the neck of the womb.

4. *Pustulous vaginitis*, where real pustules are developed

in the vagina, in persons affected with impetiginous eruptions.

5. *Glandular vaginitis*, where the follicles alone seem affected, but where the mucous membrane exhibits no trace of change, and where the secretion alone seems altered, more copious and of a yellowish-white or grayish color.

The CAUSES of these different forms of vaginitis are exceedingly varied, and it is difficult to trace them. Women of a flabby and lymphatic constitution, or such as are tainted with scrofula, chronic, cutaneous eruptions, etc., seem particularly liable to such inflammations; no age is exempt from them, even children after the second teething are more or less attacked by these irritations; among adults they are quite frequent; among old persons they become rarer, although the critical period when most women are troubled with itching at the vulva, predisposes for these diseases in consequence of the more or less inflammatory irritation which this itching causes in the vagina. Among other women there seems to exist a particular predisposition for all sorts of catarrhal inflammations, especially for inflammations of the vagina. Beside these causes, we have to note as exciting causes the friction, contusions, irritations of the vagina, caused by foreign bodies (pessaries, etc.), excessive intercourse, onanism, injections (except pure water), fatiguing walking, and recto-anul ascarides, which get into the vagina. Infection by impure coit, likewise, with individuals affected with gonorrhœa, may likewise induce a *virulent vaginitis*, of which we shall treat by-and-by.

Virulent vaginitis, also termed *blennorrhagic* or *gonorrhœal vaginitis*, has all the anatomical characteristics of acute or chronic simple vaginitis, except its origin and contagious character. In all other respects, it resembles so closely a simple vaginitis that, unless the origin of the disease were known, it would be difficult to distinguish the virulent from the other variety. Some characteristic signs seem, however, peculiar to this form of vaginitis, which we shall describe more particularly when speaking of the diagnosis.

The diagnosis of simple vaginitis, is not difficult as far as the disease is concerned; a careful exploration of the vagina, and, in some cases the simple touch, are sufficient to reveal to us the condition of the parts, either by the swelling which is seen, or by the painfulness and the heat which are ascertained by the touch; but these signs are not sufficient when we have to determine whether the inflammation is simple or gonorrhœal. The physician has to be guided in such a case by the accompanying circumstances, the time which had elapsed between the period of the infection, and the period when the disease first showed itself, and perhaps by the nature of the secretions, where, according to some authors, nothing but mucous vesicles and purulent globules are formed, when the inflammation is simple, but where *little animalculæ* (*trichomonas of the vagina*) are discovered if the inflammation is caused by the gonorrhœal virus.

In regard to PROGNOSIS, it is not at all dangerous in the *simple* or *acute* form, if the patients have a good constitution and the disease owes its origin to accidental causes; resolution is obtained promptly and without any trouble. But, if constitutional influences have slowly determined the disease, it is much more obstinate. This is likewise the case when the patients are affected with cutaneous eruptions. *Virulent vaginitis* is likewise easily cured, if it is a first attack, and the patient is of a sound constitution; but if she should be predisposed for catarrhal discharges, or have a lymphatic consitution, and be subject to cutaneous disorders, or if she should have been attacked before, the disease is much more difficult to cure, and inclines to become chronic, or, at any rate, to assume the form of a simple but obstinate chronic vaginitis.

The TREATMENT of vaginitis is generally the same as that which we have recommended for *Leucorrhœa*, Sections, 44—48, to which we refer the reader. We will give a few indications that are more particularly applicable to vaginitis. The best remedies in general are:

1. *Mercurius*, *Sepia*, *Pulsatilla*, *Sulphur*.
2. *Nitri acidum*, *Thuja*, *China*, *Kreosotum*, *Lycopodium*, *Sabina*.
3. *Alumina*, *Ammoniacum*, *Causticum*, *Conium*, *Petroleum*, *Phosphorus*, *Silicea*, *Stannum*.

And in particular:

For ACUTE vaginitis:—1. *Mercurius*, *Sepia*.
2. *Sulphur*, *Pulsatilla*.
3. *China*, *Nitri acidum*, *Thuja*, *Sabina*, *Mezereum*.

For CHRONIC vaginitis:—1. *Sepia*, *Pulsatilla*, *Conium*, *Sulphur*, *Mercurius*, *Sabina*.
2. *Calcarea*, *Alumina*, *Ammonium*, *Conium*, *Graphites*, *Kali*, *Petroleum*, *Nux vomica*, *Silicea*, *Stannum*, *Zincum*.
3. *Arsenicum*, *Cannabis*, *Carbo veg.*, *Magnesia*, *Magnesia muriatica*.

For ERYTHEMATOUS vaginitis:—*Mercurius*, *Belladonna*, *Lycopodium*, *Nux vomica*, *Kali*, *Alumina*, *Kreosotum*.

For VESICULAR vaginitis:—*Mercurius*, *Petroleum*, *Dulcamara*, *Phosphoricum acidum*, *Thuja*, *Nitri acidum*, *Sulphur*.

For VIRULENT vaginitis:—*Cannabis*, *Mercurius*, *Nitri acid.*, *Thuja*, *Sulphur*, *Sepia*, *Alumina*.

DOSE.—One or two drops of the liquid attenuation in ten tablespoonfuls of water, a tablespoonful of which solution is to be given every four or six hours.

SECTION 96.

PROLAPSUS, HERNIA AND FISTULÆ OF THE VAGINA.—By prolapsus of the vagina, we understand a protrusion of the internal membrane of the vagina within the vaginal canal, or even between the labia of the vulva, caused not by hernia of the bladder or rectum, nor by falling of the womb, but by a puffing-up of the inner lining membrane. The prolapsus may be *complete* or *incomplete*, *partial* or *general*, according as the tumor projects from the vulva or is confined to the interior of the vagina, and that it extends either over the whole of the vagina or only over a portion of this canal. The symptoms of this prolapsus vary, as far as intensity is concerned, according to the extent of the falling, and the inflammatory state of the tumor, and are generally: sense of weight at the orifice of the vagina; more or less prominent tumor, which is round when the prolapsus is only partial and looks like a circular pad when the prolapsus extends all around; impeded walk, difficulty of remaining seated; tenesmus of the bladder, dysuria; constipation, discharge of puriform mucus. If the prolapsus is complete, the action of the urine upon the tumor renders the inflammation sometimes very acute, with soreness, intense pain, and tension in the tumor as far as the loins; the swelling of the part may also produce a sort of strangulation, that may result in gangrene. Among the predisposing causes of this affection, we may number all the influences that may produce a relaxation and weakness of the tissues, such as: a lymphatic constitution, a cachectic condition, arising from bad nourishment or any other weakening cause, abuse of warm baths and relaxing beverages, inveterate and copious fluor albus, menorrhagia and frequent confinements or miscarriages. *Existing causes* are: violent friction with the hands or instruments during parturition; excessive intercourse; onanism; effort to lift heavy loads; constipation; concussions caused by leaping, falling, immoderate laughter, cough and vomiting. Sometimes the falling is caused by chronic inflammation of the mucous membrane of the vagina. The DIAGNOSIS is founded upon the existing symptoms and upon the shape of the tumor, which has transversal rugæ in partial prolapsus; whereas, in complete prolapsus, the tumor is cylindrical, with circular rugæ. The base of the tumor is united to the internal membrane of the vulva, although this is likewise, sometimes, surrounded with a cul-de-sac that is not very deep. Complete prolapsus of the vagina cannot always readily be distinguished from prolapsus of the womb. The PROGNOSIS is generally very simple; prolapsus of long standing is sometimes very obstinate. Complete prolapsus is most difficult to cure. In some cases a cure has been effected by means of accidental inflammations, which were excited in the vagina by foreign bodies, such as a pessary, for example. Cases are mentioned where pregnancy is said to have effected a cure, or at least a marked improvement. For the TREATMENT, we refer the reader to the end of this article, where the particular indications are given.

From falling of the vagina we have to distinguish *hernia*, that is descensions where other organs are engaged in a tumor in the interior of the vagina or passing out at the vulva. We distinguish three kinds: 1st, *vaginal hernia*, or incomplete hernia of the vulva, which is nothing else than intestinal hernia, where a portion of bowel is contained in the hernial sac; 2d, *vaginal cystocele*, where the bladder is engaged in the hernial sac; 3d, *vaginal rectocele*, where the rectum passes into the vagina and protrudes from the vulva. The description and treatment of these secondary descensions of the vagina, belongs rather to the pathology and therapeutics of hernia, than to those of the sexual organs; for this reason we only make a passing allusion to these difficulties here, and shall describe the treatment at the end of this paragraph.

VAGINAL FISTULÆ are *lesions of continuity*, produced by accidental wounds or by abscesses developed in the vaginal walls, in consequence of which a communication is established between the vagina and urethra, or between the vagina and bladder (*urethro-vaginal fistulæ*), or between the vagina and rectum (*recto-vaginal fistulæ*), or between some other portion of the intestines and the vagina (*intestino-vaginal fistulæ*), or between the vagina and the peritoneal cavity (*peritoneo-vaginal fistulæ*), or, finally, between the vagina and some accidental cavity, resulting from the opening of an abscess, or of some cyst that has developed itself in some neighboring organ, and has discharged its contents into the vagina.

These various lesions require the interference of the surgical art, and we should not have mentioned any of them here, if it were not proven by experience, that a well chosen remedy may sometimes enable nature to effect the spontaneous reduction of a displaced organ, of hernia, and the cicatrisation of a fistula. We have, therefore, deemed it proper to indicate the principal remedies by means of which these lesions may be cured internally, without any other surgical means than such manual assistance as is absolutely necessary.

I. For FALLING of the vagina:—1. *Mercurius*, *Sepia*.
2. *Ferrum*, *Stannum*.
3. *Belladonna*, *Nux vomica*.
4. *Calcarea*, *Ferrum*, *Kreosotum*, *Nux moschata*.

II. For VAGINAL HERNIA:—1. *Nux vomica*, *Sulphur*, *Sulphuris acid.*
2. *Ammonium muriaticum*, *Aurum*, *Cocculus*, *Lycopodium*, *Magnesia*, *Silicea*, *Veratrum*.
3. *Chamomilla*, *Clematis*, *Colocynthis*, *Nitri acidum*, *Opium*, *Petroleum*, *Phosphorus*, *Rhus*, *Staphysagria*.
4. *Aconitum*, *Alumina*, *Carbo animalis*, *China*, *Lachesis*, *Magnesia carb.*, *Thuja*, *Zincum*.

III. For VAGINAL FISTULA:—1. *Pulsatilla*, *Silicea*, *Lycopodium*, *Calcarea*.
2. *Sulphur*, *Asarum*, *Carbo vegetabilis*, *Belladonna*, *Nitri acid.*, *Conium*.
3. *Thuja*, *Petroleum*, *Causticum*, *Antimonium*, *Aurum*, *Thuja*, *Sepia*, *Lachesis*.

Moreover:—

For STRANGULATION of the parts:—1. *Aconitum*, *Sulphur*.
2. *Lachesis*, *Opium*, *Sulphuris acid.*
3. *Arsenicum*, *Nux vomica*, *Belladonna*, *Veratrum*.

INFLAMMATION:—*Aconitum*, *Mercurius*, *Belladonna*, *Sulphur*, *Nux vomica*, *Sepia*, *Sulphuris acid.*

ULCERATIONS:—*Mercurius*, *Hepar*, *Lachesis*, *Silicea*, *Sulphur*, *Chamomilla*, *Pulsatilla*, *Nitri acid*, *Thuja*, *Asarum*, *Phosphorus*.

GANGRENE:—*Arsenicum*, *Sulphuris acid.*, *Belladonna*, *Calcarea*, *Sulphur*, *Lachesis*, *Kreosotum*.

It is a matter of course that, if vaginal fistula is caused by some other disease, cancer, syphilis, etc., we have to remove this affection and select our remedies accordingly.

SECTION 97.

INDURATIONS, CONTRACTIONS, TUMORS, CYSTS, POLYPI, ULCERS AND CANCERS of THE VAGINA:—Inasmuch as these affections do not differ from similar affections of the womb, except by their locality, we shall here simply mention the characteristic symptoms which these affections develope in the vagina, and, for the rest, refer the reader to what we said of the nature and origin of these diseases in our chapters of uterine disorganizations.

Like the neck and body of the womb, the vagina may be affected with simple indurations which are neither *schirrous* nor *syphilitic*. They are engorgements or thickenings of the mucous membrane, which generally come on slowly and imperceptibly, commencing at circumscribed points rather high up in the vagina, and even round the neck of the uterus. The effect of such indurations always is to contract the vagina more or less, to render it more rigid, less dilatable, and to render the introduction of foreign bodies difficult and painful. In most cases there is not discharge, although there are cases where a profuse leucorrhœal discharge takes place from the commencement. Almost always the patients complain of pain at the outset, of smarting, itching, and increase of heat, and, in proportion as the affection develops itself, the vagina becomes contracted and sometimes entirely obliterated. What distinguishes these simple thickenings from schirrous indurations is this, that they do not present to the finger those roughnesses which characterize schirrus; that they are less consistent than schirrus, and never ulcerate. The most frequent causes of these indurations, which are most frequently met with towards the fortieth year, are:—onanism, effect of hard bodies, such as pessaries, friction by coit, or irritations caused by acrid humors, etc. As regards the TREATMENT of these indurations, we recommend the following remedies:—*Petroleum*, *Clematis*, *Pulsatilla*, *Sulphur*, *Belladonna*, *China*, *Magnesia muriat.*, *Conium*, *Lycopodium*, *Sepia*.

As regards the various TUMORS which occur in the vagina, they are:—1, *bloody tumors*, of which we shall say a few words when we come to describe the ailments incident to pregnancy; 2, *serous cysts*, resembling hydrocele; 3, *fatty tumors*, or lipoma; 4, *fibrous tumors;* 5, *polypi* and non-syphilitic ulcerated vegetations. The treatment of these lesions is the same as that of similar lesions in other parts of the body, namely purely medicinal and internal. The following remedies are the best for these affections:—

I. For BLOODY TUMORS:—*Mercurius*, *Sepia*, *Sulphur*, *Belladonna*.

II. For SEROUS CYSTS:—*Pulsatilla*, *Graphites*, *Lycopodium*, *Silicea*, *Sulphur*, *Rododendron*.

III. For FIBROUS TUMORS:—*Calcarea*, *Staphysagria*, *Thuja*, *Lycopodium*, *Mercurius*, *Nitri acidum*, *Phosphorus*.

IV. For POLYPI:—*Calcarea*, *Conium*, *Phosphorus*, *Platina*, *Staphysagria*, *Lycopodium*, *Nitri acidum*, *Mercurius*.

V. For granular vegetations:—*Nitri acidum*, *Staphysagria*, *Thuja*, *Calcerea*, *Lycopodium*.

For the treatment of simple and cancerous ulcerations of the vagina, we refer the reader to Sections 79–87, where these affections of the uterus are fully described, together with an indication of their treatment.

SECTION 98.

SPASMS AND NEURALGIA OF THE VAGINA.—These two kinds of affections, which are quite frequent, generally get well without the interference of art; however, cases which require the use of medicines, may occur, and we have deemed it ne cessary, on this account, to offer some remarks concerning them. By *spasm* of the vagina, we understand a *convulsive stricture* of the vagina, which may be so intense as to completely obliterate the canal. Sometimes this stricture is a symptom of vaginitis, but in other cases it exists idiopathically as a purely nervous disease, in which case the constriction of the vagina is exceedingly painful, intermittent, without redness, heat or swelling. Often this spasm sets in during confinement; some nervous women are attacked by it at the moment of intercourse, but it ceases as soon as the vagina secretes the seminal mucus; it may also be induced by moral causes; nervous and passionate women are more particularly liable to it. The best remedies for it, are:—*Nux vomica, Ignatia, Cocculus, Belladonna, Pulsatilla, Platina, Mercurius.*

NEURALGIA OF THE VAGINA often consists in a simple sensitiveness of this organ, but it may likewise be characterized by acute, lancing, burning, tearing pains, or even by intolerable itching. Touch is likewise painful, and most women who are attacked with this weakness, show great aversion to sexual intercourse. Sometimes they fancy that they are suffering with some serious disease, and that ulcers or cancer will break out; but on exploring the vagina we find it simple and idiopathic neuralgia, neither inflammation nor any other abnormal symptom. Such neuralgia may likewise be caused by some uterine affection, of which we have to assure ourselves by all means. Simple and idiopathic neuralgia is often caused by exhaustion consequent upon sexual intercourse, by cold injections and by other influences. The principal remedies are:—*Belladonna, Conium, Ignatia, Valeriana, Sepia, Hyoscyamus, Chamomilla, Asafœtida.*

DOSE—One or two drops of the liquid attenuation in a tumblerful of water, of which a tablespoonful is to be given every few hours.

ARTICLE XIII.

VULVITIS AND OTHER AFFECTIONS OF THE VULVA.

SECTION 99.

VULVITIS, INFLAMMATION OF THE VULVA.—Like any other inflammation, an inflammation of the vulva may be acute or chronic. In acute vulvitis the labia are more or less red on their mucous surface; there is intense heat and a distressing itching, with painful sensitiveness which does not even allow of the least contact; the swelling may be so intense as to close the vulva completely. In some cases the nymphæ are alone inflamed and swollen, so as to protrude between the labia majora; generally, however, the inflammation invades simultaneously the labia majora, nymphæ and clitoris, causing a permanent erection of this organ, and thereby exciting more or less marked lascivious desires; sometimes the inflammation spreads to the pubic region and to the inguinal glands. At the onset of the disease, the mucous membrane is dry and shining, but soon it secretes an opaque, white or yellowish mucous of a sickening smell, and excoriating acridity. In some cases, a submucous inflammation sets in which causes burning or stinging pains, and may become very extensive. Acute vulvitis scarcely ever lasts longer than eight or ten days, and the most frequent termination is a gradual dispersion of all the symptoms; in some cases the inflammation terminates in suppuration, and even in gangrene. In the latter case, the affected parts become cold, the pains cease, and the vulva exhibits a violet-colored, dark or livid border. But these cases scarcely ever happen except after violent contusions or hard labor, or in consequence of improper treatment. The most general *predisposing causes*, are:—obesity, approach of the menstrual period, pregnancy, prolonged standing, walking, dentition, piles, cutaneous affections of the vulva, uncleanliness, abuse of washes, foot-stoves, onanism, etc. Among the *exciting causes*, we have to note, irritating action of certain uterine and vaginal discharges, repeated frictions of the parts, sexual excesses, irritating injections, lacerations, various manipulations during labor, etc. Sometimes this affection results from metastasis in parotitis, otorrhœa, etc.

Chronic vulvitis has the same characteristic signs as the acute form, except that the symptoms are more marked. In most cases it is developed out of acute vulvitis, but it may likewise set in from the first as a chronic disease, especially in lymphatic persons. Often there is neither redness nor heat in the chronic form, but the parts are generally painful and slightly swollen, more or less hard and itching.

The best remedies for *acute vulvitis* are: *Mercurius, Sepia, Nux vomica, Belladonna, Conium, Nitri acid., Sulphur, Aconite.*

If the inflammation had been caused by mechanical influences, (blows, manipulations, contusions, etc.,) we give *Arnica, or Cicuta, Conium, Pulsatilla, Chamomilla.*

If PHLEGMONOUS, give:—*Belladonna, Mercurius, Sepia, Nux vomica, Sulphur.*

For SUPPURATION:—*Mercurius, Pulsatilla, Sulphur, Silicea.*

For GANGRENE:—*Arsenicum, Pulsatilla, Silicea, China.*

For CHRONIC VULVITIS:—*Sepia, Sulphur, Conium, Mercurius, Nitri acid.*

If vulvitis depends upon existing uterine or vaginal discharges, these have to be cured, of course; for which we refer the reader to the article on *Leucorrhœa.*

DOSE.—The same as at the close of the last paragraph.

Section 100.

Tumors, hernia, œdema, fistulæ, cysts, hypertrophy, varices, polypi and cancer of the vulva.—The treatment of these affections does not differ in the least from that of similar affections of other parts of the sexual organs. Our remarks bearing upon the vulva in particular will necessarily be very short.

Bloody tumors of the vulva are more or less extensive, of a violet-colored, bluish or brownish appearance, generally without pain, but occasioning a tolerably violent tension, and impeding the walk more or less. They may develop themselves spontaneously, but in most cases they are induced by blows, a fall, contusions, frictions during labor or at any other period, also during pregnancy. The principal remedies for these tumors are: *Arnica, Sepia, Nux vomica, Mercurius, Conium, Zincum.*

Hernia of the vulva is very rare; it commences like vaginal hernia, and develops itself in the substance of the labia majora, where they can easily be distinguished from vaginal hernia by the direction they take, and from a cyst or an abscess in the labia by the absence of fluctuation, by the general characters of every kind of hernia, and by the disappearance of the tumor in the horizontal posture. The principal remedies which will facilitate the reduction of hernia, are: *Nux vomica, Sulphur, Cocculus, Sulphuris acidum.* (See also *Vaginal Hernia*, Section 96.)

Œdema of the vulva may result from vulvitis, or it may come on spontaneously in consequence of the impeded circulation in the pelvic extremities, as takes place during pregnancy. What distinguishes this swelling from any other, is its softness, which causes it to retain a depression from the pressure of the finger; its decrease in the horizontal and its increase in the vertical position. The principal remedies are: *Mercurius, Sulphur, Sepia, Arnica.*

Abscessess of the vulva always result from vulvitis, or

during pregnancy. If badly managed, they may give rise to *vulvo-rectal fistulæ*, especially if the abscess is seated near the fourchette or the corresponding portion of the vagina. In regard to treatment, the best thing to be done is to prevent them, by dispersing the primary inflammations by appropriate remedies, such as: *Mercurius*, *Sepia*, *Belladonna*, *Lachesis*. After suppuration has set in, with or without fistula, we often still obtain a cure by giving: *Mercurius*, *Silicea*, *Lachesis*, *Phosphorus*, *Sulphur*, and particularly: *Silicea*, *Calcarea*, *Phosphorus*, *Sulphur*, if fistula has set in.

Cysts of the vulva are frequently met with, especially in prostitutes. They generally develope themselves on one of the labia, on the left rather than on the right. At first they are scarcely noticed at the orifice of the vagina, but they may continue to grow until they have reached the size of a nut, and even of a fist. Most frequently they are filled with a colorless liquid or a thick, yellowish substance; other cysts are stertomatous, filled with fatty matter. When the former cysts break, which seldom takes place spontaneously, their orifice remains open and continues to secrete moisture, which may irritate the parts and cause inflammations and abscesses. Under homœopathic treatment we scarcely ever need have recourse to surgical means; the internal treatment will be found sufficient to effect the dispersion of the cysts. The best remedies are:

1. *Calcarea*, *Nitri acidum*.
2. *Baryta*, *Sulphur*, *Sabina*.
3. *Graphites*, *Silicea*, *Hepar*.
4. *Kali*, *Spongia*, *Antimonium*, *Agaricus*.

Hypertrophy of the labia majorum, if supervening during pregnancy, often yields to *Sepia;* in other cases we may have to give: *Carbo vegetabilis*, *Sepia*. If the disease is caused by leucorrhœa, we have to cure this affection by the remedies indicated for leucorrhœa.

Varices and erectile tumors of the vulva likewise yield in most cases to internal treatment which may always be tried before we resort to surgical means. The principal remedies are:

1. For VARICES:—*Pulsatilla, Arnica, Carbo veget., Lycopodium, Ferrum, Arsenicum, Causticum, Sulphur, Graphites, Zincum.*

2. For ERECTILE TUMORS:—*Carbo animalis, Arsenicum, Carbo veget., Platina, Thuja, Silicea, Phosphorus, Sulphur, Nitri acidum, Lycopodium, Kreosotum.*

And if these tumors bleed a good deal:—*Phosphorus, Carbo veget., Arnica, Lachesis, Pulsatilla, Kreosotum, Sulphur.*

If they become INFLAMED:—*Pulsatilla, Asenicum, Arnica, Sulphur, Lycopodium, Spigelia, Silicea, Kreosotum.*

If they become ULCERATED:—*Pulsatilla, Lycopodium, Arsenicum, Silicea, Lachesis, Sulphur.*

POLYPI, ULCERS and CANCER of the vulva are treated in the same manner as *polypi*, etc., of the womb. (See Sections 79–87.

SECTION 101.

NEURALGIA, ITCHING, ERUPTIONS, WORMS AND LICE OF THE VULVA.—We have so little to say of these affections, that we have considered it useless to accord a special paragraph to each of them.

NEURALGIA of the vulva has the same signs as that of the vagina, often the two coalesce. The remedies are likewise the same, viz.: *Belladonna, Conium, Ignatia, Valeriana, Sepia, Hyoscyamus, Chamomilla, Asarum.*

ITCHING of the vulva, which often arises from some eruption (lichen, prurigo, eczema, etc.,) may also exist independently of these eruptions. As an independent disease, we seldom meet with it among young girls, or among women below thirty-six years old, but very often in older females, especially after the critical age. It seems induced by habitual congestion towards these parts, by a sedentary life, late rising from bed, or by continued exercise. It is especially met with among women who do not keep the sexual parts very clean. Often a proper regimen is sufficient to remove this itching. If these means are not sufficient, we may give: *Conium*, *Carbo veg.*, *Natrum muriaticum*, *Sepia*, *Sulphur*, *Calcarea*.

Among the CUTANEOUS DISEASES of the vulva, we distinguish: 1st, *erythema*, which causes efflorescences and excoriations of the vulva; it is apt to co-exist with acrid and corrosive leucorrhœa, or is frequently found in fat females; 2d, *erysipelas*, which frequently invades the labia majora, nymphæ and clitoris; the affected parts, which are hot, red and swollen, soon become œdematous, and even covered with gangrenous sloughs; 3d, *herpes*, which has the same characteristic signs as herpes præputialis, and whose vesicles leave behind them superficial excoriations, which soon become covered with crusts and heal within eight or ten days, which is not the case with the syphilitic eruptions with which they might sometimes be confounded; 4th, *eczema*, likewise accompanied by excoriations and intolerable pains, painful emissions of urine, pain during coït, and vaginal dischage, having an insipid smell; 5th, *lichen*, characterized by papulæ, occupying an erythematous base; they cause an intolerable itching, which increases towards evening or at night, and which, after scratching, is followed by excoriations that secrete a bloody serum, and then become covered with crusts; 6th, *prurigo*, characterized by papulæ that are larger and paler than lichen, occupying the mons veneris, the labia majora and the mucous membrane of the vulva; often this prurigo is accompanied by vaginitis, with a more or less copious and irritating discharge. All these eruptions often cause an intolerable itching, which leads patients to commit onanism; prurigo especially causes a tormenting desire for sexual intercourse. The best remedies

For ALL THESE ERUPTIONS, are:—*Sepia*, *Mercurius*, *Dulcamara*, *Graphites*, *Petroleum*, *Sulphur*, *Angustura*, *Kali*, *Causticum*, *Bryonia*, *Conium*, *Tartari*, *Natrum muriaticum*.

For ERYTHEMA and excoriation:—*Carbo vegetabilis*, *Causticum*, *Graphites*, *Sulphur*, *Sepia*, *Ammonium*, *Ambra*, *Lycopodium*, *Mercurius*, *Hepar sulph.*, *Nitri acidum*, *Thuja.*

For ERYSIPELAS:—*Belladonna*, *Hepar*, *Pulsatilla*, *Lachesis*, *Mercurius*, *Rhus*, *Euphorbium.*

For HERPES:—*Nitri acidum*, *Mercurius*, *Dulcamara*, *Phosphoricum acidum*, *Petroleum*, *Sepia.*

For ECZEMA:—*Graphites*, *Sulphur*, *Sepia*, *Staphysagria*, *Aconitum.*

For LICHEN:—*Aconitum*, *Sulphur*, *Dulcamara*, *Lycopodium*, *Cócculus*, *Natrum muriaticum*, *Cicuta*, *Muriaticum acidum.*

For PRURIGO:—*Aconitum*, *Nitri acidum*, *Sepia*, *Mercurius*, *Arsenicum*, *Sulphur*, *Mezereum.*

Moreover, if the itching is too troublesome, or seems intolerable, and neither *Aconitum* or *Sulphur* is of any avail, we may have the parts rubbed with *sweet oil*, or with *brandy*, especially if the itching comes on at night. This may afford relief. Washes of *camphorated alcohol* mixed with water, or *starch-flour* applied to the parts, may likewise prove serviceable. Sometimes the internal use of *Mercurius*, *Sulphur* or *Carbo veg.*, may do good, especially if the trouble comes on at night; the itching which comes on at night, after getting heated in bed, often yields to *Pulsatilla;* that which is accompanied by burning and smarting, to *Hepar*, and, if blood oozes out after scratching, we may give *Mercurius* or *Sulphur*, we refer the reader to our work on *Cutaneous Diseases*, Paris, 1850.*

SYPHILITIC affections of the vulva are: *chancres*, *flat tubercles* and *venereal vegetations.* Chancres generally occupy the internal surface of the labia majora or nymphæ; they are almost always more superficial than in the male, and sometimes disappear with an incredible rapidity, leaving behind them an indurated spot, which is exceedingly obstinate

* Translated by Charles J. Hempel, M. D., and published by W. Radde, 322, Broadway, New York.

against treatment, especially after the absurd cauterizations of the old school had previously been resorted to in the treatment. *Flat condylomata* are always a secondary symptom of syphilis. They increase prodigiously by a want of cleanliness, so that they are sometimes found in unclean individuals, scattered in large numbers, on the external and internal surface of the labia, whence they often spread towards the perinæum, as far as the anus and thighs. Cleanliness sometimes causes them to disappear, but they always incline to return as long as the general syphilis is not cured. *Syphilitic vegetations* of the pudendum are the same as those of the male prepuce. They are even more frequent in females, and are more inclined to penetrate into the female urethra. They are met with more particularly in young women and in lymphatic and fair-complexioned females. As regards TREATMENT, chancres generally yield to the continued use of *Mercurius*, second or third trituration. The same may be said of flat condylomata; *vegetations* require principally: *Nitri acid.*, *Thuja*, *Lycopodium*, *Sarsaparilla.*

The vulva is often the seat of *ascarides*, which crawl in from the lower part of the rectum, and cause such violent itchings in the vulva and such a violent desire for sexual intercourse, that a real nymphomania may be the result. The best remedies for this affection are: *Nux vomica*, *Aconitum*, *Ignatia*, *Urtica urens*, *Ferrum*, *Sulphur*, *Silicea*, *Calcarea.* Washes of diluted camphorated alcohol are sometimes very useful.

LICE are generally found among the hair growing around the parts, whence they often crawl up to the armpits, eyelids and lashes. The best and most harmless remedy is snuff mixed with oil or butter, with which the parts should be rubbed. Two or three frictions at an interval of twenty-four hours between each, are abundantly sufficient; in most cases one friction will answer. Mercurial frictions are often injurious to the health, and do not effect any more than snuff. Essence of bergamotte likewise destroys these insects very speedily, and has moreover the advantage of having a pleasant odor and of not staining the linen; this agent has, however, the inconvenience of causing a good deal of heat and smarting, for twenty-four hours or more, without however inducing any further trouble. Lastly, the *essence of turpentine* destroys these insects as speedily as tobacco, but has a rather unpleasant smell, and causes a burning and smarting on the skin.

ARTICLE XIV.

AFFECTIONS OF THE BREASTS AND NIPPLES.

SECTION 102.

GENERAL OBSERVATIONS.—Having to speak of the anomalies of the secretion of milk in the chapter on *Lactation* or *Nursing* (Chapter III., Article 9,) we shall here treat only of such diseases of the breasts and nipples as may occur at other periods than those of pregnancy or nursing. In this article we have only to treat of *inflammations, divers tumors, cancer, neuralgia, and injuries of the breasts, and of general affections of the nipples.*

SECTION 103.

INFLAMMATIONS, CATARRHAL AFFECTIONS AND ABSCESSES OF THE BREASTS.—Inflammations of the breasts present three distinct forms according to the anatomical seat of the disease:—

1. *Inflammation of the mamma proper*, or of the adipose layer, resembling inflammatory erysipelatous, with swelling, pain, heat, and a more or less intense redness of the part; the fever is proportionate to the extent of the inflammation. The causes of this inflammation are sometimes external, and at times internal. It may be caused by erysipelas, erythema, eczema, porrigo, and by any other cutaneous affection of the

chest, or by the rubbing of the corsets, a blister, burn, etc.; in all these cases the inflammation develops itself from without inwards. Inflammation may likewise be incidental to a pre-existing disease of the secretory tissue, such as milky and other engorgements, in which case the inflammatory process travels from within outwards.

2. *Deep-seated inflammation* of the breast, generally with inflammatory fever, and a good deal of swelling extending under the arm, the breast being tense, smooth, round, and traversed by full veins. This inflammation may be induced by the same causes as the preceding; it may likewise be caused by a disease of the chest, such as pleurisy, organic disease of the lungs, thoracic effusions, fracture of a rib, caries, etc. Sometimes it arises even spontaneously, or in consequence of unknown internal causes, or as a sequel of a general febrile disease.

3. *Inflammation of the mammary gland*, attacking principally women who were recently confined, wet-nurses, and being caused by a catarrhal irritation of the lactiferous parts of the breasts, or by external violence, such as blows, a fall, contusions, etc. What distinguishes this inflammation from the former is, that the pains and swelling are scattered through the substance of the breast which is not very much swollen, but where we may discover with the finger a few painful indurations. Sometimes this variety is complicated with the one or the other mentioned previously.

These inflammations almost always pursue the same course; that of the mammary gland is rather slower than the course pursued by the other varieties; but all three may terminate in resolution, induration or suppuration. If left to themselves, or under Old-School treatment, these inflammations generally terminate in suppuration, by forming *abscesses*, which it is more or less difficult to heal.

These abscesses of the breasts, which are always the result of a previous inflammation, may be as varied, as far as their locality is concerned, as the inflammations themselves; but the internal treatment of these abscesses is not affected by their divisions into classes. It may be observed, however, that whereas simple inflammatory abscesses of the mammary tissue are easily cured by proper treatment, abscesses of the mammary gland are quite obstinate. The presence of these abscesses is ascertained by the symptoms which have preceded their development, by the existing fluctuation and by the other external signs of abscesses in general. All these abscesses show a great tendency to spread and to cause ulceration of the adjoining parts, or to develope *fistulæ* of every variety, and difficult to cure.

Such *fistulæ* may be simple sinuous canals continuing after the breaking of the abscess, or canals one extremity of which terminates at the surface of the breast, and the other communicates with a milky duct. These latter fistulæ, the real *galactophorous fistulæ*, generally have a very narrow cutaneous orifice from which exudes a greater or less quantity of a seropurulent or milky fluid. These fistulæ of course are only met with among wet-nurses and women that were recently confined.

These affections can always be cured by the internal means furnished by homœopathy. In acute inflammation, no matter where seated, *Belladonna* is always the principal remedy, especially if there be hard swelling, lancinating or tearing pains, and erysipelatous redness which radiates from the center towards the periphery. Sometimes this remedy may be alternated with *Bryonia*, which is ever preferable in inflammation of the mammary gland, in the case of wet-nurses or recently-confined women, if the breasts are rigid, hard, with tensive pains, and burning heat externally.

If *Belladonna* and *Bryonia*, do not succeed in scattering the hardness and pains in the breasts, or the erysipelatous redness, we may give *Mercurius*.

If the formation of an *abscess* had to be feared, *Mercurius*, *Hepar*, *Lachesis* and *Belladonna*, may be given. *Mercurius*, often favors the breaking of the abscess, if pus has formed and resolution is no longer possible.

If the abscess is formed, give *Silicea*, *Phosphorus* and *Sul-*

phur. *Silicea* and *Phosphorus* are suitable even in the most dangerous cases, no matter where the abscess may be seated or what its nature may be.

For *induration* after inflammation, we give:—

1. *Carbo animalis*, *Conium*, *Silicea*.
2. *Chamomilla*, *Belladonna*, *Phosphorus*, *Graphites*.
3. *Sepia*, *Clematis*, *Arnica*, *Nitri acidum*.
4. *Mercurius*, *Lycopodium*, *Pulsatilla*, *Calcarea*.

For inflammations caused by contusions or external violence, we give *Belladonna*, *Mercurius* *Bryonia*, *Silicea*, *Phosphorus*, *Lachesis*; and if these remedies are not sufficient, *Conium*, *Carbo animalis*, *Arnica*.

DOSE OF ALL THESE REMEDIES.—One or two drops of the liquid attenuation morning and night in chronic cases; in acute cases mix one drop in ten table-spoonfuls of water, and give a table-spoonful of this solution every three or four hours.

SECTION 104.

TUMORS, CYSTS, HYDATIDS, LIPOMA AND HYPERTROPHY OF THE MAMMA.—We shall have to treat here of the following affections:—*Simple engorgements*, *milky and buttery tumors*, *cysts*, *fibrous*, *cartilaginous and osseous tumors*. *Milky engorgements* will be treated in the Third Chapter, where we speak of the ailments incidental to nursing.

SIMPLE ENGORGEMENTS OR CATARRHAL IRRITATIONS OF THE MAMMÆ, are transitory swellings of the breast, such as are sometimes seen after a sudden suppression of the menses. These engorgements often arise with a wonderful suddenness, so that, in one night, the breasts sometimes swell up to double or treble their normal size, and cause a good deal of trouble. But this condition, howsoever dangerous it may seem, is not serious, and generally ceases again as soon as the menses either reappear or the number of days during which they ought to have been flowing, is passed. Hence the treatment should simply aim at restoring the menses, if they do not reappear of themselves. For this purpose we give principally: *Pulsatilla, Bryonia, Conium, Sulphur, Lycopodium.*

Milky or buttery tumors always result from an infiltration of milk between the lobules or excretory canals of the gland, which may be the effect of a simple trunsudation or of some rupture. When these tumors are punctured while recent, a pure milk spirts out, which, if allowed to stand for a couple of hours, becomes covered with a layer of grease. In old tumors, the milk changes to a creamy, buttery, or cheesy substance. In most cases, these tumors form shortly after confinement, or at least during the period of nursing; and at this period, might give rise to a belief, owing to the fluctuation which is perceived in them, that suppuration is taking place, were it not that all signs of inflammation are absolutely wanting. If the milk does not flow out either through a spontaneously or artificially made opening, the tumor becomes an indurated cyst, which may continue for years without any great embarrassment to the patient. The best remedies for this affection are: *Belladonna, Bryonia,* or *Mercurius,* by the use of which a dispersion of the tumor may always be attempted in recent cases; as regards *old tumors* of this kind, we do not know whether they can be removed by internal treatment. However, if sarcomatous cysts will gradually disappear under the action of the natural forces of the organism, assisted by internal treatment, why should not such indurated milky cysts likewise yield to similar influences? At any rate, we may assist the process of natural dispersion by the use of *Calcarea, Graphites, Sulphur, Baryta, Hepar, Nitri acidum.*

The mammary CYSTS, properly speaking, differ as regards contents. We distinguish, 1st, *hydatic or serous cysts,* with fluctuation, and affecting, without any particular cause, women of all ages and constitutions; 2d, *sero-sanguineous cysts,* filled with a black or reddish fluid, having some resemblance to menstrual blood, and forming a knotty tumor where globular, elastic, and fluctuating masses are discovered; 3d, *sero-mucous cysts,* containing a gray or yellowish substance, and exhibiting tumors resembling glandular indurations. The two last-mentioned cysts often result from blows or contusions, or from any other external violence. These cysts are not dangerous; however, hydatic cysts, if left to themselves, may grow to an unlimited extent, and finally constitute a dangerous disease; as regards the first-named variety, it sometimes disappears spontaneously. In treating these cysts, we may derive benefit, in the treatment of HYDATIC CYSTS, from the use of: 1, *Pulsatilla, Graphites, Rhododendron, Sulphur, Silicia, Arnica, Lycopodium, Nux vomica,* 2, for SERO-SANGUINEOUS CYSTS: *Arnica, Conium, Sulphuris acidum, Lachesis.* 3, for SERO-MUCOUS cysts, perhaps: *Conium. Encysted hydatids,* which must not be confounded with the hydatic cysts of Velpeau that we have described just now, are encysted tumors with cavities, containing acephalogist worms; according to Cooper, they may be recognised by a fluctuation in the centre of the tumor, by the induration of the tissues that envelope the cyst, and by an absence of pain to pressure. We are not acquainted with any remedy that has been used for these cysts with success, but we will suggest: *Sulphur, Mercurius, Arsenicum, Cantharis.*

LIPOMA of the breast is a partial hypertrophy of the adipose tissue, a *fatty tumor*, having all the characteristics of lipomas in other parts of the body, and forming in the breast a lobular, well circumscribed, pendulous, and even sometimes pediculated tumor. Sometimes the lipòma is not a definitely-circumscribed tumor, but is intermediate between general and partial hypertrophy of the adipose tissue. The best medicines for these tumors are: *Baryta, Calcarea, Iodium, Antimonium, Sulphur, Lycopodium.*

HYPERTROPHY of the breast very seldom results from an excessive development of the adipose tissue of the mamma; in most cases, this hypertrophy only affects a portion of the adipose substance, thus constituting tumors which we have described before, under the name of lipoma. There are two other kinds of hypertrophy which are much more frequent; they are:—*glandular* and *cellulo-fibrous* hypertrophy. The former variety, which is almost always a characteristic of, and results in, pendulous breasts and which consists in an excessive development of the parenchyma of the mamma, is very frequently met with in America, England and Germany; it is especially observed from the age of pubescence to the age of thirty or thirty-five, and may not only lead to an enormous increase of the breasts, with excessively distressing malformations, but may likewise terminate in death. In *cellulo-fibrous* hypertrophy, which almost always results from inflammation and subsequent induration, only one breast generally becomes swollen, and tumours may form which are very much like schirrus, and cases of which have undoubtedly been reported to the world as cured under the supposition that they were schirrous tumors. We shall say something concerning the diagnosis of these tumors in our paragraph on Cancer. As regards TREATMENT, we recommend for GLANDULAR HYPERTROPHY:—*Iodine*, *Mercurius*, *Natrum*, *Spongia*, *Calcarea*, *Natrum muriaticum*, *Ambra*. For CELLULO-FIBROUS HYPERTROPHY:—*Conium*, *Carbo animalis*, *Clematis*, *Silicea*, *Phosphorus*.

For a description and the treatment of *fibrous*, *cartilaginous* and *osseous* tumors, which are more less frequently met with in the mammæ than in the womb, we refer the reader to our remarks on this subject, to Sections 75–79, where these tumors of the womb are treated of.

SECTION 105.

SCHIRRUS AND CANCER OF THE BREASTS.—Cancer of the breasts is much more frequent than is generally supposed. It occurs most frequently between the ages of thirty and fifty years, and especially at the critical period, although the disease has likewise been observed between the ages of twenty and thirty. In many cases the disease seems to have been induced by external injuries, blows, contusions, etc. Sometimes the disease sets in immediately after the injury is received; at other times at the end of three, four and twelve months. Very often the affection commences with a little induration that does not seem natural, but which does not cause any inconvenience or derange the general health. This hardness increases more and more, from the size of a small nut to that of a hen's egg; its surface becomes rough, and the edges of the tumor adhere to the skin and even to the muscular substance. At the same time painful stitches are felt in the tumor, especially towards evening and at night; the axillary glands become enlarged and painful; the mammary tumor grows more rapidly; the general health becomes altered; a general emaciation takes place; the complexion becomes straw-colored; her appetite decreases, or becomes queer and irregular. The tumor which had become sensitive to contact, begins to protrude; the skin that covers the tumor, becomes reddish, livid; the veins in the tumor become more and more apparent; the nipple retreats more and more, and finally sinks in altogether, and at the reddest part a little crack takes place, from which some serum escapes. This is the beginning of the *ulcerated* cancer; the edges of the fissure recede from each other, become thickened, everted, and the cancerous ulcer soon becomes covered with reddish vegetations and the seat of an ichorous and often very fetid suppuration, with lancinating, smarting, burning, aching or itching pains. From this moment the disease affects the whole constitution, and the general symptoms of a cancerous cachexia develope themselves with more or less intensity; the whole body assumes a wax-colored aspect; the patients experience an extreme anxiety and malaise; they are tormented by febrile motions, restless; a dry and frequent cough sets in, and in proportion as the constitutional disorder increases, the local disease becomes worse. Soon the whole breast is invaded, the pectoral muscles are destroyed, the ribs are laid bare; under the integuments deep excavations are perceived, and the angular and sinuous surface of the sore, covered with gray-colored and fetid pus, exhibits the most hideous aspect. At the same time the general symptoms continue to grow worse; the emaciation becomes excessive; an almost constant oppression of breathing torments the patient, together with the racking cough; the aversion to food becomes intolerable; a distressing constipation sometimes alternates with colliquative diarrhœa; and finally the patient perishes, exhausted by hectic fever and agonizing distress.

Open or ulcerated cancer is easily diagnosed; as long as the tumor has not advanced beyond the schirrous stage, the diagnosis is quite difficult; for there is no distinctive sign by which schirrus is distinguished from the other tumors of which mention was made in the preceding paragraph. This is particularly so at the onset of the disease. At a later period, the livid redness of the skin covering the tumor, the veins that traverse it, and which become from day to day more apparent; the adhesions which the tumor forms with the skin and muscles, are, indeed, characteristic signs which belong almost exclusively to schirrus; but before schirrus arrives at this stage, there is scarcely any difference between schirrus and other tumors of the breast. As far as the lancinating pains and the enlargement of the axillary glands are concerned, other tumors of the breast are likewise accompanied by such signs. As regards *relapses* after an operation, they simply show the uselessness of such surgical proceedings in the management of cancerous tumors. The occasional success obtained in the extirpations of ordinary tumors from the breast, does not justify a similar operation in the case of cancer. In almost every case the other breast soon begins to enlarge, sometimes after the lapse of six or eight months, and this new cancer, which develops itself after the operation, progresses towards a fatal termination with a most frightful rapidity.

As far as the TREATMENT of mammary tumors is concerned, every conscientious homœopathic or allœopathic physician should oppose their extirpation with the knife, as long as the character of the tumor is not known beyond all possibility of doubt, and more particularly in all cases of schirrous tumors. Even though we should feel convinced that the tumor cannot be cured by internal treatment, yet nothing is lost by not resorting to the operation; on the contrary, just so long as we postpone the operation, the life of the patient will be prolonged. The celebrated Doctor Walther, Professor of Surgery in the University of Bonn, told us in one of his lectures: "*I am so fully convinced of the uselessness of operations in cancerous affections, and of the impossibility of preventing relapses, that I have given up all attempts to extirpate cancer with the knife, except in cases of open cancer, where I resort to the operation simply in order to free the patient for some months at least, from such a horrible sore.*" If extirpations with the knife are pernicious, leeches, blisters, and ointments with which scirrhous tumors used to be treated by old school physicians, are no less so; more than one scirrhus which had only just commenced to show itself, has been rapidly converted into an open sore by the application of such external means. The only true method of treating cancer, is by internal specific remedies.

The principal remedies for the dispersion of schirrus, and which sometimes have effected cures, are: *Conium, Cicuta, Carbo animalis, Clematis, Silicea, Phosphorus, Rhus*, and, perhaps, also, *Mercurius bromatus.*

In OPEN CANCER we may use: *Arsenicum, Silicea, Clematis, Graphites, Kreosotum, Conium, Cicuta, Belladonna, Hepar, Lachesis.*

DOSE:—One or two drops of the liquid attenuation, in a tumblerful of water, of which solution a tablespoonful may be given every four or six hours.

SECTION 106.

MECHANICAL INJURIES OF THE BREAST.—In this paragraph we mean to treat of *external injuries*, (blows, contusions, etc.,) *wounds*, and such like accidents. Every body knows that such lesions may be attended by dangerous consequences. But here, too, the application of leeches, ointments, etc., is exceedingly pernicious. The only proper application is cold water mixed with the tincture of Arnica, 10 drops of the tincture in a tumblerful of water. Linen compresses moistened with this solution are to be applied to contusions, blows and to wounds with solution of continuity. At the same time we may give internally six globules of Arnica 15, dissolved in 6 tablespoonfuls of water, of which a teaspoonful should be given every three hours. In old wounds *Arnica* is scarcely advisable. In such cases we have to use *Conium*, *Silicea*, *Phosphorus*, *Hepar*, *Mercurius*, *Sulphur*, *Pulsatilla*, *Cicuta*, two or three globules of 15th to 30th attenuation, dry on the tongue every three or four days, changing the remedy if, after the fourth dose, no sign of improvement has become manifest. Moreover, we may use more particularly:

In simple CONTUSIONS:—*Arnica*, *Conium*, *Sulphuris acidum*, *Ruta*, *Pulsatilla*, *Hepar*, *Euphrasia*, *Sulphur*, *Cicuta*, *Iodium*.

For ECCHYMOSES:—*Arnica*, *Sulphuris acid.*, *Conium*, *Ruta*, *Sulphur*, *Hepar*, *Pulsatilla*, *Rhus*, *Bryonia*, *Dulcamara*, *Lachesis*, *Nux vomica*, *Euphrasia*, *Chamomilla*, *China*, *Plumbum*.

When the wound BLEEDS a good deal:—*Phosphorus*, *Lachesis*, *Arnica*, *Sulphur*, *Carbo vegetabilis*, *Sulphuris acid.*, *Pulsatilla*, *Mercurius*, *Hepar*, *Phosphori acid.*

When the wound is INFLAMED:—*Mercurius*, *Chamomilla*, *Pulsatilla*, *Aconite*, *Silicea*, *Arnica*, *Sulphur*, *Rhus*, *Graphites*, *Hepar*, *Sulphuris acid.*

When there is SUPPURATION:—*Mercurius*, *Sulphur*, *Chamomilla*, *Pulsatilla*, *Hepar*, *Belladonna*, *Silicea*, *Lachesis*, *China*, *Asafœtida*, *Plumbum*.

SECTION 107.

NEURALGIA AND NEURALGIC TUMORS OF THE BREAST:—This affection is characterised by keen pains, with or without swelling. In either case the pain is, if not the only symptom, but the predominant symptom of the morbid condition, and these pains are sometimes so acute, that women would rather have their breasts amputated than bear such pains any longer. The pains are generally stinging or lancinating pains, recurring or exacerbating at longer or shorter intervals. In most cases these pains are seated in the breasts themselves; at other times they seem to proceed from the uterus. They may exist without swelling, though sometimes, even if the breasts are not swollen, they are fuller, more rigid and more sensitive to pressure than usual. In case of swelling, an *induration* of the mammary gland is perceived, which feels knotty without having much increased in volume, or without the least trace of engorgement or inflammation being present. Women of twenty-five to forty are principally subject to this disease, although young girls affected with dysmenia may likewise be subject to it. This affection is not serious in itself, and often disappears again without leaving any trace behind. In other cases the induration of the mamma consists in an agglomeration of nodosities or granules scattered around the gland, and causing acute lancinating pains which are the source of much distress to those who are affected with them. This variety is peculiar to females who are near the critical period, and who often feel very uneasy in consequence of such swellings, although there is no cause for serious apprehensions. In the former variety the nodosities are so little developed that they are scarcely perceived. In this case the pains are radiating, accompanied with a little heat and numbness of the breast. Finally in other cases, we observe small rounded lenticular tumors, from the size of a coffee-bean to that of a lima-bean.

In regard to the COURSE of these neuralgic tumors, we generally see the breast enlarge, if the gland is affected by the pain; several lobes of the gland become extremely painful to the touch, and the pain which is thus excited, sometimes lasts for some hours. The lancinating and throbbing pains sometimes extend from the breast to the shoulder, axilla, elbow and even fingers, or hip on the side of the body corresponding to the diseased breast. The patient is absolutely unable to sleep on the affected side; sometimes she is even unable to lie on this side; in some cases the weight of the breast, in the bed, is sufficient to cause intolerable pains which are sometimes so distressing that they excite vomiting. At the approach of the menses the pains generally get worse, and are somewhat relieved during the menstrual flow. These sufferings may continue for weeks and even years, without any perceptible diminution; but the disease does not at all incline to degenerate into malignant tumors.

As regards TREATMENT, we have as yet no perfectly positive clinical experience. From analogy, and from experience in similar neuralgic affections, we are led to recommend the following remedies:—

1. *Graphites*, *Chamomilla*, *Aconitum*, *Spigelia*, *Mercurius*, *Arnica*, *Bryonia*, *Veratrum*, *Nux vomica*.
2. *Cocculus*, *Pulsatilla*, *Zincum*, *Phosphorus*. *China*.

And in particular:—

For VODOSITIES:—*Graphites*, *Conium*, *Chamomilla*, *Carbo animalis*, *Clematis*, *Silicea*, *Graphites*, *Baryta*, *Belladonna*, *Bryonia*, *Sulphur*.

For LANCINATING pains:—*Graphites*, *Sepia*, *Conium* *Carbo animalis*, *Aconitum*, *Spigelia*, *Mezereum*, *Phosphorus*, *Zincum*, *China*, *Cocculus*, *Veratrum*, *Verbascum*, *Belladonna*.

SENSITIVENESS to touch:—*Alumina*, *Graphites*, *Pulsatilla*, *Sulphur*, *Nux vomica*, *Sabina*, *Senega*, *Rhododendron*, *Strontiana*.

SECTION 108.

DISEASES OF THE NIPPLES.—The most frequent affections of the nipples, are:—cracks and fissures, *excoriations*, *inflammations*, *abscesses* and *exanthemata*. Excoriations are frequently met with in the case of nursing females who sometimes suffer so much from such excoriations, that they have to give up nursing. Women who nurse for the first time, are articularly liable to this difficulty, especially when the nipple is short, hard and covered with a fine and delicate skin, or when they are of a lymphatic temperament. These excoriations often give rise to cracks or fissures, which are principally seated round the base of the nipple, or in the nipple itself, or even in the areola round the nipple. In proportion as they increase, they become more painful, deeper and frequently discharge a copious quantity of blood.

The INFLAMMATIONS of the nipple are almost always limited to the areola, and are scarcely ever met with except as a sequel of the cracks and fissures consequent upon nursing. These inflammations may sometimes give rise to abscesses which are of the same nature as abscesses in other parts of the body, and which are sometimes present in considerable numbers, and scarcely ever attain to the volume of a hen's egg.

Among the EXANTHEMATA of the nipples, we sometimes distinguish *eczema*, *impetigo*, *pityriasis*, or a species of *psoriasis* or even *syphilitic eczema*.

As regards TREATMENT, we shall revert to it hereafter, at least as far as inflammations, cracks and abscesses are concerned, in speaking of the ailments incidental to nursing. All we shall do here, is to indicate most generally the principal remedies for this affection; they are:—

Pulsatilla, *Chamomilla*, *Ignatia*, *Lycopodium*, *Graphites*, *Sulphur*, *Arnica*, *Mercurius*, *Silicea*, *Sepia*, *Calcarea*, *Bryonia*, *Sabina*, *Bismuth*, *Rhabarbarum*.

And in particular:—

For simple INFLAMMATIONS:—*Chamomilla*, *Ignatia*, *Silicea*, *Calcarea*, *Phosphorus*, *Sulphur*.

For excessive SENSITIVENESS:—*Graphites*, *Zincum*, *Rhabarbarum*, *Manganum*.

For EXCORIATIONS:—*Arnica*, *Sulphur*, *Ignatia*, *Chamomilla*, *Pulsatilla*, *Calcarea*, *Graphites*, *Silicea*, *Lycopodium*, *Causticum*, *Mercurius*, *Sepia*, *Nux vomica*, *Manganum*.

For CRACKS and FISSURES:—*Sulphur*, *Graphites*, *Causticum*, *Pulsatilla*, *Chamomilla*, *Mercurius*, *Silicea*.

For ABSCESSES:—*Silicea*, *Hepar*, *Phosphorus*, *Mercurius*, *Chamomilla*, *Kreosotum*.

Afterwards:—

For exanthemata of the nipples and breasts in general:—

1. *Sepia*, *Lycopodium*, *Phosphorus*, *Plumbum*, *Carbo vegetabilis*, *Sulphur*, *Cocculus Ipecacuanha*.
2. *Bryonia*, *Belladonna*, *Hepar*, *Lachesis*, *Staphysagria*, *Silicea*, *Rhus*, *Strontiana*.
3. *Mercurius*, *Arsenicum*, *Calcarea*, *Bovista*, *Conium*, *Belladonna*, *Alumina*, *Ammonium muriaticum*, *Mezereum*, *Nitri acidum*.

In particular:—

For SPOTS in general:—*Sepia*, *Phosphorus*, *Cocculus*, *Carbo vegetabilis*, *Ipecacuanha*.

2. *Belladonna*, *Sulphur*, *Arsenicum*, *Ledum*, *Nitri acidum*, *Lachesis*, *Arsenicum*, *Ammonium muriaticum*, *Mezereum*, *Manganum*, *Squilla*.

For BROWN spots:—*Sepia*, *Carbo vegetabilis*, *Sulphur*, *Lycopodium*.

For HEPATIC spots:—*Lycopodium*, *Sulphur*, *Carbo vegetabilis*, *Sepia*, *Phosphorus*, *Arsenicum*.

For YELLOW spots:—*Sepia*, *Lycopodium*, *Phosphorus*, *Sulphur*, *Arsenicum*.

For RED spots:—*Ledum*, *Sabadilla*, *Belladonna*, *Ipecacuanha*, *Phosphorus*, *Cocculus*, *Lachesis*, *Mezereum*, *Magnesia*.

For PITYRIASIS:—*Petroleum*, *Causticum*, *Dulcamara*, *Staphysagria*, *Phosphorus*, *Arsenicum*.

For SCABS and CRUSTS:—*Lycopodium*, *Petroleum*, *Causticum*, *Arsenicum*, *Dulcamara*, *Staphysagria*.

For ITCHING:—*Sulphur*, *Alumina*, *Petroleum*, *Conium*.

DOSE.—The same as at the close of Section 105.

Section 109.

Atrophy of the nipples and breasts.—Atrophy of the nipples is not a very rare disease; in many women, in consequence of some malformation, or of the pressure of the dress, the nipple is short, flat, atrophied, so that, instead of projecting, a depression exists in its place. According to our experience, *Sarsaparilla* has the best effect on this difficulty.

We will add to this a few remarks concerning *atrophy of the breasts*, owing to which they either remain undeveloped at the age of pubescence or decrease in volume, after having acquired their full development. Either the adipose tissue or the glands, or the whole breast, may become atrophied in either way, from deficient nutrition which may induce a general atrophy, or simply from some morbid state of the breasts exclusively. This latter case sometimes arises from abuse of *Iodium* or *Mercurius*, or from pre-existing diseases of the breasts, inflammations, neuralgia, suppressed eruptions, deprivation of nursing in mothers, or from uterine affections and other influences. Whatever may be the cause of this affection, whenever the atrophy does not depend upon constitutional atrophy or marasmus, but develops itself in young girls of otherwise good health, and where, to judge from their general constitutional development, the mammæ should be well developed, the following remedies sometimes are of great use in restoring a normal condition of the parts:—

> *Iodium, Conium, Nitri acidum, Nux moschata, Phosphorus, Hepar, Silicea, Cocculus, Ignatia, Coffea, Calcarea, Nux vomica, Nitri acidum, Secale, Phosphori acid., China, Sulphur, Bryonia.*

And in particular:—

> If caused by abuse of iodine:—*Hepar, Phosphorus, Sulphur, Arsenicum, China.*

> Of mercury:—*Nitri acidum, China, Phosphori acid., Hepar, Iodium, Sulphur.*

After SEXUAL EXCESSES:—*Bryonia*, *Phosphori acid*, *Calcarea*, *Sulphur*, *Sepia*, *Ignatia*, *China*, *Nux vomica*.

INFLAMMATIONS of the breasts:—*Phosphorus*, *Silicea*, *Conium*, *Iodium*.

Deprivation of NURSING:—*Phosphorus*, *Nux vomica*, *Secale*.

SUPPRESSED ERUPTIONS:—*Calcarea*, *Sulphur*, *Arsenicum*.

With NEURALGIA:—*Cocculus*, *Coffea*, *Ignatia*.

If the mammæ develope themselves too slowly at the age of pubescence, we recommend, *Nux moschata*, *Conium*.

DOSE.—The same as at the close of Section 105.

SECTION THIRD.

FUNCTIONAL DERANGEMENTS INCIDENTAL TO PREGNANCY, CONFINEMENTS, ETC.

SECTION 110.

GENERAL OBSERVATIONS.—In this Section we shall have to treat of the following subjects:—*Pregnancy*, *Parturition*, *Confinement*, *Nursing* and *Weaning;* and we shall describe the ailments and diseases which may be incidental to each of these conditions. *Pregnancy* being, so to say, the basis from which all the other functions of maternity emanate, we shall consider it more in detail, not only as a physiological state, but likewise with regard to the ailments, be they light or serious, which may set in as a sequel of pregnancy. Our aim shall be to enable the reader to distinguish clearly between the really serious and the unimportant ailments incidental to pregnancy. *Miscarriage* being a most serious accident which may be followed by all the unpleasant consequences of real labor, we shall devote a separate article to it immediately after the diseases of pregnant females. We shall likewise consecrate a few paragraphs to the management of new-born infants, and of infants at the breast, which is a subject of the highest importance to those who are going to assume the duties of mothers. Hence, we shall have to treat in this Section of the following subjects:—1, *pregnancy;* 2, *diseases of pregnant women;* 3, *miscarriage;* 4, *regular labor;* 5, *protracted or difficult labor;* 6, *regular confinement;* 7, *diseases during confinement;* 8, *nursing;* 9, *weaning and metastasis of the milky secretion;* 10, *management of infants.* In all these articles we shall of course confine ourselves to the strictly medicinal work of the attending physician; the duties of the accoucheur as an operator are sufficiently well and fully expounded in every obstetrical treatise.

ARTICLE I.

OF PREGNANCY IN GENERAL.

SECTION 111.

SYMPTOMS OF PREGNANCY.—We shall not enter into details concerning the changes which the uterus undergoes during pregnancy; for these changes only occupy an inferior part in the work which we have proposed to ourselves to accomplish. These changes have reference to the volume, shape, situation and direction, and likewise to the tissue and properties of the uterus. During intercourse the uterus becomes erect, together with the other genital organs, and, if conception takes place, this turgescence continues, the volume of the uterus increases more and more, both in consequence of the thickening of its walls and of the dilatation of its cavity; the more it expands at the fundus, the more contracted it becomes at the orifice, so that, after a while, this orifice is no longer a linear and transversal slit, but changes to an oval opening. After the uterus has grown to a certain size, it assumes a spheroidal shape, and at its lower extremity the neck forms a sort of appendage, until, at full term, the uterus forms a complete ovoid, or egg-shaped body, the neck having become obliterated and being known only by the rim of its orifice. In the first pregnancy the lips of the neck sometimes become very thin; but among women who have had several children, they are often very much swollen and infiltrated, and are sometimes divided into several tubercles by means of fissures, that have more or less depth. This increase of volume and weight of the uterus during pregnancy, obliges it to descend in the pelvic cavity; but from the third to the fourth month, it becomes too voluminous to be contained in this narrow space; it then rises gradually, so that, at the end of pregnancy, the os tincæ is raised so high, and pushed so far backwards, that it can scarcely be reached with the finger; at the same time the uterus inclines to one of the sides of the abdomen, more to the right than the left. The uterine tissue likewise undergoes remarkable changes; the serous tissue expands, the mucous follicles become more developed, their secretion increases, the menses cease to flow after conception, although the change in the circulation, which formerly resulted in the catamenial discharge, continues to be noticed at every period by the modifications experienced in the condition of the pulse and of the general well-being of the woman. At the same time the current of blood is determined towards the uterus; the uterine circulation becomes more excited, the uterine temperature is increased, nutrition is more active, and the organ becomes so sensitive that the female perceives the least movements of the fetus, which are always more or less painful. The changes in the constitution of the uterus, are accompanied by changes in the adjoining organs. The uterus, both in its ascent and descent, drags along with it the superior extremity of the vagina; the bladder is more or less pushed backward, and the urethra is elongated and drawn out in consequence; the lesser intestines which are pressed to one side of the abdomen, most frequently to the left, push before them the transverse colon, the stomach and liver; the diaphragm becomes more concave, and the thoracic cavity being diminished from below upwards, the lungs have of course less space to breathe. At the same time, the anterior wall of the abdomen becomes quite prominent; the opening of the umbilical ring becoming enlarged, it allows a portion of bowel and of the epiploon to slip through, which explains the umbilical enlargement perceived in the third or fourth month of pregnancy; the subcutaneous veins expand, and the skin, especially on the lower portion of the abdomen, exhibits brownish or bluish ridges forming parallel curves and remaining even after confinement in the shape of fine veins of a shiny white color, like cicatrices.

Besides these local symptoms, the whole constitution becomes more or less affected owing to the mechanical or sympathetic action of the uterus upon the other organs. The *stomach* in particular is first and principally affected by pregnancy. Some women experience even from the moment of conception a loathing of food, meat; they are seized with nausea, slime on the stomach, vomiting; these symptoms generally disappear again about the third or fourth month, and are then followed by an increased appetite, and by better digestion; about the end of pregnancy they sometimes re-appear. In other cases these gastric affections only show themselves in the last half of pregnancy, whereas the functions of the stomach are perfectly natural during the first months; according to some authors this peculiarity only takes place when girls are borne, whereas, in the case of boys, the gastric disorders show themselves from the first. The biliary secretion seems to decrease; the current of blood seems to incline towards the upper parts of the body, whereas the circulation in the abdominal viscera and lower extremities is impeded; hence come varices, œdema of the legs and sexual organs; the pulse of pregnant women is generally more frequent, more animated, and sometimes fuller and harder than that of other women. The breathing is generally embarrassed and hurried during the first months of pregnancy, and sometimes an obstinate cough sets in. We have said before that the menses cease to flow after conception has taken place; some women, however, continue to menstruate during the first months, and even to the end of pregnancy; but these are rare exceptions. Defecation is generally impeded; most pregnant women are troubled with obstinate constipation. Others are attacked with diarrhœa; but this diarrhœa occurs most frequently during the last months of pregnancy, and, if the patient has not vomited any during the first months, this diarrhœa is supposed to be indicative of the birth of a daughter. At the beginning of pregnancy we sometimes notice copious ptyalism, and, at the end, many women experience frequent urging to urinate. As regards the *breasts*, they sometimes feel a change from the moment of conception; but all women very soon experience a tension, stinging and pricking in the breasts; afterwards the breasts gradually increase in volume; the nipple becomes more prominent and darker, so does the areola around the base of the nipple; the veins of the mamma become more apparent; the mammary gland secretes viscid lymph, and afterwards genuine milk, which is discharged through the nipple. The cutaneous action does not seem increased; sometimes pregnant women are affected with brownish or yellowish spots, especially in the face; some women grow quite fat during their pregnancy. Locomotion is likewise influenced by pregnancy; walking and standing become painful; the increase of weight in the pelvis compels the female to throw back her shoulders a good deal, in order to preserve her equilibrium. As regards intellect and the sentient brain, they have been supposed to be influenced by pregnancy more than is really the case; all we know for certain is, that pregnancy increases the sensitiveness of the nervous system, and induces a predisposition for nervous diseases.

SECTION 112.

DIAGNOSIS OF PREGNANCY.—Nothing is more easy than to recognize pregnancy after it has arrived at a certain stage, and particularly after the movements of the fetus have been felt; but it is exceedingly difficult to be sure of the existence of pregnancy before this period, or to know whether conception has taken place. As regards the *signs of conception*, it may be said that none of those which have been presented as such, have been sufficiently verified by experience to be fully believed in. Among these signs some authors have recorded the following: a voluptuous sensation even superior to that of coit; the retention of the seminal fluid after the act; a vermicular and painful movement in the iliac, umbilical and hypogastric regions; a sense of heaviness or swelling in the region of the womb; general spasm with shuddering, nausea, and vomiting; sometime after conception, spasmodic distension of the abdomen, anxiety, sadness, depression of spirits, pallor, languid looks, a certain diminution of the freshness of the eyelids and the features, and a bluish margin around the eyes. There are other signs no more certain than the above, such as aversion to intercourse or even to the most cherished person, a peculiar odor of the breath, and especially a slight swelling of the skin of the neck, which sign was considered by the ancients as infallible.

The only *certain signs* of the presence of pregnancy, are the movements of the fetus and *certain changes* in the development of the womb. Such are the closing of the uterine orifice, without hardness or any morbid sign; the circular shape of this orifice in women who have not yet had any children; the dilatation of the body of the uterus posteriorly; the increased weight of this organ when raising it with the finger, etc. But all these signs may exist when the uterine enlargement is due to other causes than pregnancy; unless the presumed period of pregnancy corresponds to the degree of dilatation and the uterine development takes place in regular progression from the body of the womb downwards towards the neck; to which the absence of any other morbid symptom may be added as a confirmatory sign of pregnancy. Beside these *perceptible* symptoms, there are others termed *rational* which are suggested by the reason. These are: 1st, *Menstrual suppression*, an almost certain sign when this suppression takes place without any appreciable cause in a woman of good health, nor is followed by any unpleasant consequences, except such as are incidental to pregnancy; but this suppression is not always present, and again, women who have never menstruated, may become pregnant. An increased volume of the abdomen, if accompanied by menstrual suppression, may, indeed, be a presumptive sign of pregnancy, but we ought not to forget that many other causes may likewise lead to abdominal enlargements; in pregnancy, however, the abdomen becomes progressively enlarged from below upwards; in front the abdomen projects in a marked manner, whereas the sides are flattened; but what is more important is that, in proportion as the volume of the abdomen increases, the umbilical fossa gradually fills up, and the navel actually protrudes towards the third or fourth month. The signs about the breasts and nipples are likewise observed between the periods of pregnancy, after menstrual suppression and in many other uterine affections. The signs obtained from the pulse are less reliable than any other. In some women the skin becomes of a duller white; their eyelids become soft, livid, and rings are formed round their eyes; the lustre of the eyes becomes less and the look is more languid; there is aversion to exercise, sexual intercourse and work; the patients become capricious, morose; they are seized with fancies for the strangest things, and the memory is sometimes weakened, These signs, however, may likewise exist in many other diseases. In order to make up our minds whether pregnancy exists, we have to put all the perceptible and rational signs together, and draw our conclusions accordingly; but, in order to establish our diagnosis upon a firm basis, we have to depend upon the *movements of the fetus*, and upon the signs furnished by auscultation, by the application of the stethoscope to the abdomen, By this means we discover two kinds of *pulsations* in the abdomen, those which belong to the fetal heart, and which are double and more frequent than those of the pulse of the mother; the other pulsations are isochronous with the pulse of the mother, and accompanied by a blowing sound. As soon as we hear these double pulsations we may rest assured that pregnancy has taken place.

Section 113.

Hygienic rules during pregnancy.—Pregnancy is not in itself a pathological state. On the contrary, it is a perfectly normal state which would not require any sort of particular care, if the marked changes which this condition induces in the sensibility and in the different functions of the female, did not predispose her for a variety of derangements which may either be avoided by a proper mode of life, or cured by the application of suitable remedies. In the article where we shall treat of the different diseases which pregnancy may induce, we shall indicate the simplest and most efficient means of removing them; in the present instance where we consider pregnancy only in its physiological aspect, we have simply to mention the hygienic means which will prevent the advent of such ailments and preserve to pregnancy its character as a strictly physiological function.

Among these means we number above all things a pure air free from excessive heat or cold, dampnes or dryness; but this is very difficult to attain, and yet the privation of fresh air, or air of a normal temperature causes more suffering to pregnant women than is generally supposed. As soon as a woman has reason to believe that she is pregnant, she ought to dress according to the season, not expose herself to disturbing atmospheric influences, avoid all sudden changes of temperature, and not sacrifice herself to the exigencies of fashion or social gallantry. She ought to consider it her highest duty to devote herself physically and mentally to the little being to whom she is to give birth, in order to secure to its physical, moral and intellectual development the most favorable constitutional disposition.

At the same time she ought to dress loosely, without compressing the abdomen or chest, which might injure the growth of the nipples, or impede still more the action of the lungs. Pregnant women should abandon corsets and belts; undue pressure upon the waist by such means is exceedingly injurious. Busks do not, as is generally supposed, prevent the fetus from ascending too much, but they keep the uterus in an obilique position, which may afterwards become an exceedingly active cause of prolapsus. Corsets and belts, by their habitual compression, impede the portal circulation, which may cause incalculable inconveniences to the mother and child, such as miscarriage, uterine affections, heart-disease, pulmonary or cerebral affections, false positions of the fetus, varices, etc. Such improper modes of dressing may perhaps also be a remote cause of hydrocephalus by inducing an abnormal development of the head.

The habitual sensitiveness of the digestive organs during pregnancy, and the wants of the fetal being, show that the nourishment of pregnant females should be easily digestible, wholesome and sufficiently nourishing. Aliments that do not possess these properties, should be excluded from the table of pregnant women. In most cases women are rightly guided by their desires for particular kinds of food; if a few of them have to be restrained, there is no doubt that, generally speaking, the woman may be allowed to indulge her appetite. Sometimes these desires are natural indications, especially if they continue in spite of the patient's own wish. The most suitable food for pregnant women is meat boiled or roasted, beef, mutton, venison, and in general meats furnished by the mammalia, whatever may have been said to the contrary by Old School experimenters. White meat, such as veal, poultry, fish, etc., is generally much more difficult to digest; this is shown by the diarrhœa and the digestive derangement they cause, if persons unused to this kind of nourishment live on such articles of diet for some days in succession. Farinaceous and vegetable diet, ripe fruits of the season, if eaten in moderate quantities, not between meals, but by way of dessert, likewise constitute an agreeable and useful diet. As a beverage nothing is better than fresh water, or if the water of the place where the patients reside is not good, water united with about one-fifth claret. Pure wine, alcoholic liquors, spices, coffee and tea should be prohibited in most cases. Coffee not only injures the mother, but also the child, predisposes her for hæmorrhage, difficult labor, toothache during pregnancy, and while nursing the infant; it is the cause of a good many difficulties which infants experience during dentition, and develops a nervous state of the system which may remain for life. Chamomile-tea, of which such enormous quantities are used by pregnant women, is as hurtful as coffee. As a general rule, *warm drinks* and *decoctions* are more hurtful than useful, owing to the debilitating and relaxing action which they exercise upon the digestive organs. *Ice-beverages* should likewise be avoided; they have been known to cause miscarriages; in cases of gastralgia or vomiting, where such drinks are sometimes resorted to as sedatives, they have to be taken in small quantities as if they were medicines.

BODILY EXERCISE, especially in the open air, on foot, and moderately enjoyed, so as not to cause any weariness, is likewise necessary during pregnancy; it prevents the developement of many diseases to which this condition predisposes the female, and is frequently a means of curing them and securing an easy confinement. But as useful moderate walking may be to pregnant females, as injurious riding in a carriage, or on horseback, dancing, etc., may prove to them in consequence of the violent shaking which the body undergoes, and which may induce hæmorrhage and miscarriage. Keeping late hours at night is likewise hurtful during pregnancy; women in this condition should sleep a little longer than usual. The use of warm baths which are so generally recommended by Old School physicians and nurses, is an improper practice, such bathing should only be resorted to for purposes of cleanliness, and the patient should not remain in her bath longer than from five to ten minutes; if used too frequently and too long, they weaken the constitution and cause a good deal of trouble to feeble, lymphatic women, or such as are disposed to œdema or uterine hæmorrhage. It is particularly towards the end of pregnancy that warm baths are hurtful and therefore condemnable. Foot and hip-baths should likewise be strictly forbidden; they facilitate or even cause uterine hæmorrhages and miscarriages.

Some women unfortunately continue to entertain the pernicious Old School error, that SANGUINEOUS DEPLETIONS in the first months of pregnancy tend to prevent the phenomena of plethora which sometimes trouble females from the third month of pregnancy. This is a great mistake; for the supposed plethora exists only in appearance; no pregnant woman ever has one drop of blood too much; all the blood she has, is necessary to her for the development of her infant, and blood-letting will invariably injure the constitution of the little being. Dr. Croserio said some time ago:—"*Bleeding a pregnant woman is a double attempt of homicide which the laws should prevent; both the mother and child may be destroyed by this practice.*" What has been said of blood-letting, may likewise be said of the emetics and cathartics which alloeopathic physicians prescribe for the gastric derangements and the constipation of pregnant females. Whatever tends to weaken the organs and the constitution is prejudicial to the health of the mother and child, and should be avoided as a wrong.

We have said above that the sensibility of pregnant women is increased, that their imagination is more lively, and that they are more liable to start as if in affright. This susceptibility is sometimes so excessive, that a mere odor, the sight of some repulsive object, the least fright, a fit of anger, an unexpected joy, a moderate pain may produce convulsions, hæmorrhages, miscarriages and other serious accidents. Philosophical physicians do no longer admit the theory that the image of such things as were strongly desired by the mothers, becomes impressed upon the fetus. We know of but one case where this happened; it is the case of a young female who was frightened at a ball by a black mark, and who from this instant, became so keenly impressed with the idea that her child would be injured by her fright, that, at the end of six months, she gave birth to a child whose face was as black as that of a negro. We have no disposition to draw any inference from this isolated fact; but it certainly shows the propriety of guarding the mother against all impressions that tend to disturb or impress her nervous system or imagination in an unfavorable manner. All violent emotions, be they agreeable or otherwise; the sight of wild animals, of athletic exhibitions, monstra, serious wounds, or the narration of frightful events should be kept away from them altogether.

As regards SEXUAL INTERCOURSE, it is rather forbidden than allowed by most practitioners. If enjoyed too frequently, especially by newly-married persons, it may undoubtedly become a cause of miscarriage. It should be abstained from by women who have miscarried, or where a miscarriage may be apprehended, or by women of a nervous and sensitive temperament, who are subject to leucorrhœa, to profuse menstruation, or to menses that last either too long or are too frequent. Nature will sometimes indicate the true course to follow. Some women, especially such as have not had any children, experience immediately after conception such an aversion to sexual intercourse, that they would not consent to it even if they loved their husbands ever so much. This should always be respected as a sacred indication of nature. Generally, such an aversion lasts until the fourth or fifth month of pregnancy. Intercourse during the last months of pregnancy has never been known to be injurious; some authors pretend that it secures an easy confinement.

ARTICLE II.

DISEASES OF PREGNANT FEMALES.

SECTION 114.

GENERAL OBSERVATIONS.—The diseases peculiar to pregnancy are nothing else than the divers physiological phenomena, depending upon it carried to an intense degree of exhaltation. Several authors have classified these diseases according to the period of pregnancy when they manifest themselves; but inasmuch as several of these affections may occur at any time of life, this classification, which is not without its advantages, seems nevertheless to present practical difficulties which prevent us from adopting it in this work. Other authors classify these diseases agreeably to the physiological functions involved in the disturbance, and it is this arrangement which, with some slight modifications suggested by the plan of our work, we shall likewise adopt in its general features. We shall therefore treat successively: 1*st*, *of the derangements of the digestive organs; 2d, of the derangements of the circulatory system; 3d, derangements of the respiratory organs; 4th, derangements of the secretory functions; 5th, derangements causing pain; 6th, convulsions and mental derangements; 7th, cutaneous derangements; 8th, derangements of the uterus and its appendages; 9th, influence of pregnancy upon existing diseases.* Before treating of each of these disorders specially, it seems proper that we should offer a few remarks concerning the ADMINISTRATION OF REMEDIES during pregnancy. It is supposed by many women, that any kind of medicine taken during pregnancy, exposes them to the danger of miscarrying. This is undoubtedly true as regards allœopathic medication, or even the use of massive doses of homœopathic tinctures or first attenuations, of which they order whole drops dissolved in a few ounces of water, to be taken in table-spoonful doses. Aconite, Calcarea, Sepia or Sabina, administered in this manner, have often caused a good deal of harm during pregnancy. We should never give more than two or three globules either dry on the tongue every day, or even every two or three days, or dissolved in about ten table-spoonfuls of water, a tea-spoonful of which solution should be given every two or three hours even in the most acute and rapidly progressing cases. *Discite moniti.*

Section 115.

Digestive derangements.—The diseases which belong to this category, are, *anorexia* and *strange tastes; vomiting* (nausea, mucus on the stomach); *colic, constipation, diarrhœa.* We shall say sometimes about each of these various conditions, and at the same time mention the treatment to be pursued in each.

Anorexia and strange tastes are extremely frequent during the first months of pregnancy; they generally cease of themselves towards the fourth or fifth month, and are followed by a better appetite and by easier digestion than usual. Either of these derangements will sometimes yield to a small dose of *Sulphur;* if this remedy should not suffice, we may prescribe:—

For desire for sour things:—*Aconitum, Arnica, Pulsatilla, China, Arsenicum, Veratrum.*

Bitter:—*Digitalis, Natrum muriaticum.*

Coffee:—*Arsenica, Bryonia, Carbo veget., Conium, Aurum.*

Chalk, clay:—*Nitri acidum, Nux vomica, Calcarea, Hepar, Ignatia.*

Charcoal:—*Cicuta, Conium.*

Sourcrout:—*Carbo vegetabilis, Chamomilla.*

Brandy: — *Lachesis, Sulphur, Hepar, Arsenicum, China.*

DAINTIES:—*China, Ipecacuanha, Calcarea, Natrum, Petroleum, Rhus.*

COLD food:—*Sulphuris acid., Veratrum, Pulsatilla, Ignatia, Tartarus.*

FAT:—*Nux vomica, Nitri acidum.*

HERRINGS:—*Nitri acidum.*

PIQUANT things:—*Pulsatilla.*

COOLING:—*Pulsatilla, Rhabarbarum, Cocculus, Causticum.*

SALT:—*Conium, Calcarea, Causticum, Nitri acidum, Carbo vegetabilis, Phosphorus.*

SWEETS:—*China, Lycopodium, Sulphur, Calcarea Carbo vegetabilis, Nux vomica, Kali.*

SMOKED meat:—*Causticum.*

WINE:—*Calcarea, Staphysagria, Aconitum, Bryonia, Hepar, Lachesis, Sulphur.*

For AVERSION to food:—*Pulsatilla, Arnica, Nux vomica, Bryonia, Ipecacuanha, China.*

TO BROTH:—*Rhus, Chamomilla, Arnica, Graphites, Arsenica, Belladonna.*

WATER:—*Belladonna, Stramonium, Nux vomica, Bryonia, Natrum muriat., Lycopodium, China, Causticum, Sulphuris acid.*

MILK:—*Sepia, Calcarea, Pulsatilla, Guaiacum, Bryonia, Silicea, Sulphur.*

BREAD:—*Natrum muriat., Conium, Sepia, Lycopodium, Pulsatilla, Nux vomica, Sulphur.*

SOLIDS:—*Ferrum, Angustura, Mercurius, Staphysagria.*

MEAT:—*Sulphur, Sepia, Calcarea, Rhus, Carbo veget., Muriatic acid, Silicea, Petroleum.*

VOMITING, NAUSEA, MUCUS ON THE STOMACH, are likewise very common in pregnancy, and they sometimes increase to a real disease. As a general rule, they cease after the third or fourth month of pregnancy, but sometimes they continue longer, or recur periodically during the whole course of pregnancy, or they discontinue at the end of the fourth month, and reappear again at the close of pregnancy. Most frequently the patients are attacked in the morning, and vomit a viscid or slimy fluid; at other times they break out after a meal, and in this case, the food is rejected by the vomiting; in other cases again, the women reject every thing they take into the stomach, be it solid or liquid food. In most cases, the best remedy for this trouble is *Nux vomica*, especially if the vomiting takes place in the morning, and the patients only vomit a viscid liquid; or *Ipecacuanha*, especially if the vomiting continues all the time, and the patient rejects every thing she takes into her stomach, both solids and fluids, with or without bile or mucus. If neither of these remedies should prove sufficient, we may often derive benefit from *Pulsatilla*, especially if the vomiting comes on in the evening or at night; *Ferrum*, if the patients, a few hours after eating, suddenly vomit up the food taken into the stomach; *Sepia*, especially for vomiting of milky mucus, the patients are sad, subject to hemicrania, leucorrhœa or uterine derangements; or *Conium*, suitable to patients affected with engorgements or induration of the neck of the womb or breasts. In a case where no other remedy seemed of any avail, two globules of *Sulphur*, dry on the tongue, has removed the whole trouble in twenty-four hours. *Petroleum*, *Arsenicum*, *Natrum muriaticum*, may likewise be useful.

Colic is as frequent in pregnancy as anorexia and vomiting; generally the trouble consists in abdominal spasms that set in during the first months of pregnancy, and which ought not to be confounded with the false labor-pains of which mention will be made hereafter. The best remedy for these colics, in most cases, is: *Chamomilla* (two globules dry on the tongue,) especially when there is much wind in the bowels that cannot be passed, and anguish and pressure in the pit of the stomach; or *Nux vomica*, if *Chamomilla* is not sufficient, and if the bowels are very costive; or *Belladonna*, if the bowels feel a pain as if clutched with nails or crushed between stones; or *Colocynthis*, if the pains are extreme, not allowing the patient any rest, and feeling better by walking. *Pulsatilla, Sepia, Bryonia, Arnica,* may likewise be tried.

CONSTIPATION troubles pregnant women, especially towards the end of pregnancy; if continuing too long, the appetite gets lost, digestion becomes difficult, and the patients become restless and do not sleep well; not to mention the danger of hæmorrhage and miscarriage to which the straining at stool occasioned by the expulsion of hard and large fecal messes, give rise. Constipation of pregnant women should be attended to with great care by the practitioner. But cathartics, even ever so mild, are the very worst means to remove the difficulty. Often a change of diet, a little more vegetables or fruit, a little more exercise in the open air, or a good drink of fresh water, after rising in the morning, and two or three times during the day, are sufficient to bring about a cure. If these dietetic measures are not sufficient, we may resort to *Nux vomica*, two globules dry on the tongue, which should be allowed to act for three or four days in succession, especially when the patient's complain of dull headache, heat in the abdomen, pressure towards the anus, with frequent but ineffectual urging to go to stool, and congestion of the head with red face. If *Nux* is not sufficient, we may have recourse to *Sulphur*, one dose, or to *Bryonia*, likewise one dose. If none of these remedies help, *Sepia* is often extremely useful. In obstinate cases we may give *Lycopodium* and *Alumina; injections* are only serviceable, if the constipation has lasted two or three days, with frequent urging to stool, but inability to expel the fæces on account of their hardness or size. In such a case, we may resort to an injection of tepid water, in which a little castile-soap had been dissolved. It would be wrong to take injections every day; this would fatigue and irritate the bowels and anus.

Diarrhœa is an untoward symptom in pregnant women, not so much in itself, as because it may bring on miscarriage. The best remedy for this trouble is *Chamomilla*, which should be given first, especially if the patient complains of violent colic, with yellow, greenish stools, or resembling stirred eggs; or *Pulsatilla*, if the stools are greenish or watery, preceded by colic, with slimy, bitter mouth, chilliness, loss of thirst, nocturnal stools; or *Dulcamara*, when the diarrhœa results from a cold, with colic, slimy, greenish stools; if these remedies do not suffice, we may give *Sulphur*, followed by *Calcarea*, or *Sepia*. We may also try *Antimony*, *Phosphorus*, *Petroleum*, *Hyoscyamus*.

SECTION 116.

DERANGEMENTS OF THE CIRCULATION.—The morbid conditions of which we shall have to treat in this Chapter, are:—*Plethora*, *abdominal congestions*, *palpitations of the heart*, *syncope*, *hæmorrhage*, *piles*, *varices*, *œdema of the legs*.

Plethora is present in every case of pregnancy, so that several physicians have regarded it as the principal, if not the only cause of all the accidents to which pregnancy may give rise, and have recommended blood-letting as the sovereign remedy for this condition. We have stated before that this plethora of pregnant women is only an apparent symptom. What is supposed to be owing to a general increase of the volume of blood, is caused by a certain embarrassment in the circulation. These phenomena of supposed plethora generally set in about the sixth or seventh month of pregnancy. With a full and hard pulse, females suffer with heaviness of the head, somnolence, vertigo when stooping, a sense of fulness and embarrassment in the limbs, sometimes slight nose-bleed, congestion in the pelvic vessels, and sometimes pains in the gums. These symptoms may continue for a good while without the general health being disturbed; but sometimes congestions or hæmorrhages take place, the most frightful of which are cerebral hæmorrhage and metrorrhagia. The adoption of a suitable regimen, such as we have indicated in the previous Chapter, is generally sufficient to prevent every unpleasant accident and to scatter all these symptoms little by little. But if these symptoms should nevertheless become too fatiguing, or should cause any apprehension in the patient's mind, a dose of *Aconitum*, six globules dissolved in half a tumblerful of water, and a tea-spoonful of this solution administered every three hours, will remove the unpleasant condition more promptly, more safely and more radically than all the blood-lettings in the world could do. After Aconite a dose of *Belladonna* may be given, two globules dry on the tongue, if two or three days after the administration of the Aconite, the patient still feels some heat and pain in the head; or a dose of *Nux vomica* may be given, if the digestive functions are deranged, or the bowels are constipated.

ABDOMINAL and UTERINE CONGESTIONS, generally develope themselves in the first weeks and even days of pregnancy. The patient experiences a more or less painful tension, and a sense of weight in the hypogastrium, behind the pubes, with frequent urging to urinate, lassitute in the limbs, anguish, palpitation and depression, and uneasiness of spirits. These symptoms sometimes disappear of themselves, by adopting a suitable regimen, but in some cases they may have to be acted upon by medicinal means, lest they should lead to miscarriage. The best medicine is *Belladonna*, especially if the face be red and warm, with congestion of the head, sensation as if the weight felt in the bowels would press through the parts; or *Nux vomica*, if Belladonna is not sufficient, with frequent desire to urinate, and ineffectual urging to go to stool. *Pulsatilla* is suitable to women of a delicate and feeble constitution, with disposition to leucorrhœa and other mucous discharges, occasional shiverings, pale face and soft features.

PALPITATION OF THE HEART is generally an accompaniment of general plethora; *Aconite* is the best remedy for this symptom. If unaccompanied by symptoms of general plethora, *Pulsatilla* may be given for palpitation, if Aconite remains without effect. Beside these two remedies we may also give *Lycopodium*, *Sulphur*, *Sepia*, *China*, *Spigelia*, *Natrum mur.*

FAINTING FITS often assail pregnant women without any

known cause from the moment of conception; in some cases they are caused by dresses that are too tight around the waist; sometimes they depend upon a certain general or partial plethora, or they may result from a general debility occasioned by hæmorrhage, deficient nourishment, or some previous sickness. The best remedies for these fainting turns, when happening WITHOUT ANY KNOWN CAUSE, are, *Ignatia*, two globules dry on the tongue, especially in the case of hysteric or sad and melancholy women; *Chamomilla*, suitable to women of an irritable temperament; *Nux vomica*, suitable to women of an irascible disposition; if the fainting depends upon a GENERAL PLETHORA, *Aconitum*, *Belladonna*, *Bryonia;* if caused by tight clothes impeding the circulation, *Aconitum*, *Opium*, *Bryonia*, *Arnica;* if caused by DEBILITATING LOSSES, *China*, *Carbo vegetabilis*, *Veratrum*, *Nux vomica*, *Sulphur.*

The various kinds of HÆMORRHAGE occur quite frequently during pregnancy, from the *nose* (epistaxis,) *lungs* (hæmoptysis, blood-spitting,) *stomach*, (hæmatemesis, vomiting of blood,) *uterus* (metrorrhagia, flooding.) This last is the most dangerous, both because it may lead to miscarriage and to the mother's death. Having treated these accidents in detail, together with the remedies to be used for them (Sections 39 and 43,) we shall here simply mention the medicines that are most suitable for flooding during pregnancy: *Crocus*, *Platina*, *Sabina*, *Belladonna*, *Chamomilla*, *Bryonia*, *China*, *Hyoscyamus*, and more particularly, if miscarriage is to be apprehended; *Sabina*, *Chamomilla*, *Crocus*, *Kreosotum*, *Platina*, *Secale;* if the flooding is caused by a *strain*, *wrong step*, *blow* on the abdomen or small of the back: *Arnica*, *Bryonia*, *Ruta*. However, not every loss of blood from the womb during pregnancy need cause apprehension. As long as the blood only flows as during the menses, we can easily arrest the hæmorrhage by *Belladonna*, *Ipecacuanha*, *China*, *Sabina;* and if the inflammation should become suddenly acute and dangerous, give *Ipecacuanha*. NOSE-BLEED during pregnancy is often relieved by *Aconitum*, *Arnica*, *China*, *Bryonia*, *Conium*,

Belladonna. For BLOOD-SPITTING, if not caused by disease, but resulting from a simple determination of blood to the lungs, we give *Aconitum*, *Arnica*, *Ferrum*, *Ipecacuanha*, *Chamomilla*, *Phosphorus*, *Sulphuris acidum*. For VOMITING OF BLOOD: *Ipecacuanha*, *Arnica*, *Ferrum*, *Sulphur*, *Aconitum*. See the article, *Metrorrhagia*, (Sections 39–43,) where detailed symptomatic indications of every remedy may be found. As regards dose, six globules may be dissolved in half a tumblerful of water, and a teaspoonful of this solution may be given every fifteen minutes or half hour, or even less frequently, according as the danger is more or less imminent.

PILES of pregnant women seem to originate in habitual constipation rather than in impeded circulation of the pelvic vessels. These engorgements of the hæmorrhoidal veins cause sometimes such violent pains, that the patients wish to be freed from their trouble at any price. It would not be advisable, however, to combat these piles by external applications; the true treatment is to give a dose of *Pulsatilla* internally, two globules dry on the tongue, which may be repeated every four or six days if necessary. If Pulsatilla is not sufficient, we may give *Nux vomica*, especially if the bowels are always bound, or the patient has used much coffee, wine or other heating beverages: *Arsenicum*, *Carbo veget.*, *Chamomilla*, *Natrum muriat.*, are likewise excellent remedies for piles.

VARICES which are bluish enlargements of the subcutaneous veins, and are sometimes found at the vulva and thighs, are caused in consequence of the circulation of the pelvic veins being impeded by the volume and weight of the uterus, and by the pressure of this organ upon the veins of the pelvis and abdomen. Often one side is alone affected, or at any rate more than the other. The varices generally cease after confinement; but as long as they continue, they are hurtful by the pain which they cause and by the impediment which they occasion during exercise. Sometimes they rupture and give rise to serious hæmorrhage. Old school physicians employ blood-letting as a remedy for varices; but the remedy is worse than the disease. The most efficacious homœopathic remedy for varices is *Pulsatilla*, or we may try *Carbo veget.*, *Lycopodium*, or *Silicea*. According to Croserio the *South pole of the magnet* applied for a few minutes is very efficacious. For rupture of the varices and subsequent hæmorrhage may be recommended: *Arnica*, *Carbo veget.*, *Lachesis*, *Phosphorus*. It is necessary to a cure, that the patients should not stand too long at a time, and that all compression by tight lacing, tight garters and the like should be avoided.

Œdema of pregnant women is caused by the same influences as varices, to which a peculiar constitutional predisposition and an improper mode of life may be added. This trouble generally sets in about the sixth or seventh month of pregnancy, especially if the patients lead a sedentary life, or have a lymphatic constitution. Sometimes retrocession of some cutaneous disease may cause the swelling. At times the swelling extends to the lower abdomen, giving the pelvic extremities enormous dimensions. If the œdema is not very considerable, it disappears over night, and a little walking generally removes it entirely. But if the thighs are involved these hygienic means are no longer sufficient; we then have to give *Bryonia*, six globules in half a tumblerful of water, a teaspoonful morning and night, and if *Bryonia* is not sufficient, *Sulphur*, two globules dry on the tongue, a dose every other day, three doses at most. *Arnica* is sometimes useful. For œdema of the vulva, if occasioned by the same causes, we have to give *Sepia*, *Mercurius*, and *Nux vomica*.

Section 117.

Derangements of the respiratory organs.—These are *oppression* or *dyspnœa* and *cough*.

Dyspnœa which is caused by the crowding upwards of the diaphragm in the last months of pregnancy, generally affects women of small size, and in whom the uterus has acquired very large dimensions. If the thorax is badly shaped, or the lungs and heart are diseased, the dyspnœa may sometimes reach a very high degree. In every case it is rather troublesome and accompanied by digestive derangements. It is generally after a meal that females are attacked by the distress for breath, with anguish, congestions of the head, red face. The best remedy is undoubtedly *Nux vomica;* two globules dry on the tongue will often dissipate the trouble. In some cases *China*, is an excellent remedy, especially if flatulence and distention of the abdomen after eating, are present; or *Aconitum*, a few globules dissolved in half a tumblerful of water, in teaspoonful doses every three to six hours, in cases of plethora, with palpitation of the heart, red face, vertigo and anguish; or *Arsenicum*, for great weakness, swelling of the legs, pale and puffed face, or yellow and greenish face; or *Pulsatilla* for difficult digestion, with pale face, bitter taste in the mouth after eating, frequent mucus on the stomach, and chilliness; or *Ipecacuanha*, for desire to vomit, with pale or bluish red face, disposition to faint. If old pulmonary disorganizations are present, give *Phosphorus*, *Sulphur*, *Kali*, *Lachesis*.

COUGH is not always a necessary accessary of pregnancy; it may be caused by a cold or some other exposure independently of pregnancy. There is a cough, however, which results from the compression of the larger vessels and consequent determination of blood to the lungs. This cough is dry, frequent, fatiguing, and continues to the end of pregnancy. It often leads to a sudden spirting out of the urine, and may cause hæmorrhages and miscarriage. The best remedy for this cough is *Aconitum* in half a tumblerful of water, in teaspoonful doses every three or four hours; or *Sepia*, if aconitum should not be sufficient; or *Belladonna*, if the cough should set in in the evening or night; *Nux vomica*, if the cough happens in the morning or after a meal, with pain, as if bruised in the hypochondria or head, when coughing; *Ipecacuanha* or *Pulsatilla*, if the cough excites vomiting; *Conium* or *Dulcamara*, if the cough is accompanied by obstinate tickling in the throat and chest; or *Natrum muriat.*, (*Causticum* or *Phosphorus*,) if the cough comes on involuntarily, and sudden spirting out of the urine. If an ordinary catarrhal cough should set in, it has to be treated like any other catarrh.

Section 118.

Derangements of the secretory and excretory functions.—Having spoken of constipation and diarrhœa, and likewise of vomiting of pregnant women, we have to treat now of *ptyalism*, *derangements* of the *urinary functions*, such as *dysuria*, *stranguria*, *ischuria*, and *incontinence of urine.*

Ptyalism of pregnant females proceeds from the same cause as vomiting. It incommodes them very much, and is incurable by Old School treatment. Generally it ceases of itself, about the end of the fourth or fifth month of pregnancy. The best remedy for it is *Sulphur*, or *Mercurius*; if Sulphur is not sufficient or the ptyalism is very profuse. If accompanied by nausea and aversion to food, *Pulsatilla* and *Ipecacuanha* are very useful; or *Veratrum* and *Arsenicum*, if the patients are very feeble and chilly.

Dysuria and stranguria are equally frequent among pregnant females, in consequence of the pressure of the uterus upon the bladder and urethra, and likewise in consequence of the irritation of the mucous lining caused by this pressure. Hence a frequent urging to urinate, sometimes without result or with frequent emissions of a few drops of burning urine and tenesmus of the bladder. The best medicine for this trouble is *Pulsatilla*, or *Nux vomica*, if Pulsatilla is not sufficient, and dysuria is caused by displacement of the uterus. In some cases *Cocculus*, *Phosphori acid.*, *Sulphur*, and even *Aconitum* may be of great use.

In complete retention of urine, it may sometimes be necessary to depend upon the catheter before administering the suitable remedy. Previously, however, we may try *Camphor*, or *Nux vomica*, or *Pulsatilla;* however, if the retention has already continued for twenty-four hours, and the remedies have no effect, the catheter should be resorted to, after which we may give *Nux vomica* or *Pulsatilla.*

INCONTINENCE of URINE during pregnancy, consists in a frequent desire to urinate, which is sometimes so violent that a few drops of urine will escape before the patient is able to reach the vessel. Sometimes the vulva and thighs are very much irritated by the continual dribbling of the urine. The principal remedy for this difficulty is *Pulsatilla*, or *Sepia*, if Pulsatilla is not sufficient. Sometimes we may give *Aconitum, Belladonna, Natri muriat., or Causticum.*

All the remedies mentioned in this paragraph may be given as follows:—Dissolve six globules, or one drop of the liquid attenuation in half a tumblerful of water, and give the patients a dessertspoonful of this solution every three or four hours.

SECTION 119.

DERANGEMENTS THAT ARE PAINFUL.—We unite in this paragraph all those derangements, the principal symptom of which is *pain*, except colic, of which we have spoken before. Here we treat of *toothache, pains in the breasts, pains in the small of the back, painful stitches in the abdomen, false pains* and *cramps in the calves.*

TOOTHACHE occurs quite frequently among pregnant females; some women lose a tooth during every pregnancy. This toothache lasts sometimes from the moment of conception to the end of pregnancy, and often is very troublesome indeed. The best remedy for it is *Sepia*, two globules dry on the tongue, or *Chamomilla*, if the pain proceeds from a single carious tooth; *Pulsatilla*, if a whole side of the jaw is affected, or the pain shifts about; *Coffea*, if the pain is violent, comes on in paroxysms, and the patient cries out with pain; *Nux vomica*, if the pain proceeds from a decayed tooth to the facial bones, and gets worse by wine, coffee and mental work; *Aconitum, Belladonna* or *Hyoscyamus*, for violent congestion about the head; *Staphysagria* for toothache, in carious teeth, if neither *Chamomilla* nor *Nux vomica* helps. The specific remedy affords instantaneous relief, if two globules are given dry on the tongue; if no improvement follows in a couple of hours, another remedy will have to be chosen; it would be useless to give a second dose of the same remedy.

PAINS IN THE BREASTS generally come on in the first weeks of pregnancy, owing to the rapid development of the mammary gland, the copious afflux of fluids to this organ, and the tension that results from it. But the patients sometimes feel a good deal of pain in the last months of pregnancy; caused by excessive distension of the breasts and cracking of the skin. The best remedy for this condition, for which allœopaths bleed their patients, is *Bryonia*, especially if the tension is very painful; or *Belladonna*, if there is erysipelatous or inflammatory redness. For distensive pains, *Secale*, *Auricular*, *Nux vomica*, *Sepia*, are excellent remedies.

PAINFUL STITCHES during pregnancy are principally felt in the lower part of the thorax, false ribs, in one side or in the inguinal region; they seem to be induced by the pulling of the muscular fibres caused by the extreme tension of the abdominal integuments. These pains are confined to narrow localities; they do not hinder respiration, but often become more acute by pressure, motion, and by various positions of the body, and sometimes do not cease until after confinement. The best remedies for these pains, are:—*Nux vomica*, *Belladonna*, *Bryonia*, *Arnica*, *Pulsatilla*.

THE PAINS IN THE SMALL OF THE BACK during pregnancy, may be owing to various causes, such as the pulling of the large ligaments, compression of the lumbar nerves, engorgement of the pelvic or uterine vessels, excessive distension of the uterus, and weariness of the spinal muscles. When the pains are caused by the pulling of the large ligaments and the compression of the lumbar nerves, they increase by walking and standing, but decreased in a recumbent position; when the vessels are full, a sense of fulness and weight in the hypogastrium and pelvis is experienced; the pains caused by a distension of the uterus, are characterized by a sensitiveness in the region where the pains are felt, and the pains which are caused by weariness of the muscles, are distinguished by their locality and by an exacerbation of the pains when pressing upon the muscles. The chief remedies for these pains are, *Nux vomica*, when there are symptoms of abdominal plethora; *Belladonna*, or *Pulsatilla*, or *Nux vomica*, when there is great sensitiveness, hardness and tension in the uterine region; *Rhus* or *Arnica*, if the pain is caused by muscular fatigue or by a strain.

FALSE PAINS come on at various periods during the last months of pregnancy, especially at the end of the seventh month, or eight or ten days before confinement. The pains set in suddenly as if labor would come on, but when exploring the uterus with the finger, the neck is found closed and soft during the whole of these pains. The best remedy for false pains is generally *Pulsatilla*, two globules dry on the tongue, or *Coffea* and *Nux vomica*, if *Pulsatilla* is not sufficient. In some cases *Chamomilla*, *Belladonna*, *Nux moschata*, *Hyoscyamus*, *Sepia*, may prove useful.

CRAMPS IN THE CALVES AND FEET often torment pregnant women day and night, and fatigue them by depriving them of sleep and rest. The best remedy for this trouble is *Veratrum*, two globules dry on the tongue, or *Sulphur*, or *Colocynthis*, if Veratrum does not help. Sometimes we may give with success, *Camphor*, *Secale*, *Chamomilla*, *Sepia*, *Cuprum*, *Calcarea*, *Lycopodium*.

SECTION 120.

NERVOUS AND MENTAL AFFECTIONS.—In this paragraph we have to mention *sleeplessness* of pregnant women, *convulsions*, *fear of death*, which sometimes haunts them in a very fatiguing manner, and *moral emotions*.

SLEEPLESSNESS may be in a great measure removed by a suitable regimen, and by regular exercise in the open air. If the want of sleep should continue without any other ailments, a dose of *Coffea* or *Belladonna* will often bring back sleep. If night-mare should occur, we may give *Aconitum* or *Sulphur*, two globules dry on the tongue.

We shall return to CONVULSIONS when speaking of confinement and labor, at which period convulsions occur much more frequently than during pregnancy. If convulsions occur during pregnancy, they are always dangerous, and may result in miscarriage. *Belladonna*, six globules in half a tumblerful of water, a dessertspoonful every three hours, will remove the danger in most cases. If Belladonna should remain powerless, we may resort to *Chamomilla* or *Ignatia*, or even *Hyoscyamus* or *Ipecacuanha*. In other cases we might give *Cicuta*, *Cocculus*, *Platina*, *Moschus*, *Stramonium*, *Veratrum*.

The best remedy for FEAR OF DEATH which so often haunts pregnant women, is *Aconitum*. Recent critics have undertaken to show that the symptoms 540 of Hahnemann's Materia Medica; *moaning, with apprehension of impending death*, (from two to twelve hours); 541, *apprehensions lest some misfortune should happen to him;* 538, *apprehension of impending death* (Richard); are false, and that they should be blotted out from our collection of symptoms. But we have more faith in the numerous practical experiments of the large majority of homœopathic practitioners than in the baseless criticisms of a few neophytes, and the experience of all the best practitioners of our school shows that whenever *dread of death* is a symptom in mental or nervous diseases, *Aconitum* is a specific remedy for such affections. We shall therefore insist upon recommending *Aconitum* as a specific remedy for fear of death during pregnancy, unless the totality of the symptoms should indicate a different drug.

As regards MORAL EMOTIONS, we have a good many remedies by means of which their unpleasant effects may be safely and gently prevented or removed. For the effects of FRIGHT or FEAR, *Opium* will always be found efficacious, if the remedy can be employed immediately, or if there be trembling, anguish and dyspnœa, with red face and congestion of the head or chest; or *Aconitum*, if Opium does not help, if there is beating of the heart, pale face, fainting fits; or *Veratrum*, if there be diarrhœa with general coldness of the body, after an attack of fear; or *Belladonna*, if the fright causes convulsions, heat of the head, red and sweaty face; or *Hyoscyamus*, if Belladonna is not sufficient to stop the convulsions; or *Platina*, if fright is followed by uterine hæmorrhage. For the consequences of GRIEF, *Ignatia*, especially when there is much sadness, pains in the stomach, headache, vomiting and vertigo; or *Phosphori acid.*, or *Staphysagria*, if Ignatia is not sufficient; for violent ANGER, *Chamomilla*, especially when there is dyspnœa, weight about the heart, bilious symptoms with bitter vomiting, or yellowish, greenish diarrhœa; or *Nux vomica*, if Chamomilla is not sufficient; or *Bryonia*, if the patient feels chilly all over, with irascible mood; or *Staphysagria* or *Colocynthis*, when anger and indignation go together, with a sense of horror of what causes the anger; for EXCESSIVE and SUDDEN JOY, *Coffea*, or *Aconitum*, if Coffea is not sufficient. We always give two globules dry on the tongue, of any of these remedies; the dose should not be repeated until the symptoms get worse again.

SECTION 121.

CUTANEOUS DERANGEMENTS.—These are freckles and cracking of the skin of the abdomen.

FRECKLES are generally seated in the face; they are dirty-yellow or yellowish-brown spots. The best remedy is *Sepia*, when the spots occupy the upper part of the face, forehead or nose, where they form a sort of saddle across the nose; in other cases, *Sulphur* is the best remedy, or *Lycopodium* or *Antimony*.

CRACKING OF THE SKIN OF THE ABDOMEN.—A little blood becomes effused into these cracks which generally occur about the seventh month of pregnancy, in consequence of the distension of the abdomen by the uterus. We do not like to recommend Arnica washes for this trouble, for the drug is too readily absorbed by the torn skin, and might produce medicinal symptoms; we prefer frictions with almond-oil, and we recommend pregnant women to keep the abdomen perfectly free and easy, in order not to interfere with the gradual expansion of the integuments.

Section 122.

Local derangements of the sexual organs.—These local diseases are: *acute metritis*, *hydrometra*, *moles*, *false pregnancy* and *tumors of the vulva.*

Metritis of pregnant women is so little known, that we cannot say any thing about it here. If, however, the womb should become inflamed during pregnancy, we have to treat the inflammation precisely as any other metritis, see Sections 63–71.

Hydrometra or uterine dropsy differs from this disease when supervening in the unimpregnated womb, in such a marked manner that we will describe it here more minutely. The affection arises from an excessive abundance of the amniotic fluid, whence metritis develops itself in some cases, and which leaves even traces of inflammation in the placenta and ovum. In other cases this dropsy seems to come on after an inflammatory action in the uterus. It may befal women of any age, temperament or condition of life; sometimes it coincides with twin-pregnancy; at other times it has been seen to come on after a blow on the epigastrium. The symptoms of this increase are too rapid a growth of the uterus, a dull pain in the hypogastric region, and a more or less marked sense of weight in the pelvis, sometimes with swelling of the legs, thighs, face and hands, weakness, difficult digestion, oppression, often obliging the patients to spend the night on a seat. The signs which distinguish hydrometra of pregnant women from common uterine dropsy, are those of pregnancy having preceded the state of dropsy or coexisted with it; moreover the balloting of the fetus that can be perceived in most cases. The prognosis, though not serious for the mother, is always unfavorable to the fetus which always perishes if the amniotic liquid escapes through the uterine orifice. It is not always easy to treat this affection, especially on account of the obscurity of the symptoms at the onset of the disease, and afterwards on account of their limited number, and the absence of particular indications; nevertheless, if the disease is well marked, we may always commence the treatment with *Sulphur*, six globules in half a tumblerful of water, a dessert-spoonful of which solution should be given three times a day; or with *Arsenicum*, if there be a marked dyspnœa, swelling of the legs, face and thighs. Sometimes we may give *China* with success, especially if the patients have been weakened by loss of blood or deficient nourishment; or *Nux vomica*, if there be constipation, frequent urging to urinate, difficult digestion and vomiting of food.

FLESHY MOLES which must not be confounded with *false pregnancy*, where a germ is always wanting, are an affection of pregnant women consisting in a degeneration of the product of conception. Unfortunately this condition cannot be recognized by any characteristic sign before the expulsion of the mole; and, if some signs should lead us to suspect the presence of a mole, the expulsion is generally close at hand and cannot be prevented. We have indicated Section 75, the best remedies to facilitate expulsion if it should go on too slowly; hence we refer the reader to this passage.

FALSE PREGNANCY which has nothing in common with pregnancy but the name, is a species of *hydatic hydrometra*, occasioned by acephalocyst worms in the womb that may simulate an incipient pregnancy most perfectly. We refer our readers to Section 76, where we have given a full description of this affection and of its treatment. The treatment of such disorders as may set in after the expulsion of moles, such as *lochia*, *milk-fever*, or even *metroperitonitis*, is the same as that which we have indicated in the paragraphs concerning the ailments that may complicate labor and confinement. Sections 130–135.

The TUMORS OF THE VULVA which occur during pregnancy, are the *phlegmonous swelling* and *œdema* of this organ. For a description of these diseases and of their treatment, we refer the reader to Sections 99–101. The best remedies for INFLAMMATION of the vulva during pregnancy, are *Sepia* and *Mercurius*, and for ŒDEMA of the vulva, *Bryonia*, *Sulphur*, *Mercurius*, *Sepia*.

SECTION 123.

INFLUENCE OF EXISTING DISEASES UPON PREGNANCY.—We have to examine in this paragraph: 1st, *the influence which diseases exercise over pregnancy;* 2d, *the influence which pregnancy exercises over diseases;* 3d, *the treatment to be followed in case unpleasant consequences should result from either.*

As regards the influence which DISEASES EXERCISE OVER PREGNANCY, it is generally admitted, that acute epidemic or other diseases when befalling a pregnant female, easily lead to miscarriage, and often result fatally; but this termination may be owing to the heroic treatment pursued by old school physicians rather than to the disease itself. We have treated measles, variola, scarlatina, dysentery, etc., supervening during pregnancy, without having ever had a fatal result to deplore. *Chronic diseases* scarcely ever modify the course of pregnancy; consumptive persons, or women affected with aneurisms or dropsy, or with other chronic diseases, generally go their full term. So do women affected with abdominal tumors, nervous diseases, mental derangements, and other affections of the same sort; syphilis, however, will often produce miscarriage, after destruction of the fetus.

The INFLUENCE OF PREGNANCY OVER DISEASES is likewise well known. In some cases certain epidemic diseases seem to spare pregnant women, whereas other epidemic diseases seem to attack them more readily and more dangerously than other persons. It seems certain that the high functional vitality of otherwise healthy pregnant women preserves them from, rather than exposes them to, acute diseases; whereas weakly females become more liable to the invasion of acute diseases than previous to pregnancy. On the other hand, pregnancy sometimes slackens the course of chronic maladies and even suspends the development of the symptoms. This is especially applicable to pulmonary phthisis; although there are likewise cases of pregnancy where consumption was hastened onward to a fatal issue. Generally, however, consumptions that seemed to be arrested during pregnancy, break out again with a redoubled fury after confinement; and tubercles which had remained in a state of crudity previous to pregnancy, sometimes become inflamed and ulcerated immediately after confinement. Old ovarian tumors and other tumors of the sexual organs sometimes disappear entirely under the influence of pregnancy. In Section 58, about displacements of the uterus, we have said all that we have to say concerning the pretended curative influence of pregnancy over prolapsus of the womb. Mania and dementia are sometimes favorably affected by pregnancy; but as far as a radical cure of these affections goes, it cannot be effected by pregnancy except where these affections depend upon accidental disorders of the menstrual functions, or upon certain uterine disorders of the same sort.

Diseases which supervene during pregnancy, have to be treated in the same manner as if they occurred at any other period. As regards chronic diseases, the period of pregnancy is exceedingly favorable to their treatment, inasmuch as the female organism is never more sensitive to the action of the drugs than during pregnancy, it is at this time that the germs of disease are most easily extinguished in the human body. Both the mother and the child which she bears in her womb, are benefitted by a wisely directed treatment. We recommend with others, and with Croserio in particular, the administration of two globules of *Sulphur*, which are to be allowed to act for six weeks, after which a dose of *Calcarea* is to be given, and to be allowed to act for the same period; a strict homœopathic regimen is to be pursued all the while. Mothers that had always given birth to poorly looking children, bore perfectly healthy and robust children under the invigorating influence of such a treatment. *Sulphur* and *Calcarea*, however, are not the only remedies adapted to this condition; other remedies will very often have to be chosen. The rule is to select them in accordance with the perceptible symptoms; in order to enable the mother to bear healthy children, it will very often be sufficient to treat her for the ailments that may successively develop themselves during pregnancy. By invigorating the constitution of the mother, we benefit the child she is to give birth to; hence the mother should be watched during the whole period of pregnancy, not only with a view of regulating her diet, but likewise in order to remove the unpleasant symptoms, weaknesses, pains, etc., that may set in previous to her confinement.

ARTICLE III.

MISCARRIAGE.

Section 124.

Symptoms and course.—By miscarriage is understood the expulsion of the fetus from the womb before it is able to live separately from the mother. This accident may take place at any period during pregnancy, but it occurs much more frequently during the first three months, and especially during the third. In the two first months, the ovum which is yet very small, is often expelled without pain or any considerable flooding. The patients often fancy that they have simply been laboring under temporary suppression, followed by increased flooding, whereas in reality there was a miscarriage. The pains and the flooding which accompany the miscarriage, increase in proportion as the pregnancy is more advanced, and the flooding which accompanies the miscarriage, is often much more violent than the loss of blood that occurs after confinement at full term. The other symptoms vary according to the causes that have given rise to the miscarriage. If resulting from chronic weaknesses, the accompanying symptoms generally are: loss of appetite, thirst and nausea; shuddering followed by heat; pains in the small of the back, lassitude, fainting turns, palpitation of the heart, coldness of the extremities, depression of spirits, prostration, pallor, livid and bloated eyelids, dull eyes; foul breath; sense of weakness in the abdomen, cold feeling towards the pubes, weight on the anus and vulva, flabbiness of the breasts with serous discharge from the nipples; ichorous and bloody discharge from the vagina, followed by discharge of a thin and grumous blood, slackening and sudden cessation of the fetal movements, sinking-in of the hypogastrium, increased frequency of the uterine pains; progressive dilatation of the uterine orifice and membranes; lastly expulsion of the amniotic liquor and of the fetus, followed after some time by expulsion of the placenta. Miscarriage which is induced by accidental causes, is frequently preceded by pains in the small of the back, weight in this region, sense of heavy pressure on the lower portion of the vagina, with general malaise, gastralgia and shivering. These symptoms are often from the first accompanied by a little show of blood, followed by discharge of a sero-sanguineous liquid, which increases to flooding some time previous to the miscarriage taking place. In other cases the accidental cause immediately excites a copious hæmorrhage; frequent and lancinating pains in the abdomen from the umbilicus to the vulva set in, the uterus becomes the seat of expulsive efforts, and the fetus is discharged. Hæmorrhage may cease after the expulsion, or may continue sometime after. If miscarriage takes place at an advanced period of pregnancy, it is accompanied by similar phenomena as confinement at full term, such as lochia, secretion of milk, and milk-fever.

Section 125.

Causes of miscarriage.—These are *predisposing* and *exciting* causes.

The predisposing causes are partially peculiar to the mother, and partially to the fetus. Those that are peculiar to the mother consist either *in a vicious conformation* of the organs of the mother opposing a sufficient expansion of the uterus and consequently preventing the growth of the fetus, or in some constitutional taint which affects both the womb and its contents. Among such causes we may enumerate the excessive rigidity of the fibres of the uterus, or else an excessive degree of contractility and sensibility of this organ; weakness or laxity of the neck of the uterus; atony of the uterus caused by copious leucorrhœa or by previous unfavorable confinements; chronic metritis, scirrhus, carcinoma, various tumors, polypi, dropsy of the womb, presence of several fetuses. Among the general constitutional causes we have a sanguine temperament, plethora, piles, profuse and irregular menstruation; great weakness, extreme sensitiveness, cachexia, syphilis, hysteria, scurvy and other chronic maladies, an hereditary disposition, tendency to miscarriage induced by previous miscarriages even accidental. Prolonged watching, deficient food, misery, tight dresses, may also become predisposing causes of miscarriage. Sometimes a peculiar epidemic condition of the atmosphere may favor miscarriage. The predisposing causes inherent in the fetus are weakness, monstrous development and disease; feeble adhesion of the placenta, placental presentation at the uterine orifice, various organic defects (scirrhus, hydatids, aneurisms, varices, etc.,) hypertrophy or atrophy; excessive shortness, length, thinness, hypertrophy or atrophy or other defects of the umbilical cord; thinness of the membranes of the ovum; disproportionate quantity of amniotic liquor.

The *exciting* causes are so numerous that they can scarcely be enumerated. The most common of these are uterine diseases, acute diseases, fevers; diarrhœa, dysentery, colic, constipation, urinary diseases, moral emotions, acute pains, strong odors, sexual intercourse, shocks, violent emotions, dancing, riding in a carriage or on horseback, laughter, cries, coughing; vomiting; falling, blows on the abdomen and small of the back; abuse of cathartics, emmenagogues, blood-letting (especially from a vein of the feet,) foot-baths, etc. It is particularly towards the menstrual period that these causes are most to be dreaded. They affect the fetus and its appendages as much as the uterus, either by destroying the former and thus compelling its expulsion, or by exciting the uterus into expulsory movements before the full term and while the fetus was alive. Abortive means, such as bleeding at the feet, drastics, emmenagogues, puncturing the membranes of the ovum, are likewise to be numbered among the exciting causes. These criminal measures do not always lead to the desired result, especially if the patients are of sound health, so that intentional miscarriages are much less frequent than those which are the result of accident. These exciting causes are scarcely ever sufficient to produce miscarriage, if there is not a predisposition that favors their action. Even the mechanical means which are resorted to for the purpose of puncturing the membranes, frequently lead to serious injuries of the womb without producing expulsion of the fetus.

Section 126.

Diagnosis and prognosis.—In diagnosing miscarriage it is not sufficient that the general character of the pathological process that we are called upon to treat, should be recognized; we have to determine how far the danger has become imminent, and what causes have led to it. As regards the *causes*, most of them are easily ascertained, or are revealed without any obscurity by the general state and constitution of the patient, particularly to the homœopathic physician who is in the habit of observing every symptom. As regards the imminence of the danger, we may suppose that a miscarriage is to be apprehended, if, after the operation of one of the above mentioned exciting causes, some of the precursory symptoms of miscarriage make their appearance, and if these symptoms should be accompanied by labor pains, softening and gradual dilatations of the uterine orifice, protrusion of the membranes during the pains, discharge of the amniotic fluid, we may consider the process of miscarriage as having actually commenced. The *prognosis* depends upon the fact whether miscarriage has actually set in, or whether we have only the precursory symptoms to contend against. Many accoucheurs regard actual miscarriage as much more serious than confinement at full term. This may indeed be true, if the accident was caused by violence, intentional or unintentional. In such a case the danger is proportionate to the unexpected suddenness of the attack. If the accident takes place spontaneously and without any apparent cause, it is often painless and unattended by unpleasant consequences; but relapses are apt to take place in such cases, and their frequent recurrence may finally develop many inconveniences, such as menstrual irregularities, chronic metritis, hysteria, etc. The prognosis also depends upon the accessory symptoms. If violent flooding takes place, the danger is of course considerable. Convulsions, diarrhœa, dysentery, acute inflammations, fevers, eruptive diseases, likewise complicate the trouble, and render the prognosis more doubtful. If we have only the precursory symptoms to combat, the prognosis under homœopathic treatment is of course much more favorable than under old-school treatment. Nevertheless, in spite of the excellent means which our school possesses to prevent or arrest miscarriage, this is not very easy, if some internal dyscrasia, uterine disorganization, vicious mode of living, etc., is the cause of the disorder; the nature and seriousness of the exciting cause likewise determines in a measure the chances of a favorable issue; the intensity of the accompanying symptoms which are more immediately traceable to the accident, is likewise to be considered. But whatever may seem the amount of the danger, the homœopathic physician need not despair until the miscarriage has actually taken place. Even where the most violent flooding or convulsions had already set in, or in placental presentation, or after the discharge of the amniotic fluid, the use of homœopathic means has often prevented the occurrence of miscarriage.

Section 127.

Preventive treatment.—The main point is to prevent the miscarriage, especially where there is a predisposition for such mishaps. To this end we have to acquaint ourselves with the hygienic conditions of our patient, and to remove all the predisposing and exciting causes which, in her case, might lead to miscarriage. We have said above (Section 113) every thing that we had to say concerning the mode of life to be pursued during pregnancy, clothing, dwelling, exercise, food, etc. In respect to these things every necessary precaution has to be observed by females disposed to miscarry; they should take moderate exercise in the open air, especially walking; their food should be plain and substantial; coffee, tea, drugs of every description, herb-teas, decoctions, warm baths, etc., should be strictly avoided, and the mind should be kept easy. Riding on horseback or in a carriage is likewise hurtful. Such old-school means as sleeping in extension-chairs, are likewise condemnable, for the reason that the constitution of the patient is weakened in consequence, and the disposition to miscarry is increased rather than diminished.

After regulating the hygienic conditions of the patient, and removing the predisposing and exciting causes, we have to examine the sanitary condition of the patient generally, inquire into her previous sicknesses, the character of her catamenia, her most common indispositions, and then institute a treatment in conformity to the information which we have obtained. Some beginners in homœopathy imagine that there are medicines which prevent miscarriage absolutely, in any constitution, and they prescribe a whole string of such medicines, simply because the repertories recommend them as efficacious. This species of treatment is a great mistake. The best means of preventing miscarriage is to invigorate the patient's constitution, to cure her of all constitutional weaknesses, and the medicines which affect this object best, will likewise prove the best preventive medicines as far as miscarriage is concerned. It is evident that we cannot mention a remedy for every individual case of constitutional suffering that may occur among pregnant women, for the symptoms by which such weaknesses are characterised are too numerous. Nevertheless the following remedies will in general prove efficacious against the chronic ailments of women predisposed to miscarriage:

1. *Calcarea, Camphora, Sabina, Sepia, Pulsatilla, Sulphur, Carbo veg., Ferrum.*
2. *Asarum, Camphora, Cocculus, Hyoscyamus, Nux v., Plumbum, Ruta, Silicea.*

And in particular:

CALCAREA, in the case of plethoric women of full habit, with profuse and premature menstruation, disposed to leucorrhœa, painfulness of the breast, colic, pains in the small of the back, frequent congestions of the head and the chest, vertigo, varices of the genital organs, etc.

CAMPHORA, suitable to females of a feeble constitution, subject to leucorrhœa, colds on the chest or in the head, or catarrhal discharges generally, with pale, loose and cold skin, sensitiveness to open or cold air; indifference to sexual intercourse, little enjoyment during intercourse, etc.

SABINA, suitable to plethoric women with profuse and long-lasting menses, or where the patients had been in the habit of miscarrying in the third month. If this medicine is indicated, the patient may take three globules dry on the tongue, a dose every forty-eight hours, during the week preceding the period when the menses ought to have set in; this treatment has to be repeated until after the time when the previous miscarriages took place.

SEPIA, suitable to feeble, soft constitutions with a delicate and sensitive skin, dingy color of the skin, brownish or yellowish spots in the face, slender waist; disposition to leucorrhœa, with soreness, eruptions and itching of the parts; menses generally too scanty or premature, with sadness, weeping, headache or toothache; frequent attacks of megrim; tendency to perspire; frequent colic; disposition to cold in the head and bronchial catarrh.

PULSATILLA, for the same conditions as *Sepia*, or in alternation with *Sepia*, and preferable to this agent if the patient is chilly, averse to drinking, disposed to bilious diarrhœa, derangements of the stomach, with pale face, gentle disposition.

SULPHUR, often at the onset, before *Calcarea* or *Sabina;* the menses are premature, profuse; or after *Pulsatilla* or *Sepia*, when the menses are scanty and retarded, with leucorrhœa, itching, burning and soreness of the parts; eruptions or tetter on the skin; disposition to piles, bronchial catarrh or other mucous discharges; weariness, nervous debility, loss of appetite; frequent headach with pressive pain and congestion of blood about the head.

CARBO VEGETABILIS, in some cases when the menses are too pale and too scanty, or too copious and premature, with varices at the parts, frequent pains in the small of the back and headaches, spasmodic colic, etc.

FERRUM, suitable to chlorotic patients with leucorrhœa and amenorrhœa; or suitable to plethoric females, with vascular excitement, red face, full and strong pulse, premature and copious menses.

LYCOPODIUM, profuse and long catamenia, with itching, burning and varices of the parts; dryness of the vagina; disposition to melancholy and tears; leucorrhœa, headache, pains in the small of the back, fainting turns.

Moreover:—

ASARUM, suitable to females who are subject to megrim; menses too early and long, with discharge of black blood and pains in the small of the back; nervous sensitiveness, especially of the hearing.

CANNABIS, suitable to females who had been affected with virulent gonorrhœa; sensitive disposition; weariness after the least exertion; hysteric ailments; scrofulous constitution; disposed to constipation, etc.

COCCULUS, difficult menstruation, with colic and uterine cramps; weakness and frequent hysterics; aversion to open air; scrofulous engorgements; gentle and phlegmatic disposition; sad.

HYOSCYAMUS, copious menses with hysteric ailments; disposed to have boils; brownish spots and freckles all over; *jealous*, *quarrelsome* and talkative.

NUX MOSCHATA, suitable to hysteric females who are disposed to fainting turns, convulsions or uterine cramps; irregular menses, with pains in the small of the back and discharge of a thick and dark blood; sensitiveness to the open, cold and damp air; cold and dry skin; no perspiration; changing mood; disposed to feel chilly, with pale face.

PLUMBUM, suitable to patients who are fond of sexual intercourse, with yellowish or blueish color of the skin, and brownish spots on the body; habitual constipation; dryness and falling off of the hair; pale face; chlorotic symptoms, etc.

RUTA, suitable for irregular catamenia either too profuse or too scanty, preceded or followed by acrid leucorrhœa.

SILICEA, when the catamenia are generally too early and profuse, with disposition to corrosive leucorrhœa.

Predisposing causes arising from chronic metritis, leucorrhœa, scirrhus, carcinomatous tumors, polypi, etc., have to be met by treating these diseases in the manner indicated in previous paragraphs.

But whatever pathological condition we may have to act upon in order to prevent miscarriage, it is always well to be very cautious in not giving too much medicine. A single dose of two or three globules dry on the tongue is sufficient at a time; and this dose should not be repeated without a positive indication by the symptoms.

SECTION 128.

ACTIVE TREATMENT OF THE PRECURSORY SYMPTOMS.—If, in spite of our preventive measures, miscarriage will threaten, and precursory symptoms of it develop themselves, such as pains from the umbilicus to the genital organs, or real labor-pains coming on in regular succession and accompanied by discharge of blood or bloody mucus, we have at once to give a remedy corresponding to these symptoms and to the exciting cause. The patient should be kept perfectly quiet in her bed, avoid warm drinks and warm solid food, or any thing that may excite the abdominal viscera. The best remedies for this purpose are:—1. *Arnica*, *Ipecacuanha*, *Sabina*, *Belladonna*, *Chamomilla*, *Hyoscyamus*, *Secale*, *Nux vomica*, *Bryonia*, *Pulsatilla*, *Rhus*, *Cinnamon*. 2. *Chamomilla*, *China*, *Cinnamon*, *Cocculus*, *Crocus*, *Nux vomica*, *Platina*, *Ruta*. And more particularly,

ARNICA, when, after a blow on the stomach, fall, or after violent movements, labor-pains with discharge of blood or bloody mucus have set in.

IPECACUANHA, for acute hæmorrhage with continuous flow of bright red blood, colic, cutting pains at the umbilicus, violent pressure on the womb and rectum, nausea, weakness, pale face, shuddering, or even convulsions without loss of consciousness. If *Ipecacuanha* does not help, we may give *Platina* or *Cina*.

SABINA, if the precursory symptoms of miscarriage show themselves during the first months of pregnancy, especially in the third; but, also at any other period, and particularly when the following symptoms occur:—discharge of dark-colored coagulated blood; pressive and drawing pains from the small of the back to the sexual parts; soft and flat abdomen; continual urging to stool, with diarrhœa, nausea and vomiting; fever, with shuddering and heat.

BELLADONNA, for pressive and tensive pains in the whole abdomen, with sense of constriction or distension, lumbar pains as if the sacrum would break; pressure downwards in the abdomen and private parts, as if every thing would fall through.

CHAMOMILLA, for discharge of dark or black and foul blood, with coagula; *violent cutting colic from the small of the back to the hypogastrium, with frequent desire to go to stool or to urinate;* sense of heaviness in the abdomen; frequent yawning; shivering and shuddering; restlessness and convulsive movements.

HYOSCYAMUS, for convulsions, restlessness, loss of consciousness, stupefaction, vanishing of sight and hearing, delirium, etc.

Secale cornutum, when the uterus is organically diseased, or for deficient vitality of the womb; suitable to feeble, exhausted, cachectic females, with disposition to passive hæmorrhage or convulsions; pale and earthy complexion; pulse small and almost extinguished; fear of death; profuse discharge of black and thin blood.

Nux vomica, for obstinate constipation with violent cramp-pains, congestion of the womb, suitable to women who have abused coffee or alcohol; scanty flow of blood, but accompanied with great weakness and pale face.

Bryonia, if Nux is not sufficient for the violent pains, constipation, congestion of the head, dry mouth and thirst.

Pulsatilla, for intermittent hæmorrhage, recurring every now and then with redoubled violence, accompanied with expulsive pains and discharge of a dark blood with coagula.

Rhus, when the attack is caused by violent efforts such as lifting a weight, or by a strain of the side or a false step.

Cinnamonum, if Rhus is not sufficient, or if the effort is followed by profuse flooding.

As a general rule we may give—

For violent hæmorrhage:—*Ipecacuanha, Arnica, Sabina, Pulsatilla, Cinnamon.*

Continuous:—*Ipecacuanha, Sabina, Arnica, Cinnamon.*

Intermittent:—*Pulsatilla.*

With bright-red blood:—*Ipecacuanha, Arnica.*

Dark-red:—*Sabina, Chamomilla, Secale.*

Convulsions:—*Ipecacuanha, Hyoscyamus, Chamomilla, Platina, Cinnamon, Secale.*

Blows on the abdomen:—*Arnica.*

A strain:—*Rhus, Cinnamon.*

The dose should be six globules in half a tumblerful of water, of which solution a dessertspoonful may be administered every two or three hours.

Section 129.

Treatment of the consequences.—If the accident cannot be prevented, and the physician is called after the expulsion of the fetus has already commenced, we will have to treat the patient in the same manner as if actual confinement had taken place. We refer the reader in this respect to Sections 130–133. If the accident should occur previous to the seventh month of pregnancy, we should abstain as much as possible from interfering by manual manipulations with the natural process. If the fetus should be expelled, we have to hold it in a manner that will prevent the tearing of the cord. For, if the placenta should remain in the womb, after the expulsion of the fetus, it may still continue to grow and give rise to the symptoms of false pregnancy, or to fleshy moles. Moreover, the expulsive pains in miscarriage are always more violent and protracted than in natural confinement, so as to frequently occasion convulsive movements. In this case, manual interference would be of no use. A dose of *Coffea*, *Pulsatilla*, or *Secale* (three globules dry on the tongue) will facilitate the expulsion of the fetus, if it cannot be avoided.

After the miscarriage, we proceed in the same manner as after *confinement* and *labor*. Sections 130–153.

ARTICLE IV.

OF NATURAL CONFINEMENT AND OF THE DUTIES OF THE PHYSICIAN ON SUCH OCCASIONS.

Section 130.

Symptoms and course of labor.—At the approach of the natural term the organs of generation become moist, the uterus descends sometimes a fortnight before confinement, the epigastrium becomes disembarrassed, the breathing easier, the digestive functions less difficult; on the other hand, a sense of weight in the lower portion of the pelvis, a sense of numbness in the uterus and frequent urging to urinate often set in, until labor commences. First the patient feels short, transitory and slight pains in the hypogastrium, during which the uterine tumor becomes harder, whereas the orifice which had been somewhat dilated, contracts and becomes more rigid all around, and mucus is discharged from the vagina. Soon the pains become sharper, occur more frequently and last longer, every pain sometimes being ushered in by a sort of internal trembling or even a slight chill. At the same time the pulse becomes hard, frequent, raised; the heat of the body increases, the face becomes redder, the lips and tongue become dry; the patient feels thirsty, restless, sick at the stomach, and even vomits; the orifice of the womb opens and dilates, the borders of the orifice become stretched and thinner; the membranes pass into the orifice in the shape of a spherical segment, the dimensions of which augment at each pain; the abdominal muscles contract; at last the pains cease, and all these symptoms disappear except the dilatation of the orifice which increases more and more until the uterine cavity forms a continuous canal with the vagina, the superior portion of which becomes dilated correspondingly to the neck of the womb. After the dilatation of the uterine orifice is completed, the first part of the process of labor is accomplished, and the second part commences with the same symptoms as the former, only more intensely; the restlessness of the patient increases sometimes even to delirium; the pains become more acute, more frequent, but are followed by a period of more complete repose during which the patient shows a disposition to sleep. At the same time the patient experiences in the lower portion of the pelvis a sense of heaviness, a sort of tenesmus, which determines the contraction of the abdominal muscles and of the diaphragm; the amniotic fluid which is pushed downwards by these contractions, forces the inferior portion of the membranes which break and allow the fluid to escape, sometimes with so much force that the patient utters a cry of surprise. After the expulsion of the fluid, the head of the fetus presents at the orifice which becomes stopped up in consequence, so as to prevent any further escape of the amniotic liquid. At each new pain the head of the fetus descends a little lower in the vagina, protrudes through the orifice, and passes into the vagina which dilates accordingly, and at the same time, becomes elongated, the vulva opening a little at the same time; the labia majora and minora are stretched out into one fold, the mons veneris sinks in, the perinæum becomes distended and thinner; the anus protrudes, dilates and the fæcal matter which the rectum happened to contain, escape; the urine is likewise expelled spontaneously. The more labor advances, the more the efforts of the patient increase; the patient is seized with a convulsive trembling, and the pains extort cries from her. Lastly, a most violent expulsive pain presses the head out of the vulva; this is followed by a moment of rest, then a new and less violent pain takes place, which propels the body of the infant out of the vulva, and with it the remainder of the amniotic fluid. Labor being over, a delicious calm is experienced by the mother after these excessive exertions and pains; and she enjoys the sweet thought of having given birth to a new being that is to be the pride and joy of her earthly existence. After this calm has lasted for a while, the phenomena of placental delivery begin to develop themselves; of this mechanism we shall treat by and by, after having described the attentions which it behooves the accoucheur to bestow upon the mother both during natural and præternatural labor.

Section 131.

Diagnosis and prognosis.—The object of diagnosis in confinement is to find out whether labor has really set in, or how long it may possibly be before it does set in; and secondly, whether the existing conditions justify a favorable prognosis. As regards the beginning of labor, we have hardly a right to say that labor has actually set in before the neck of the womb is entirely effaced, no matter how far the orifice of the womb may otherwise be dilated; if the complete disappearance of the uterine neck is accompanied with regularly increasing pains, a progressive dilatation of the uterine orifice and tension of the membranes during the pains, discharge of mucus from the vulva: we may rest assured that labor has actually set in. In regard to the pains we have to distinguish false from real pains. Real pains are those which depend upon uterine contraction during which the uterine orifice becomes more and more dilated; the false pains are entirely foreign to the process of labor, and are generally located in some part adjoining the uterus; often these pains are inflammatory or spasmodic colicky pains, not accompanied by any other sign of labor, and leaving a sense of pain during the intermission, provided there be such a period. As regards the conditions of a spontaneous termination of natural labor, they are revealed to us by the position of the fetus, and by an exploration of the straits through which the child has to pass. The canal through which the fetus is transmitted into the outer world, must have the necessary dimensions; the fetus has to pass through this canal in such a manner that the various dimensions of the fetus are in exact co-adaptation to the various diameters of the straits; the orifice of the uterus has to be sufficiently dilated to allow the fetus to pass; and lastly, the muscular contractions of the women have to be strong enough to effect the expulsion of the fetus. Having ascertained these various points, we can easily determine how long the process of labor may last. The prognosis depends upon the constitution of the patient, the strength she possesses, the shape of the pelvis, the softness or hardness, the thinness or thickness of the uterine orifice, the dampness or dryness, flexibility or rigidity of the genital organs, the probable size of the child, and the position in which it presents; the intensity of the uterine contractions, and their effect upon the progress in the expulsion of the fetus, likewise the number and character of her previous confinements. Most of these signs are ascertained by the *touch*, which has to be resorted to as soon as the first signs of labor have become apparent.

Section 132.

Hygienic attentions during confinement.—The first care of the accoucheur should be to enable the patient to keep up her strength, and to prevent the untoward consequences of such external influences as might effect her unpleasantly; next, he has to assist and watch nature, in order to bring about a favorable termination of the process of labor. In this paragraph we will treat of the hygienic conditions of the patient, and in the next paragraph we will describe the particular medicinal measures which the physicians may have to adopt to help his patient through.

The hygienic regulations constitute one of the most important points in obstetric therapeutics; many unpleasant ailments may be prevented by wise precautions. The external conditions must be adapted to the patient's wants in order to enable her to have an easy confinement. As soon as she experiences the first pains, she ought to remove every species of clothing that feels tight on the body, and especially around the neck, in order to be freed from every embarrassment that might be disagreeable to her, and might impede the liberty of respiration and of the circulation of the blood. The air that she inhales, should be pure and of moderate temperature; neither too warm, lest the patient should become restless and the circulation should become excited; nor too cold, lest she should take cold to her great detriment. The woman's strength should be kept up by nourishment of easy digestion, which is taken in small quantity; but pure wine, stimulants or icy beverages should be strictly prohibited; pure water or water with sugar are the best drinks for our patient; and if the patient should be so weak as to require something strengthening, we may resort for this purpose to broths or soups. In order to prevent the involuntary emission of urine, or the involuntary evacuation of fæcal matter, or, on the other hand, the excessive accumulation of fæces in the rectum, the patient should be advised to go to stool as long as the labor is not too far advanced to render this impossible; in case of constipation with difficulty of evacuating the bowels, we may administer an injection of tepid water. Whatever has a tendency to excite the patient or to depress her spirits, should be kept away from her; perfumes, strong odors, noises, loud conversation, etc., should likewise be removed as hurtful. A little walking about in the room facilitates the process of labor; but during the pains the patient should lean against something, and take a position that will prevent all useless straining. After the discharge of the amniotic fluid, the patient should be fixed in the position in which she is to be confined, upon a bed prepared expressly for this purpose, where the head is somewhat elevated, and the body gently inclined. The bed should be sufficiently provided with pieces of linen to receive the blood which is discharged from the vulva; the covering of the patient should be adapted to the season. The head and shoulders should be gently raised, the thighs flexed upon the abdomen, and the legs upon the thighs, the knees being at the same time spread apart from one another. All mechanical means to dilate the organs of generation preparatory to labor, are absolutely condemnable; they irritate the parts and are moreover useless; for nature is amply able to achieve this work. The finger should not be introduced in the vagina any more frequently than is absolutely necessary to discover the position of the child, and to ascertain whether any manual interference is required. Hip-baths, tepid injections, fumigations, etc., are likewise condemnable; if any medicinal assistance is to be tendered, the following paragraph will explain more fully what is to be done.

Section 133.

Attentions of the accoucheur during the process of labor.—Having devoted the following paragraph to the details concerning præternatural labor, we shall here simply confine ourselves to the means by which labor can be facilitated, or else restored in case it should have been arrested. The accoucheur should therefore keep an eye upon the *muscular contractions that have to bring about the expulsion of the fetus;* 2, *the dilatation of the uterine orifice and of the canal through which the fetus has to pass;* 3, *the more or less favorable positions of the fetus.*

We have alluded above to the false pains during which the uterine orifice remains closed, whereas it dilates and becomes rigid during the real labor-pains. Hence, if a pregnant woman begins to feel pain, the physician has to inquire into the period of her pregnancy, and if it should appear that the patient has gone her full term, the pains should not be interfered with. But if, in spite of the full term, the pains do not progress, and the uterine orifice does not become rigid or contracted during the pains, we may administer three globules of *Pulsatilla* dry on the tongue, or a similar dose of *Coffea*, or *Nux vom.*, or *Belladonna*, or perhaps *Chamomilla*, or *Nux mos.*; the pains will either cease or else progress in regular order.

Sometimes the pains continue properly and regularly; but the uterine orifice remains closed; this may be owing to a wrong position of the fetus, or to an excess of resistance on the part of the neck. If the neck does not resist sufficiently, or does not become thinner, a dose of *Pulsatilla* may remedy the defect; for Pulsatilla seems to be endowed with a faculty of changing the wrong position of the fetus as long as it is still floating in the amniotic fluid. If the neck should remain closed and a hard rim should be felt all around the orifice, three globules of *Belladonna* dry on the tongue will bring about the regular evolution of the process of labor.

In other cases the orifice dilates regularly during the pains, but the watery tumor does not seem disposed to make its appearance. This may likewise be owing to a false position of the fetus, which may be remedied by a dose of *Pulsatilla.*

Sometimes every thing goes on favorably, pains, muscular contractions, progressive dilatation of the uterine orifice and of the whole canal through which the child has to pass, and the watery tumor seems to present properly; but the pains are too violent, and the patient fancies that she cannot bear them any longer. In this case, three globules of *Coffea,* dry on the tongue, will afford great relief, especially if the patient is very nervous and sensitive, restless and utters loud cries; or we may give a dose of *Nux vom.*, when there is frequent urging to stool or to void the urine, with irascible and impatient mood; or *Chamomilla* when the pains are accompanied by anguish, with twitching of the limbs, fear, weeping, disconsolate and vehement mood; or *Belladonna* if none of the other medicines help.

In spite of the most favorable course of the process of labor, the patients are sometimes seized with a *dread of death,* inexpressible anguish and terror; especially primiparæ who are attacked in this way as soon as the pains commence; no reasoning, no encouragement, no assurance on the part of the accoucher succeed in dispelling this symptom. A single dose of *Aconite* (three globules dry on the tongue) will do all that is required.

There are other symptoms which sometimes intervene during the course of labor and require the interference of the accoucheur: such symptoms are: *absence of labor-pains, fainting, cerebral congestions, convulsions, hæmorrhage,* etc.; we have united all these accidents by which the regular process of labor is sometimes interrupted or interfered with, in a special chapter under the heading of *difficult and protracted labor*.

ARTICLE V.

OF DIFFICULT OR PROTRACTED LABOR.

SECTION 134.

GENERAL OBSERVATIONS.—Labor may be protracted by: 1st, obstacles existing in the passage through which the child has to pass; 2d, obstacles offered by the fetus; 3d, accidents that may happen to the mother during labor. Several of these obstacles are of the domain of instrumental labor, and we shall content ourselves with simply mentioning them here, inasmuch as we have only to deal with the medicinal treatment which the condition of the patient may require.* Several conditions, however, which it was supposed required the interference of operative obstetrics, can be remedied much better by internal homœopathic treatment, so that the domain of medicinal obstetrics is much more extended now-a-days than it was formerly. Hereafter we shall explain the various accidents that appertain to each of the above mentioned categories, and at the same time furnish a description of the treatment required by each.

* See the *Practical Treatise on Obstetrics* by Chailly-Honoré, Member of the Imperial Academy of Medicine, Professor of Obstetrics, former head of the Obstetrical Clinique of the College of Medicine in Paris. Third edition, considerably increased. Paris, 1853, one Vol. in 8vo., 1050 pages, with 275 wood cuts.

Section 135.

Obstacles inherent in the mother.—These obstacles are: *deformities of the pelvis, tumors in the body or the appendages of the uterus, tumors of the vulva and vagina, contractions of the vagina and vulva.* Evidently some of these affections cannot be removed during the process of labor, and the accoucheur, as soon as he is called for a pregnant female, has to explore the condition of the passage in order to determine whether any interference of art is required for their removal previous to the period when labor will set in.

The deformities of the pelvis are all of them inaccessible to the ministering agency of art; but as long as there is barely space sufficient to admit the passage of the child's head (two inches and a half,) the accoucheur should not despair. A dose of *Secale*, two globules second attenuation, in half a tumblerful of water, a dessertspoonful at a dose, taken each time that the pains seem to flag, or a similar dose of *Pulsatilla*, will sometimes conquer every difficulty, and bring about a happy termination of labor. Osseous excrescences and tumors in the orifice or neck of the womb, or membranes in the vagina or vulva are likewise incurable by medicine. Deformities which prevent the passage of the fetus, belong to the domain of operative obstetrics, and need not be mentioned here.

It is different with tumors in the soft parts, neck of the womb, vagina or vulva. Most of them can be treated during pregnancy, provided their formation is known in season, and the proper treatment can be pursued. But even if they cannot be removed by treatment, they do not necessarily prevent the regular process of labor, for they may be pushed out of the way of the fetus by a suitable management of the parts, or the uterine contractions may be strengthened by a dose of *Secale* or *Pulsatilla*, sufficiently to enable the fetus to overcome the obstacles alluded to. *Nux vomica* may be given in case of vaginal hernia. If labor is interfered with by falling or protrusion of the umbilical cord, *Pulsatilla* will be found very useful.

As regards CONTRACTION OR STRICTURE OF THE VAGINA, this condition may either be congenital or accidental. If congenital, without any other organic defect, labor is not prevented by it, and the parts dilate gradually so as to admit the passage of the fetus. But if this dilatation should proceed too slowly or be too painful, a few doses of *Coffea*, *Secale*, *Pulsatilla* or *Nux vom.*, will remedy this trouble. But if the stricture is accidental, owing to some tumor, we should treat it during pregnancy by appropriate remedies. Inflammatory swellings of the vulva and vagina generally yield to a few doses of *Mercurius*, *Sepia*, or *Thuja*. If the excessive tenderness of the vulva or vagina should prevent the dilatation of these parts on account of the acute pains excited by this process, which sometimes render the danger of convulsions imminent, a few doses of *Coffea* or *Nux vomica*, will sometimes prove an efficient remedy.

SECTION 136.

OBSTACLES PRESENTED BY THE FETUS.—These are: *false positions*, *excessive size of the head*, *shortness of the umbilical cord*, *death of the Infant*.

We have stated that, if these positions can be known while the fetus is still enveloped in its membranes in the interior of the uterus, a dose of *Pulsatilla* will often be sufficient to change them. But if they are found out too late, or *Pulsatilla* remains without effect, we have to resort to the operations which are fully described in obstetric treatises for such occasions.

As regards the EXCESSIVE SIZE OF THE HEAD, some homœopaths advise the employment of *Pulsatilla* or *Secale*, in very small doses, in order to obtain the natural expulsion of the fetus in spite of this inconvenience. We have no clinical observations concerning this phenomena except one, which is the case of a mother who, on three successive occasions, gave birth to children with such enormous heads that instrumental delivery had to be resorted to in every case; during her fourth pregnancy, I gave her *Calcarea*, *Sulphur* and *Silicea*, and the child was brought to life without any instrumental interference whatever.

The SHORTNESS OF THE CORD is not necessarily a dangerous obstacle to delivery, provided the physician is made aware of it in season. If the head should not descend with a promptitude proportionate to the force of the uterine contractions, which often cease at the very moment when they should be the most powerful, and if the patient feels at every pain as if the bowels would be torn out, we may be certain that the cord is too short. A dose of *Pulsatilla* or *Secale*, a dessertspoonful of a solution of six globules in half a tumblerful of water, to be given at every contraction, will assist the efforts of nature and bring about a favorable termination of labor.

The DEATH OF THE FETUS does not prevent its expulsion, but renders the labor often less effective, the more so the longer the fetus had been dead. *Pulsatilla* and *Secale* will likewise be of great use to the patient.

SECTION 137.

ACCIDENTS THAT MAY HAPPEN TO THE MOTHER DURING LABOR. These accidents by which the process of labor may be more or less retarded, are: *absence or cessation of the pains*, *fainting*, *cerebral congestion*, *convulsions*, *hæmorrhage*.

ABSENCE OF PAINS may depend upon constitutional weakness, or upon transitory causes, such as passion, contrarieties, etc. *Secale*, *Pulsatilla* or *Opium*, in small doses will always prove useful.

SECALE is particularly suitable to feeble and cachectic women, or to such as have become exhausted by hæmorrhage. PULSATILLA, when the pains set in slowly in females of good constitution; or when the pains only affect the small of the back without benefitting the labor; in one word, when the absence of pains seems to be caused by inactivity of the uterus rather than by a general weakness of the constitution. OPIUM is suitable for robust women, the pains cease suddenly in consequence of a fright or some other violent emotion, with congestion of the head, red and puffed face, coma, etc. If the pains do not cease entirely, or are not entirely wanting, but are only slow and feeble, and do not progress regularly, without any known cause, and in the case of otherwise healthy patients, the best thing to be done is, not to give any medicine, but to wait patiently. However, if after the discharge of the amniotic fluid, the pains should still remain feeble and slow, we may give a dose of *Pulsatilla.* If the pains should have become suspended by some accidental cause, such as an unpleasant impression, the presence of a disagreeable person, strong odors, etc., all that is generally required is to remove these obstacles, after which the labor will resume its natural course.

FAINTING is an unpleasant symptom during labor, especially if it occurs at every pain; such an accident seriously threatens the patient's life. In most cases it is induced by an extreme dilatation of the uterus, but it may also be caused by deficient nourishment, previous hæmorrhage or other sickness, nervous debility, etc. The best remedies for this trouble are: *Nux vomica*, *Aconitum*, *Veratrum*, *Ignatia*, *Pulsatilla*, *Secale.* NUX VOMICA, in the case of feeble women, with nausea, pains in the stomach, anguish, trembling, pale face, etc. ACONITUM, for congestion of blood to the head, violent palpitation of the heart, alternate paleness and redness of the face. VERATRUM, if the patient is very weak, with coldness of the whole body and extremities, the attack comes on after the slightest effort, with anguish or convulsive movements. IGNATIA, especially for hysteric women, of a delicate constitution. PULSATILLA, if the attack depends upon an excessive distension of the womb, with inactive pains, signs of internal hæmorrhage. SECALE, if Pulsatilla is insufficient, or at the onset in the case of feeble and exhausted women.

CONGESTIONS OF THE HEAD which occur during labor, may become very serious and degenerate into real cerebral congestions or apoplexy. The best remedies are: *Aconitum*, *Pul-*

satilla, Opium, Belladonna, Arnica. ACONITUM, for headache, as if the head would split, with drowsiness, heaviness of the head, oppression, red and puffed face even during the intermission. PULSATILLA, for sopor, absence of muscular contraction, blueish-red face, violent palpitation of the heart, loss of pulse and stertorous breathing. OPIUM for heaviness of the head, vertigo followed by drowsiness, red, hot and bloated face, hot and sweaty head, red eyes with dilated and insensible pupils, slow and rattling breathing, convulsive rigidity of the body, twitching and trembling of the limbs, froth at the mouth. BELLADONNA, vertigo with the loss of consciousness and speech, twitching of the limbs and facial muscles, paralysis of the right side of the tongue, dysphagia, dilated pupils, red and puffed face. ARNICA, for full and strong pulse, symptoms of paralysis of the left side, loss of consciousness, dizziness, involuntary stool and urine. Dissolve in all these cases three globules in half a tumblerful of water, and give the patient a dessertspoonful of this solution every two or three hours according to circumstances.

CONVULSIONS are a most dangerous accident if occurring during labor; if increasing in intensity by any cause whatever, they become complicated with loss of consciousness and delirium, and are soon followed by the death of the mother and child. Nervous, timorous and sensitive women are most liable to such accidents, and such patients require to be watched with great care, in order that the attack may be arrested at the very onset. Encouraging advice will do a good deal towards quieting the patient; if medicines should be required, we may use *Aconitum, Coffea, Belladonna, Chamomilla, Opium* or *Ignatia*, which will often arrest the attack at once. But even if the physician should not arrive until the most violent convulsions have broken out, he will still be able to afford relief by an appropriate remedy, especially by ACONITUM, at the onset, if the face remains red between the paroxysms, with headache, glistening and sparkling eyes, impatience, restlessness, shortness of speech, etc. COFFEA, if Aconite does not quiet the patient at the beginning of the attack, especially suitable to sensitive women. CHAMOMILLA, sometimes after Coffea or Aconitum, if these remedies do not arrest the convulsions at the commencement, or if they set in in consequence of a fit of anger, with convulsive twitching during sleep, redness of the face on one, and paleness on the other side, hot sweat about the head and the face, convulsive motion of the eyes, lids and tongue, restlessness, irritable mood. BELLADONNA, congestion of the head, red and puffed or pale face, dilated pupils, convulsive twitching of the corners of the mouth, eyes and facial muscles, the attack is excited by the least contact or disappointment, with comatose sleep or sleeplessness between the attacks. IGNATIA, when the attack is caused by grief or chagrin, with throwing back of the head, alternate paleness and redness of the face, or redness of one and paleness of the other cheek, frequent yawning, twitching of the limbs, eye-lids and facial muscles. OPIUM, when the attack is caused by fright, with violent motion of the limbs, deep, comatose sleep, cries, choking turns. HYOSCYAMUS, blueish and bloated face, protruded eyes, convulsive jerking of the whole body, comatose drowsiness, delirious, tertorous breathing, or sleeplessness with anguish and restlessness.—STRAMONIUM, risus sardonicus, gaping or loss of speech, smiling face, or frightful visions, cries, moaning, desire to escape; the attacks are excited by touch or by the sight of shining objects.—Dissolve three globules of 12th to 18th attenuation, in half a tumblerful of water, and give a dessert-spoonful of this solution at every attack; if no improvement takes place after the second or third dose, select another remedy.

HÆMORRHAGE during labor may be external or internal. External hæmorrhage is readily perceived, but internal hæmorrhage sometimes attains to a very high degree of intensity before its existence is known. It is generally occasioned 1st, by the insertion of the placenta over the uterine orifice; 2d, by the tearing of the placenta; 3d, tearing or some other injury of the uterus; 4th, rupture of the umbilical vein or arteries; in any of these cases the blood may remain enclosed within the uterine cavity or be discharged externally. If it remains within the cavity, the patient experiences a sensation of heaviness or tension in the uterine region, which swells perceptibly, whatever be the cause of such an hæmorrhage, it is always a most formidable occurrence, and may terminate fatally. However, success may crown our efforts to assist the patient; whatever be the kind of hæmorrhage that we have to combat, three globules of *Arnica* in half a tumblerful of water, a dessertspoonful every fifteen or thirty minutes, will generally remove all immediate danger. If Arnica does not help soon, *Pulsatilla* will speedily bring about a suppression of the hæmorrhage and evacuation of the uterine cavity from all foreign contents. For other remedies we refer the reader to *Metrorrhagia*, (Sections 39, 43.)

ARTICLE VI.

DELIVERY OF THE PLACENTA.

Section 138.

Natural Delivery.—The delivery of the placenta terminates the process of labor. First, the placenta is detached from the womb by means of the uterine contractions during the expulsion of the fetus, on that the placenta is sometimes found completely detached and resting upon the neck of the uterus, as soon as the fetus is expelled. The presence of the detached placenta in the womb causes new contractions which are similar to, but weaker and longer than labor-pains. The neck of the uterus dilates, and the placenta passes into the vagina and rests upon the rectum. The final expulsion takes place by means of contractions of the diaphragm and of the abdominal muscles, and by the pressure which the abdominal viscera exercises upon the placenta. Sometimes this expulsion takes place immediately after the birth of the fetus: at other times there is an interval of fifteen minutes or several hours. As a general rule, delivery of the placenta takes place more promptly in robust than in feeble and exhausted women. In most cases the placenta comes down into the vagina without the assistance of the accoucheur; in other cases it has to be extracted by the accoucheur. Care should be had not to tear the placenta by unseasonable tractions; such injuries might give rise to violent hæmorrhage. If resistance is met with in gently pulling the cord, we have to wait until the placenta is entirely detached. Should this take place too slowly, we may give a small dose of *Pulsatilla* or *Secale*, three globules in half a tumblerful of water, a dessertspoonful every fifteen minutes; this would induce stronger and more successful contractions, and bring about a speedy delivery without any accidents.

SECTION 139.

DIFFICULT OR COMPLICATED DELIVERY.—In the preceding paragraph we have mentioned inertia of the uterus which may retard delivery; here we have to speak of *adhesions of the placenta*, *hæmorrhages*, *convulsions* and *fainting turns*, by which placental delivery is sometimes complicated in a serious manner.

PLACENTAL ADHESIONS may give rise to violent uterine hæmorrhages and inflammations, if the placenta remains in the uterus, or is only partially detached; for this reason some accoucheurs advise to remove the placenta on any account, even in pieces rather than to leave it in the uterus. Under homœopathic treatment a few globules of *Pulsatilla* or *Secale* will be sufficient to detach the placenta, or, if necessary, *Belladonna* and *Placenta* may be administered.

UTERINE HÆMORRHAGES during or after placental delivery may be caused by adhesions of the placenta, inertia of the uterus, insufficient uterine contractions leaving the mouths of the bleeding vessels open. Such hæmorrhage may likewise be internal or external. *Pulsatilla* and *Secale* will remove the difficulty, or we may have to give *Platina*, *Cocculus*, *China*, *Ipecacuanha*, *Chamomilla*, *Crocus*, *Ferrum*, *Sabina*, *Belladonna*. PLATINA, flooding, voluptuous tingling in the inner parts, with painful pressure in the small of the back and lower abdomen, as if the menses would appear. CROCUS, black and viscid blood, with movements in the abdomen, as of a living fetus. CHINA, thin, impoverished blood, weakness by previous losses. IPECACUANHA, flooding every now and then, with discharge of a red and thin blood. CHAMOMILLA, dark-red blood. FERRUM, profuse flooding with red blood mixed with black coagula, vascular excitement, and burning redness of the face. SABINA, bright-red blood, with pains like labor-pains. BELLADONNA, bearing-down upon the parts as if every thing would fall through. See *Metrorrhagia*, (Sections 39–43.)

CONVULSIONS which occur during or after delivery of the placenta, have to be treated like those occurring during labor, (Section 137.)

For FAINTING, we refer the reader to fainting during labor, (Section 137.)

ARTICLE VII.

OF REGULAR CONFINEMENT AND ATTENTIONS REQUIRED IN THE SICK-CHAMBER.

SECTION 140.

PHENOMENA AFTER PARTURITION.—After the expulsion of the fetus and the placenta, the uterine contractions still continue more or less until the uterus has resumed the conditions which it had before conception. This generally takes place in from twelve to fifteen days. The effect of these contractions is to expel the coagula or fluids which may have remained within the cavity or parenchyma of the uterus. These contractions or *after-pains* generally commence immediately after delivery of the placenta, soon reach their highest degree of intensity, and cease with the appearance of the milk-fever. Their intensity is sometimes proportionate to the number of confinements, and primiparæ are generally free from them. After an easy confinement they are likewise more severe than after tedious labor. They are readily distinguished from other pains by this, that they recur at regular intervals and are always followed by the expulsion of a coagulum or of a quantity of fluid.

Together with the after-pains the *lochial discharge* takes place, which is an expulsion of the fluids, blood and mucus that impregnated the walls of the uterus. The lochia generally commence shortly after the placental delivery; first a pure blood is discharged for twelve or fifteen hours; gradually this loses its consistence and dark color, and changes to a sanguineous serum, until the milk-fever sets in, during which the lochial discharge is generally interrupted, but after the termination of which the lochia resume their flow as a yellowish-white more or less thickish liquid. Hence we term them *sanguineous*, *serous*, *milky*, etc. The smell of the lochia is first insipid, but afterwards it becomes peculiarly fetid. They flow from two to four weeks, and among women who do not nurse their infants, they generally flow until the menses have resumed their course. In this case the lochia are generally more copious.

In consequence of these continued contractions and expulsions of fluids, the uterus gradually resumes its natural form and size. The uterine orifice which had remained dilated some time after confinement, contracts again upon itself, but remains a little larger, and the lips show the cicatrices of the fissures which the passage of the child had occasioned. The vagina becomes shorter, contracts again to a certain point, the rugæ reappear, and it resumes its original form but not as perfectly as the uterus. The vulva and the abdominal walls likewise experience the same changes, except that they retain the streaks which had formed during pregnancy, and which look like white veins traversing the abdominal walls.

At the same time the physiological condition of the woman undergoes a series of remarkable changes. The pulse which, shortly after the labor was contracted and frequent, becomes soft and large; the woman is feeble and prostrate, she feels weary in her whole body, is exceedingly sensitive to impressions, and a mild moisture breaks out upon the skin, which sometimes changes to a profuse sweet, having a sourish smell and causing a stinging sensation on the skin. At the end of two days, the milk-fever sets in; the breasts swell and become indurated, and towards the close of the fever, the distension of these parts reaches the highest degree. After this, the breasts become smaller, the secretion of milk goes on continuously and regularly during the period of nursing; but it decreases little by little if the woman does not nurse her infant.

Section 141.

Hygienic rules during confinement.—A strict and well regulated regimen during confinement may keep off a good many unpleasant accidents. The first thing to be attended to after parturition, is the comfort and cleanliness of the patient. The parts should be bathed with tepid water to which a few drops of the tincture of Arnica may be added, especially if the parts have been violently contused and torn during labor. After this we change the linen and other garments of the patient, taking care to dry and warm every article of clothing thoroughly before using it; lastly, we put her in a fresh bed, with her head sufficiently raised, and neck and arms covered so as to enable her to keep them outside of the bed-cover without being exposed to the danger of taking cold. As regards the bandage which is put on the patient by most accoucheurs in order to prevent the determination of fluids to the uterus and consequent inflammations of this organ or of the abdominal viscera, all we have to say is that inasmuch as the bandage keeps shifting all the time, it might just as well be omitted. The air of the sick-room ought to be neither too warm nor too cold, (about 52° F.) so as neither to give rise to any excessive sweating nor to check the gentle cutaneous moisture which is so useful to women in confinement; ventilation should not be neglected, but care must be had not to expose the patient to the direct contact of the air; exposure to strong light or to loud noise should likewise be avoided. The patient should be kept perfectly clean; the parts have to be bathed very frequently; every day the linen should be changed likewise. The food should be of easy digestion, moderate in quantity, not stimulating; a little soup three times a day until the milk fever sets in;

during this fever, the patient may take some broth ; gradually the quantity of nourishment may be increased until the usual mode of life can be permitted again without any danger to the patient. Wine, coffee, tea, stimulating drinks which are supposed to promote the secretion of milk, should be avoided as injurious ; most of these preparations predispose for fevers, and give rise to copious sweats and even inflammations ; the abuse of chamomile tea, which is unfortunately so universal and so inveterate, occasions flooding, inflammation of the abdominal viscera, convulsions, etc, ; coffee not only deranges the nervous system of the mother, and excites the circulatory organs, but likewise prepares the way for a difficult digestion and for all the ailments inherent in this trouble. Water, either pure or with a little sugar or a few drops of claret, is the best beverage for women in confinement. Fomentations of warm vapors to the sexual parts for the purpose of removing the dysuria by which the patients are so often troubled, or the use of cathartics in order to keep the bowels open, should likewise be avoided, inasmuch as we possess excellent means to obtain these results, without resorting to any of the above contrivances. In order to prevent uterine prolapsus which is apt to be occasioned by the laxity of the parts and the weakness of the ligaments, the patient should keep quiet until the parts are restored to their former strength. The patients should certainly be kept in bed for nine or ten days at least. Sleep is an excellent restorer of strength in the case of confined women. The old school resorts to opium to procure it ; in homœopathy we have other and better means of which we shall treat by and by. The most precious thing for such patients is internal tranquillity ; hence, their senses, imagination or feelings should be left undisturbed ; frequent visits and social gatherings around her bed would fatigue her, and should never be permitted during the first ten days.—Lastly, is it necessary to remind the young mother of the duty imposed upon her, of nursing her infant ? Nursing is too intimately interwoven with the whole organism of the mother to be neglected without injury to both mother and child. Only if the mother is too feeble, or the milk is wanting, other means of feeding the infant, may be resorted to.

Section 142.

Medical attentions during confinement.—These attentions consist in 1st, *repairing the injuries* which the parts may have suffered after confinement, such as *contusions of the vulva, rupture of the perineum! prolapsus of the womb, piles, contusions of the neck of the bladder and of the urethra, etc.;* 2d, in attending to the *after-pains, lochia* and, if the patients do not nurse their infants, to the *secretion of milk;* 3d, *in restoring the exhausted strength of the patient,* we shall treat of each of these subjects, uniting in the next article all that we have to say concerning the accidents which may occur during confinement, such as *puerperal fever, metritis, phlegmasia alba, miliaria, etc.*

In regard to contusions of the vulva, we have already said, (Section 141,) that the parts may be bathed with tepid water, in which a few drops of the tincture of Arnica are mixed. If inflammatory symptoms should have developed themselves, *Mercurius, Belladonna* or *Thuja*, may be given internally. If an abscess should have formed, *Mercurius* will favor its coming to a head, unless *Belladonna* or *Lachesis* should have brought about its dispersion.

Rupture of the perinæum is not near as terrible an accident under homœopathic treatment as it is under the old school management. As soon as the accident is known we should bathe the parts with Arnica-water, brings the edges the wound in contact, and apply a pad of lint thoroughly soaked with pure Arnica. Over this pad thick compresses moistened with Arnica-water may be applied, over which two bands are to cross each other, proceeding from a large bandage around the pelvis and coming down to the thighs, which bands cross each other opposite the perinæum and are fastened to the main bandage, one on each side near the groin, in such a manner as to hold the edges of the wound necessarily juxtaposed. The patient should be kept quiet, in bed, on one side, and the bandage should be frequently changed during the first days, in order to facilitate the lochial discharge; afterwards, after the lochia are decreased, the bandage need only be renewed if the patient wants to urinate. Croserio advises the use of the strong tincture of Arnica, which is sufficiently diluted by the water that is discharged from the uterus in tolerably copious quantity and is imbibed by the compresses; but as soon as the lochial discharge decreases, Arnica-water may be resorted to. By continuing this treatment for some six weeks with care, the wound will be found healed perfectly.

PROLAPSUS AND INVERSION OF THE UTERUS, accidents that happen pretty frequently after tedious labor, are likewise readily cured by internal homœopathic treatment save such manual operations as are absolutely indispensable to replace the womb in its natural position. The patient should be kept quiet as we stated in Section 62, and a small dose of *Nux vomica*, or *Sepia*, in case Nux should not help, may be given, three globules of 30th attenuation, in half a tumblerful of water, in dessertspoonful doses, morning and evening, this treatment will help, provided the patient is kept on her back as long as she feels a weight in the uterine region when rising. If neither Nux nor Sepia should be indicated, we may have to resort to *Thuja* or *Platina*.

CONTUSIONS OF THE NECK OF THE BLADDER AND OF THE URETHRA, caused by the pressure which the head of the child in the pelvis makes upon these parts, sometimes cause retention or incontinence of urine during confinement. Either of these difficulties yields to *Belladonna* in small doses. If insufficient we may give for RETENTION, *Pulsatilla;* for INCONTINENCE OF URINE, *Sepia* or *Sulphur*.

PILES yield most generally to *Pulsatilla*, three globules of 12th attenuation in half a tumblerful of water, a dessertspoonful of which solution should be given every three or four hours.

AFTER PAINS, though resulting from the necessary contractions of the uterus after parturition by means of which this organ returns to its normal condition, may be modified, in case the pain should be too acute, by a small dose of *Coffea*, especially in the case of nervous women who are sensitive to pain and deprived of their usual sleep. If Coffea should not suffice, *Nux vomica* may be resorted to, especially if the pains bear upon the rectum or bladder, with frequent desire to evacuate the bowels or bladder ; or *Chamomilla*, in the case of women who have drank a good deal of coffee, and if Nux does not afford any relief; *Pulsatilla*, if fragments of the placenta have remained in the uterus.

The LOCHIA may either be too scanty or too profuse, or altered in their quality. If too scanty or suppressed, and if this condition does not depend upon any other cause, *Aconitum* will restore them, if they were still red, and a cold or sudden emotion caused the suppression; or *Chamomilla*, if the suppression is followed by diarrhœa and colic, or by headache, toothache or other aches. If the suppression is symptomatic, arising from metritis, peritonitis, enteritis, or from some other disease, or if inflammatory symptoms threaten to develop themselves in consequence of the suppression, the remedies which have been prescribed for these affections, will have to be indicated ; we may likewise give *Aconitum*, if there are symptoms of inflammatory fever ; *Colocynthis*, if the abdomen is distended ; *Belladonna*, *Hyoscyamus* or *Stramonium*, if the brain is deranged, with frightful visions, delirium, etc. ; *Platina* or *Zincum*, if the symptoms of nymphomania set in.

As regards EXCESSIVE LOCHIA, we have to distinguish between the periods when the excessive flow takes place. If it takes place while the lochia are still red, we have to prescribe the remedies that have been indicated for metrorrhagia or for excessive menstruation, such as, *Platina*, *China*, *Calcarea*, *Rhus*, or *Secale*, unless the symptoms should indicate *Bryonia*, *Crocus*, *Hepar*, *Conium*, or *Bromium*. If the white or mucous lochia are excessive, this symptom indicates an irritation in the lining membrane of the uterus, and has to be treated like leucorrhœa, with *Pulsatilla*, *Sepia*, *Sulphur* or *Calcarea.* If the red lochia continue too long, *Calcarea* or *China* will hasten their transformation into mucous discharges. If the excess of red lochia depends upon wrong diet, a change of diet will remove the difficulty; if this should not be the case, we may give *Coffea, Ignatia* or *Nux vomica,* if the patient have used much Chamomile tea; *Arnica* or *China,* if the difficulty arises from excessive bodily exertions; *Nux vomica,* if the patient has indulged in coffee, or alcoholic or heating beverages and aliments.

ALTERED LOCHIA, black, purulent, etc., indicate an irritation of the uterine lining membrane, and require no other treatment beside the general uterine affection. In some cases some special remedy may be indicated, such as *Calcarea* or *Sepia,* if the mucous lochia become again bloody; *Sepia, Mercurius* or *China,* if they become purulent; *Carbo animalis, Belladonna, Secale, Kreosotum* or *Sepia,* if they have a putrid smell. Black lochia, which generally arise from the decomposition of patches of membrane or bloody coagula in the uterus, do not require any treatment, unless there should be a peculiar foul smell or other symptoms denoting putrefaction or gangrene of the uterus.

MILK-FEVER, which generally commences on the second or third day after confinement, does not require any treatment, especially if the woman nurses her infant, and the milk can be drawn out as soon as it commences to flow. If the woman does not nurse her infant, the fever may become complicated with other ailments which it is necessary to prevent. For this purpose we use *Aconitum, Bryonia* or *Belladonna*; ACONITUM, if there be much fever with marked heat, full and strong pulse, violent headache and a good deal of thirst. BELLADONNA, if symptoms of cerebral inflammation set in, with stupefying headache, more or less marked delirium, glistening eyes, red and hot or else very pale face; BRYONIA, if the breasts become too much distended by the milk, with painful oppression of the chest; or PULSATILLA, if after the cessation of the fever and the adoption of a somewhat more nutritive diet, the milk still continues to increase in the breast.

If the milk should continue to flow out in spite of Pulsatilla, we may give *Calcarea* or *Lycopodium*. The accessory ailments which may occur during lactation, will be described in Sections 149–153, in a continuous series.

As regards the RESTORATION OF STRENGTH after confinement, no particular treatment is required for such a purpose; if no serious derangement has taken place, the strength will speedily return by means of a good diet and rest; and if existing diseases prevent the restoration of strength, these have to be treated with suitable remedies. If the patient should have become exhausted by FLOODING or by excessive SWEATS, we may give her six globules of *China* dissolved in half a tumblerful of water, a dessertspoonful of which solution is to be given every twelve hours; or *Calcarea*, *Kali*, *Sulphur*, *Nuxv omica*, *Phosphori acidum*, *Veratrum*. If the weakness should cause excessive SWEATING, we may give *Carbo vegetabilis*, *Aconitum*, *Arsenicum*. *Sambucus*. The FALLING OFF OF THE HAIR which sometimes cannot be prevented after confinement even by the greatest care, soon ceases after using *Sulphur* or *Calcarea*, three globules dry on the tongue, which are to be allowed to act for four or five weeks. If these remedies do not help, we may try *Natrum muriaticum*, *Lycopodium*, *Hepar* or *Silicea*. Another inconvenience which sometimes befals women who have had several children, is an enlargement of the abdomen, vulgarly termed pot-bellied; this defect requires to be treated with *Sepia*, *Colocynthis*, three globules every week.

ARTICLE VIII.

DISEASES OF WOMEN DURING CONFINEMENT.

SECTION 143.

GENERAL OBSERVATIONS.—The peculiar sensitiveness to external impressions which child-birth excites in the organism of the young mother, exposes her more at this than at any other period to the action of the epidemic type of disease or to other disturbing influences which develop diseases characterised by symptoms peculiar to the changed condition of the system. Such diseases are inflammatory affections which principally invade the parts that have suffered most during the process of labor and during pregnancy. Hence the frequency of metritis, peritonitis, ovaritis, enteritis and other similar affections during confinement; even the thoracic organs and the brain are frequently attacked with inflammatory diseases. These affections generally run a rapid course, and show a tendency to terminate in suppuration or effusions of purulent serum; in most cases these inflammations are accompanied by suppression of the milk and lochia, thus complicating the existing inflammation by other affections. The arrest of perspiration likewise, becomes the frequent cause of acute or chronic rheumatism which may attack the articulations of the pelvic bones; or such a suppression of the perspiration may cause an inflammation of the pelvic veins known under the name of phlegmasia and alba dolens, or an inflammation of the ganglious and lymphatic vessels of the extremities. To these diseases we have to add some neuroses, such as hysteria and mania, and the so-called *milk-affections*. In the following chapters we will treat of: — 1st, *puerperal fevers;* 2d, *local diseases of the uterine tissue;* 3d, *abdominal affections;* 4th, *cerebral affections;* 5th, *external diseases of women in confinement*, omitting for the present the affections of the milk which will be treated in the chapter on *lactation.*

Section 144.

Puerperal fevers.—The affections of this class, with marked febrile symptoms, are:—*puerperal peritonitis, uterine phlebitis* and *adynamic fevers* during confinement. Acute metritis and phlegmasia alba dolens do not belong to this category, inasmuch as neither of these affections has the characteristic signs of a puerperal inflammation. In this Article we will describe the symptoms of each of these fevers, and then proceed to indicate their causes and treatment.

Puerperal peritonitis is the most frequent and one of the most dangerous of puerperal fevers. It generally develops itself the first eight days after parturition, and it is sometimes preceded by a general malaise with a slight diarrhœa. Most frequently, however, it comes on suddenly, with vague shiverings or a violent chill, followed by heat, more or less frequent paroxysms of vomiting, and an acute stinging pain, increased by pressure, touch, straining when vomiting, or at stool, or when voiding the urine, or by the least motion in bed. The pain is at first confined to the hypogastrium and remains most violent in this region, even if the pain should extend to other parts of the abdomen. At the same time the lochia become less, or are entirely suppressed; the breasts do not expand, or they sink in after having been filled with milk; the secretion of milk either does not come on or stops; the abdomen acquires in a few days a considerable volume in consequence of the effusion that takes place in this cavity, and we generally perceive there the same fluctuation as in ascites. In ordinary cases, puerperal peritonitis does not last very long, and if it terminates successfully, the volume of the abdomen decreases as rapidly as it had increased previously; the lochia reappear, the breasts swell, and the secretion of milk sometimes resumes its course.

Uterine phlebitis is much more serious, but fortunately

much less frequent than puerperal peritonitis. It generally commences about twenty-four hours after parturition with a more or less acute pain in the region of the womb, accompanied or followed by violent shiverings, with suppression of the lochia, quick pulse, headache or slight delirium, sense of distress all over, and sometimes nausea and vomiting. These symptoms are sometimes followed by heat and muscular twitches in the face and extremities, hurried and feeble pulse, anxious and hurried breathing, intense thirst, brown and dry tongue. Sometimes effusions of pus take place in the lungs, pleural cavities, cellular tissue, etc. Under Old-School treatment, this frightful disease generally terminates fatally.

ADYNAMIC FEVER, which is the most serious fever that befals women during confinement, generally sets in on the second or third day after parturition, and the danger is so much greater the nearer to this period the invasion of the disease takes place. Sometimes the fever commences like a simple puerperal peritonitis, but soon after cerebral symptoms supervene, the sight becomes obscured, sparks are seen before the eyes, and a buzzing in the ears is felt; the muscles and lower extremities begin to twitch, delirium, twitching of the tendons and picking at flocks set in. At the same time the mouth becomes dry, the tongue becomes covered with a thick and brownish coating, the features become altered, the nose looks pointed, the breathing is hurried, sighing and moaning, and the patient is tormented by an unquenchable thirst. In some cases petechiæ, miliaria alba, convulsions and furibond delirium supervene. Towards the close, the face becomes excessively pale, the look becomes fixed and fierce, the mouth exhales a stream of hot and foul air; colliquative, clammy sweats break out; a watery, greenish-brown, foul-smelling diarrhœa sets in, and death finally takes place by paralysis of the abdominal or cerebral nerves, or by gangrene of the affected parts.

The most frequent CAUSES of these fevers are:—violent irritations of the uterus by tedious and hard labor; manual or instrumental operations for turning or destroying the child;

astringent injections, sudden suppression of the lochia and milk by any physical or moral cause, exposure to cold air, violent emotions such as fright, joy, anger, etc. Dietetic transgressions, excessive eating on the part of women who do not nurse their own children, heating or stimulating food, purgatives, chamomile-tea, infusions of juniper-berries, irritations of the urinary passages by diuretics, etc., may likewise be considered as exciting causes of this fever. In lying-in hospitals the disease sometimes becomes epidemic without any apparent cause. It is as an epidemic disease that the fever exhibits the dangerous character of cerebral typhus described above.

These fevers can sometimes be prevented by proper diet and a careful removal of all disturbing influences either physical or moral. But if the disease has set in in spite of our precautions, we often succeed in breaking the fever, if we give at the very onset of the disease *Aconitum*, six globules of eighteenth attenuation, in half a tumblerful of water, of which solution a dessert-spoonful should be given every three hours until the disease is conquered, especially if the following symptoms are present:—excessive dry and burning heat, glowing redness of the face, bilious vomiting, unquenchable thirst, excessive sensitiveness to pain, disconsolate anguish with restlessness and moaning, and especially *dread of death*, warm baths, etc., should of course be avoided. Pure water should be the patient's only drink, and a strict diet should be enjoined. If we should be called too late for *Aconitum*, or if Aconitum should prove ineffectual after twenty-four, or, in very acute cases, after twelve hours, we have to resort to *Belladonna*, *Mercurius*, *Nux vomica*, *Bryonia*, *Rhus*, *Chamomilla*, *Cocculus*, *Hyoscyamus*, *Platina*, *Arsenicum*, *Carbo vegetabilis*, *Sulphur*, *Pulsatilla*, *Arnica*, *Opium*.

And particularly:—

In simple PUERPERAL PERITONITIS:—*Mercurius*, *Bryonia*, *Chamomilla*, *Belladonna*, *Sulphur*, *Hyoscyamus*, *Platina*, *Nux vomica*, *Colocynthis*, etc.

In UTERINE PHLEBITIS:—*Belladonna, Mercurius, Arsenicum, Rhus, Bryonia, Pulsatilla, Arnica, Nux vomica*, etc.

In ADYNAMIC FEVER:—*Belladonna, Bryonia, Rhus, Mercurius, Hyoscyamus, Arsenicum, Carbo vegetabilis, Sulphur*, etc.

But independently of names, the homœopathic physician will have to be guided in the selection of his remedy by the following symptomatic indications:

BELLADONNA, for distension of the abdomen with tympanitic resonance on percussion, stinging and digging pains, *or as if the bowels were grasped by claws or nails;* violent pressure towards the genital organs, as if every thing would be pressed out there; sensitiveness of the abdomen to contact; partial shuddering, with burning heat of the head and face, redness of the face and eyes, frontal headache with pressure, throbbing of the carotids; dry mouth, with thirst and red tongue; *dysphagia and spasms in the fauces;* cerebral symptoms such as furibond delirium and comatose sleep, or complete loss of sleep; also, scanty watery or mucous lachia; or *uterine hæmorrhage* with discharge of coagulated and fetid blood; empty and flabby breasts or else swollen and inflamed.

MERCURIUS, in many cases where Belladonna is not sufficient, or in alternation with Belladonna, especially when the cerebral symptoms are less marked than the symptoms of the abdomen, or when signs of effusion are developed, with lancinating, pressive and boring pains; constant moaning; excessive sensitiveness of the abdominal integuments to the least touch and motion; burning and unquenchable thirst; altered, yellowish or earthy countenance; profuse ptyalism; mucous and bloody stool with tenesmus; dark and fetid urine; sweat all over, profuse and weakening, with nocturnal aggravation of all the symptoms.

NUX VOMICA, sudden suppression of the lochia, with weight and burning in the abdomen and sexual organs; or profuse lochia, with violent pains in the small of the back; strangury and burning urine; *constipation, nausea and vomiting;* red face; rheumatic and crampy pains in the thighs and legs, with numbness of these parts; pressive headache with vertigo, buzzing in the ears, fainting turns and vanishing of sight; especially suitable to women who have indulged in spirits and chamomile-tea.

BRYONIA, sometimes after *Aconitum*, if this is not sufficient, or at the onset for the following symptoms; *sensitiveness of the abdomen* to the least touch or motion, with constipation; lancinating pains in the abdomen, worse by pressure; violent fever, with burning heat all over, burning thirst and desire for cold drinks, irritable, irascible mood, with dread of the future, and concern about her sickness.

RHUS, sometimes indispensable if cerebral or typhoid symptoms exist from the first, with aggravation by the least unpleasantness, return of bloody lochia in the place of mucus, discharge of coagula.

CHAMOMILLA, flabby and empty breasts with whitish diarrhœa, scanty lochia, distention and sensitiveness of the abdomen to touch; colic like labor-pains; heat all over with red face and thirst; nocturnal aggravation of the pains, followed by sweat: restlessness, impatience and nervousness; the disease was caused by anger or exposure of the body to cold.

COLOCYNTHIS, if Chamomilla is insufficient in cases where the disease was caused by a fit of anger, especially for the following symptoms: violent pains in the abdomen, dry and burning heat, diarrhœa and colic after the least drink; hard, full and hurried pulse; hot head and red face; delirium alternating with comatose sleep; symptoms of cerebral paralysis, with the lower jaw depressed.

HYOSCYAMUS, if Belladonna is insufficient for the cerebral and typhoid symptoms, with frightful visions or loss of consciousness, frequent discharge of coagulated blood, convulsions and spasms in the throat.

PLATINA, excited sexual instinct, signs of nymphomania with voluptuous crawling in the parts; painful pressure at the hypogastrium and on the parts, like labor-pains; discharge of a thick and black blood; sensitiveness of the parts; headache, restlessness and weeping; especially suitable to women of a proud disposition.

Arsenicum, if Mercurius is insufficient in cases where effusion in the peritoneum has taken place, with great weakness; pale, earthy and altered countenance, frequent desire for cold drinks, of which the patient only takes a little at a time.

Carbo vegetabilis, sometimes in the last extremity, if neither Arsenicum nor Mercurius help in cases of effusion.

Sulphur, suitable to women who are subject to chronic eruptions, or when the following symptoms occur: violent colic, excessive distension of the abdomen and pains in the small of the back; suppression or decrease of the lochia; tenesmus of the rectum and bladder; violent pains in the hypogastrium, with heat, shivering and epileptiform convulsions.

Of all these remedies dissolve three globules of 6th or 12th attenuation, in half a tumblerful of water, and give the patient a dessert-spoonful of this solution every three hours.

Section 145.

Local derangements of the uterine system.—The most frequent of these affections during confinement are; *acute metritis, ovaritis, uterine hæmorrhage and gangrene of the uterus.* To what has been said concerning these affections in other parts of this work, we have to add the following:

Puerperal metritis generally requires the same treatment as parenchymatous metritis, Sections 70–71. The disease is most frequently induced by the following causes: dietetic transgressions, cold drinking soon after confinement, exposure to a draught of air, moral emotions, premature resumption of sexual intercourse, violent exercise and mechanical injury during confinement, astringent injections, suppression of the lochia, and any physical or moral cause by which such a suppression may be induced. If no peritonitis is as yet developed, three globules of *Nux vomica*, 18th attenuation, dry on the tongue, will generally prove sufficient to arrest the disease. If other affections should complicate the disease, or if Nux should not be sufficient, we may give the following remedies: *Belladonna*, *Bryonia*, *Chamomilla*, *Rhus*, *Colocynthis*, *Aconitum*, or: *Hyoscyamus*, *Mercurius*, *Platina*, *Pulsatilla*, *Secale*, *Arsenicum*, *Stramonium*, *Veratrum*, *Arnica*, *Lachesis*.—For special indications concerning the use of these remedies, we refer the reader to Sections 70–71.

PUERPERAL OVARITIS does not differ from acute ovaritis, described Section 92, with the treatment. During confinement the disease may be treated most successfully with *Belladonna*, *Platina*, *Mercurius*, *Sabina*.

UTERINE HÆMORRHAGE during confinement requires to be treated like hæmorrhage during labor, Section 139. If resulting from general debility, *China* is an excellent remedy. In other cases *Sabina*, *Platina*, or *Crocus* will prove efficient. See, also, the remedies mentioned Section 139, and Metrorrhagia, Sections 42–43.

GANGRENE OR PUTRESCENCE OF THE UTERUS, is the most dreadful accident that can occur during confinement, and is often not perceived until it is too late to do any good. For the symptoms and treatment of this disease, we refer our readers to Section 89.

PROLAPSUS AND INVERSION OF THE WOMB, have been spoken of in detail, Section 142.

SECTION 146.

ABDOMINAL AFFECTIONS.—The abdominal affections that may take place during confinement, are: *deep-seated enteritis, superficial enteritis or diarrhœa, and constipation.*

DEEP-SEATED OR PHLEGMONOUS ENTERITIS, does not occur very frequently as a sequel of confinement; if it should, however, we may give three globules of *Aconitum*, in half a tumblerful of water, a dessert-spoonful of which solution should be administered every three hours until the fever ceases; or, if *Aconitum* should not prove sufficient, we may give *Belladonna*, *Bryonia*, *Nux vomica*, or *Colocynthis* If peritonitis should supervene, we have to use the remedies recommended for puerperal peritonitis, Section 144.—For COLIC during confinement we give: *Chamomilla*, *Bryonia*; or, *Belladonna*, *Hyoscyamus*, *Pulsatilla*, *Sepia*, *Veratrum*, *Arnica*, *Lachesis*, *Nux vomica*.

SUPERFICIAL ENTERITIS OR DIARRHŒA during confinement is less to be dreaded for its inherent intensity than for the derangement it causes in the milky secretion. If the patient has not indulged too freely in chamomile tea, the best remedy for this trouble is *Chamomilla*, especially when there is colic, watery, greenish or yellowish stools, the latter looking like stirred eggs. Women who have used much chamomile tea or who have deranged their stomachs by overeating, should take *Pulsatilla*. If the stools are papescent, fermented, having a marked sour smell, we give RHUBARB. Sometimes *Antimonium* will help, especially when there are gastric symptoms, white-coated tongue, nausea, eructations, sticky mouth, etc., or *Dulcamara*, if the diarrhœa is caused by a cold; or *Hyoscyamus* for painless, watery and mucous stools.

CONSTIPATION occurring the first week after confinement, is a sign that the patient is getting better and stronger, and should therefore be left undisturbed by treatment. If the constipation should continue beyond this space of time, a few globules of *Bryonia* may be given one evening and another dose the next. If *Bryonia* should not help, we may give *Nux vomica*, six globules in half a tumblerful of water, and a dessert-spoonful of this solution every evening until the patient is quite easy; Nux is particularly indicated by piles, distension of the abdomen and loss of appetite; or *Opium* for inertia of the bowels, with complete absence to all urging to stool; or *Sulphur* if none of the other remedies help; in some cases *Platina* may be useful. If the constipation is owing to the hardness and size of the excrements, an injection of tepid water may remove the difficulty.

Section 147.

Cerebral affections.—These affections during confinement, are: *puerperal meningitis* and *mental derangement.*

Puerperal meningitis is never an idiopathic disease, but only occurs as a distressing accessory of one of the above-mentioned puerperal fevers. It is characterised by the usual cerebral symptoms, such as furibond delirium, sopor, twitching of the tendons and muscles, grasping at flocks, loss of sight, sparks before the eyes, buzzing in the ears, dry mouth, brown-coated tongue, etc., and generally violent headache and vertigo. The best remedies for these symptoms are: *Aconite, Belladonna, Bryonia, Rhus, Colocynthis, Sulphur,* etc.; for the particular indications concerning the use of these remedies we refer the reader to Section 144.

Mental derangement generally commences already during pregnancy; the patient is sad, has sinister forebodings and shows a good deal of restlessness without any appreciable cause. The face is generally pale; she complains of pain in the uterine region; the pulse is small, feeble, contracted. The real dementia generally develops itself during confinement and the period of nursing. The patient is altogether irrational, has frequent hallucinations during which the patient sees her child consumed by fire or drowned; the strangest fancies sometimes chase each other with the most wonderful rapidity. In some cases the dementia is complicated with furious mania, nymphomania, etc.; whereas in other cases we observe a deep, taciturn melancholy; sometimes there is complete dementia. The most frequent causes of this derangement are: a cold, fright, domestic trouble or other unpleasant emotions, sudden weaning, suppression of the lochia and milky secretion. This derangement may last from one to six months, and may have frequent relapses. If not radically cured, the patients sometimes remain for ever subject to hysterical or other convulsions, or to fixed ideas, melancholy or attacks of dementia with or without paralysis. This affection is rather easily cured by *Aconite, Aurum, Bel-*

ladonna, *Pulsatilla*, *Platina*, *Sulphur*, *Veratrum*, *Stramonium*, *Zincum*. ACONITUM is indicated by fear of death, and if the derangement was caused by fright; AURUM, anguish with thoughts of suicide, weakness of memory and intellect; BELLADONNA, restless and uneasy nights, fear of ghosts, fright with desire to escape or to hide herself, paroxysms of rage and fury; PULSATILLA, sad thoughts, weeping mood, taciturn disposition, the patient remains in one corner, embraces her knees and gesticulates like a crazy person, acid stomach, gastralgia; PLATINA, excessive sexual desires, with voluptuous crawling in the parts; SULPHUR, disposition to meditate on religious subjects, with despair of salvation; forgets the names and words she wants to use; VERATRUM for religious melancholy or nymphomania with desire to embrace every body; STRAMONIUM for nymphomania, with obscene gestures and language, the body smells like that of a goat; ZINCUM for nymphomania or melancholy during confinement, with fear of thieves, demons and other frightful figures; HYOSCYAMUS for nymphomania with furor, loss of modesty, desire to uncover one's self, etc.

Dissolve any of these remedies in half a tumblerful of water, 6 globules of 6th or 12th attenuation, and give a dessertspoonful of this solution every three hours.

SECTION 148.

EXTERNAL AFFECTIONS.—These are *phlegmasia alba dolens* and *miliaria*.

PHLEGMASIA ALBA DOLENS is considered by many authors a symptom of puerperal fever, and is characterised by a white, smooth and hot swelling, sometimes affecting one limb only, and consisting in an inflammation of the veins of these extremities or of the veins of the pelvis. It is a species of external phlebitis having the same characteristic signs as uterine phlebitis and depending upon similar influences which, however, produce different symptoms owing to the difference in the tissues and organs affected. Phlegmasia generally runs a slow course and exists without fever; but in some cases it may give rise to acute inflammations and even terminate in gangrene. If treated improperly, the trouble may last from six to nine months, and even if the disease terminates favorably at the end of this period, the affected limb preserves for a long time afterwards a great weakness and sensitiveness to contact and motion. Bleeding is a highly improper proceeding in this disease, and although the homœopathic treatment is not free from danger, yet if the remedies are well chosen, a cure is generally effected by ACONITUM, if the phlegmasia has an acute character, with violent inflammatory fever, heat all over and violent pains;—ARNICA, if the phlegmasia sets in after tedious labor, violent manipulations or mechanical injuries of the vessels;—BRYONIA, drawing or *lancinating pains from the hip to the foot*, with copious sweat and excessive *sensitiveness to touch or motion;* pulling in the abdomen and legs as if the menses would appear; painful rigidity and tension and pale swelling of the leg;—*Belladonna*, stitches as with knives; heaviness in the thighs, hypogastrium and sexual parts; creeping in the limbs, with paralytic weakness; violent fever with burning thirst, violent pains disturbing her sleep, and not permitting either motion or contact;—PULSATILLA, if Belladonna or Bryonia have effected no improvement. We may also recommend *Rhus*, *Sulphur*, *Nux vomica*, *Arsenicum*.

MILIARIA during confinement is not very dangerous in itself, but may become so by improper treatment with sodorifics, purgatives, warm infusions and other debilitating decoctions and herb-teas. Too much covering in bed or an excessive temperature in the sick chamber excites copious sweats and consequently such an eruption as the one here mentioned. By avoiding every thing that might excite such sweats, and by simply preserving a little gentle moisture upon the skin, the miliaria generally disappears of itself in a day or two. Should it nevertheless prove obstinate and troublesome, we may give *Bryonia*, three globules dry on the tongue, which may be allowed to act for twenty-four hours.

ARTICLE IX.

OF LACTATION AND OF THE ATTENTIONS REQUIRED BY THIS FUNCTION.

SECTION 149.

GENERAL PHENOMENA.—The secretion of milk continues during the whole period of pregnancy; the breasts become harder and larger, discharging sooner or later a serous fluid which is the first appearance of the future milk, and immediately after confinement, becomes changed into a yellowish liquid of a sweetish taste, and known under the name of *colostrum.* Forty-eight hours after parturition, the breasts swell and harden in a marked manner; the patient experiences slight chills followed by heat of the skin, and in few hours, by a profuse perspiration; the face becomes red and animated; there is headache, loss of appetite, white-coated tongue, suppression or diminution of the lochia and hurried pulse. This fever which must not be confounded with puerperal fever, is the *milk-fever* which, from a slight fever of some twelve hours duration, may increase to an inflammatory fever of some three or four days. It can be distinguished from puerperal peritonitis by the fact that the abdomen is never painful to pressure. At the close of the fever, the breasts which had become very much distended, become softer, the milk flows out spontaneously, the lochia return, and the mother whose condition has again become normal, is able to nurse her infant.

The SECRETION OF MILK, if once established, goes on uninterruptedly; but various circumstances may induce an excessive secretion of milk, with a tingling and stinging sensation in the breasts, the milk sometimes spirting out from the nipples with considerable force. This will sometimes take place as soon as the child is held near the breast, or even at the mere sight or thought of a child. This rush of milk may likewise take place without its cause being known; but it almost always takes place as soon as the child commences to nurse. The act of nursing is an indispensable excitant by means of which the secretion of milk is kept up. In women who from one cause or another do not nurse their little ones, the milk soon dries up, whereas by nursing the child, the secretion of milk may sometimes continue for several years. It appears, moreover, that it is an infant's mouth that has to draw out the milk; for if the milk be drawn by an adult or by some mechanical contrivance, the breasts are indeed emptied, but the secretion soon ceases. By the act of nursing infants have been able to excite a flow of milk for months even in females who were still far remote from the period of confinement, or in women of sixty years old, or even in young girls and males. Nevertheless there are cases where the secretion of milk ceases even if the nursing be steadily continued. Some wet-nurses have been able to have children at the breasts for seven years and longer, but there are likewise cases where the milk ceased to flow at the end of a month in spite of nursing.

As regards the milk itself, it may vary both in quantity and quality. The quantity especially varies a good deal in different women. Some have milk enough to nurse several children at once, whereas others have scarcely milk enough for one. In some cases scarcely any milk is secreted. As a general rule, after a first confinement, less milk is secreted than after subsequent confinements; on the other hand, there are women with large breasts who secrete less milk at every subsequent confinement, until the secretion ceases altogether after the third or fourth. As regards quality, the milk of some women is too watery to serve as nourishment; in other women, the chemical constituents of the milk are altered, imparting to the milk a saltish or bitter taste, beside other alterations not perceptible to external observers, but sufficient to excite an aversion in the child. Even good and healthy milk will sometimes vary in its nutritive properties, being in the course of twenty-four hours more or less creamy and consistent. It is generally supposed that lymphatic women have more milk, but more serous and less nourishing than others. Moreover, the more actively the secretion of milk is going on in consequence of excitable influences, the thicker and fatter does the milk become. There is probably no secretion which is more influenced by the general causes that affect health and nutrition, than the secretion of milk. The nature and quantity of the food which is used by the mother, affect the milk; the odour, taste and color, and even the medicinal properties of the substances which the mother takes into her stomach, impart similar conditions to the milk; chagrin, fright, anger and other moral emotions suddenly alter both the quantity and quality of the milk, so as to cause the most serious accidents in the child that nurses it. The diseases by which the nursing mother happens to be attacked, likewise affect the milk. If the catamenia reappear during the period of nursing, or the mother should again become pregnant, the quantity and consistence of the milk are likewise lessened; in most cases pregnancy stops the secretion of milk, or alters the milk to such a degree that the child is unwilling to nurse or is made sick by the milk. It seldom happens that pregnancy leaves the milk unchanged.

Section 150.

Hygienic attentions during lactation.—It is of great importance that nothing should occur which might impede or arrest the secretion of milk, or alter and diminish the nutritive qualities of this fluid. It follows from what we have stated in the preceding paragraph concerning the influence of food on the qualities of the milk, that the mother has to be very particular in the choice of her nourishment in order to impart to the milk such properties as will make it a wholesome and nutritive agent. Plain and wholesome food is generally sufficient to effect this result, and if this should not be the case, there is undoubtedly something wrong in the mother's constitution, which has to be removed by treatment. The means which are ordinarily recommended by nurses and even by accoucheurs under these circumstances, are pernicious, such as quantities of coffee, anis, caroway and other drugs. The medicinal qualities which these things impart to the milk, exercise an unpleasant influence over the child; a difficult dentition, nervousness, colic, sleeplessness, crying and tossing about, are generally the effects upon the child, of the coffee which so many nursing mothers use in such large quantities. Tea likewise disposes people to become nervous; many young girls would have stronger nerves if their mothers had used less tea during their nursing time. The same remark applies to all the other herb-teas and decoctions which are so frequently recommended by Old School practitioners, but which every mother who is anxious to bring up healthy and robust children, should avoid. The poor little beings suffer enough, forsooth, without being tormented by such improper management. As regards the alcoholic and other stimulating beverages which are used by so many nursing mothers, by the recommendation of nurses, we are of opinion that the use of these things is a crime, inasmuch as both the physical and intellectual faculties of the child are impaired thereby. We cannot forbear raising our voice against the horrible custom of some nurses to use drugs for every little trouble they may experience; they seem to forget that they inflict incalculable injury upon their nurslings by such indiscretions. A nurse should never take any medicine without the advice of a physician, even under homœopathic treatment; nor should the physician prescribe any thing without considering the condition of the infant and the probable effect which the medicine may have upon it.

In the preceding paragraph we have likewise spoken of the influences which moral emotions may exercise upon the quality of the milk and the health of the infant. It may not be possible for nursing mothers to avoid all opportunities of getting angry or sad; but it is certainly possible to avoid every violent and artificial excitement, such as theatres, novel-reading, or even any other exciting amusement or serious business. It is not only the diet that should be attended to, but the condition of the breasts and of the secretion of milk should never be lost sight of. How many women render themselves diseased for life by exposure to draughts of air or other causes while they are nursing their children. The breasts and every other part of the body should be kept in an uniform temperature; too much heat around the breasts, or exposure to cold is injurious to the milk.

The homœopathic regimen prescribed by Hahnemann in his Organon is more particularly applicable to nursing females. A mother who avoids salt and young meat, strong spices, sausage meat, acids and heating substances, herb-teas, drugs, except such as are necessary on given occasions; in one word, everything that might injure the body and spirit of the child, and who contents herself in the place of all this with plain and healthy nourishment, will have the satisfaction of raising a healthy and vigorous offspring. A true mother will be willing to conform to our demands; she will be willing to sacrifice her coffee and tea, her social dissipations and theatres, for the benefit of her child. As long as the mother is not yet aware of her pregnancy, such excitements may seem pardonable; but as soon as the child is born, and its sweet smile has greeted the young mother's eyes, she cannot, if she is a true mother, find our rules too strict, or the privations which we recommend, too fatiguing.

Section 151.

Medical attentions during nursing.—The accidents or morbid conditions that may require the attention of the physician during the period of nursing, are: *agalactia*, or loss of milk; *dysgalactia*, or bad milk; *galactirrhœa*, or involuntary flow of milk; *diseases of the nipples; diseases of the breasts, and phthisis of the nurse.* We shall speak of each of these conditions in succession.

AGALACTIA or loss of milk, may be total or partial, primary or accidental, according as the milk fails entirely or is not secreted in sufficient quantity, and according as the milk fails from the beginning, or the secretion decreases or stops in consequence of some accidental cause. The most frequent causes of agalactia are deficient nourishment, a constitutional weakness caused by debilitating moral affections, sickly pregnancy or other chronic affections, and finally, the bad condition of the breasts, their atrophy, organic disorders or insufficient development. If this condition is owing to a temporary want of food, the best means to restore the proper secretion of milk is to give the patient suitable nourishment as often as she requires it. If the trouble is caused by CONSTITUTIONAL DEBILITY, the best remedies are: *Agnus*, *Calcarea*, *Causticum*, *Pulsatilla*, *Rhus; Agnus*, especially deserves a preference, unless the symptoms indicate some other remedy; for NODOSITIES IN THE BREAST we have to give, *Dulcamara*, *Agnus*, *Belladonna*, *Chamomilla*, *Rhus*, and if no appreciable cause can be discovered, we may prescribe: *Dulcamara*, *Agnus*, *Zincum*, *Calcarea.* In case of ACCIDENTAL SUPPRESSION of milk, we will always find the following remedies efficacious, according to circumstances: *Belladonna*, *Bryonia*, *Pulsatilla*, *Dulcamara*, or *Calcarea*, *Chamomilla*, *Coffea*, *Mercurius*, *Aconitum*, *Rhus*, *Sulphur;* and more particularly, if the suppression is induced by a cold; *Dulcamara*, or *Pulsatilla*, *Belladonna*, *Chamomilla*, or *Aconitum*, *Mercurius*, *Sulphur;* after a fit of GRIEF: *Ignatia*, *Causticum*, *Phosphori acidum;* after a fit of ANGER: *Chamomilla*, *Bryonia;* after a FRIGHT: *Aconitum*, *Belladonna*, *Opium*, *Coffea;* after AMOROUS JEALOUSY: *Hyoscyamus*, *Pulsatilla*, *Lachesis*, *Causticum;* after a sudden JOY: *Coffea.*

DYSGALACTIA, or bad milk takes place if, in spite of a sufficient supply of milk, the child refuses to take the breast either because the milk is too bad, or the child finds it too troublesome to draw it out. We have spoken above of the various changes that the milk may undergo in its nutritive and other qualities. The best remedies for BAD MILK are:

Sulphur, Mercurius, China, or *Borax*; *Silicea, China*, or *Pulsatilla, Rhabarbarum, Carbo animalis, Lachesis, Nux vom., Sambucus*; and more particularly, if the milk is too SEROUS, NOT SUFFICIENTLY NUTRITIVE, and if the child does not thrive from it: *China* or *Sulphur*, or *Cina, Mercurius*; if the milk COAGULATES READILY: *Borax* or *Lachesis*; if it TURNS SOUR READILY: *Rhabarbarum, Pulsatilla*; if the child REFUSES TO TAKE THE BREAST, without any appreciable cause: *Mercurius, Cina, Silicea*; if the child VOMITS after nursing: *Silicea, Cina, Mercurius*. If the milk should be secreted in sufficient quantity, but cannot be readily drawn out by the child, there is generally too much action in the lactiferous tubes, and a state of plethora bordering upon inflammation, owing to which the excretory canals are, so to say, stopped up by a species of partial orgasm. This condition, which is often met with in the case of plethoric young females overflowing with health, yields to *Aconitum, Bryonia, Chamomilla, Belladonna, Mercurius*.

GALACTIRRHŒA, or involuntary flow of milk, takes place when the milk is secreted in excessive quantity, and the breast is unable to retain it. If this loss should continue and become excessive, it must necessarily be injurious to the health of the mother, and may even induce a considerable degree of emaciation and loss of strength. In most cases this condition yields to the following remedies: *Pulsatilla*, or *Calcarea*, or *Belladonna, Borax, Bryonia, Rhus*, or *China, Conium, Phosphorus, Stramonium*. Sometimes the milk, though secreted in excessive quantity, nevertheless remains in the breast in spite of nursing. The mammæ swell, become painful and knotty, the knots forming strings from the breasts as far as the armpits. For this trouble, *Bryonia* or *Calcarea*, if Bryonia should not suffice, will prove an excellent remedy; sometimes *Belladonna, Phosphorus, Pulsatilla*, may be useful.

The DISEASES OF THE NIPPLES which may prevent nursing, are deficient development and soreness of the nipples. We refer the reader to what we have said concerning these affections, Sections 108–109. If the nipples are not sufficiently prominent, the child being unable to take hold of them, of course, cannot nurse. If such a difficulty exists, it has to be attended to even during pregnancy. The simplest way to remedy this defect is to draw the nipple out by applying to it a small vial or the bowl of an earthen pipe, after having previously expelled the air from either, by holding the flame of a piece of burning paper or spirit-lamp over it. The nipple having been drawn out, a little cup of soft India rubber cloth may be tied over it, in order to prevent its being chafed by the pressure or friction of the clothes. In order to prevent the soreness of the nipples, the patient will do well to bathe them even during her pregnancy with a little brandy; this strengthens the skin, and diminishes its liability to tear. If this means should not prove sufficient, and the nipples should become sore, they may be bathed with a solution of a drop of Arnica-tincture in 100 drops of water; if this remedy is applied at once, a cure will soon follow. If *Arnica* does not help, *Chamomilla*, or *Ignatia*, and sometimes *Pulsatilla* will prove efficient, if the nipples are simply inflamed without being either raw or cracked. If they are cracked or excoriated, *Sulphur*, or, perhaps, *Graphites*, *Calcarea*, or *Lycopodium* will be found sufficient.

The DISEASES OF THE NIPPLES with which nurses may be attacked, are: *phlegmonous inflammation* and *abscesses* of the nipples. We refer the reader to Section 103. These accidents generally result from a cold, accumulation of milk, stoppage of the lactiferous vessels or from a blow upon the breasts. If the physician is called as soon as the disease shows itself, with a little inflammation and swelling, *Aconitum* will sometimes prove sufficient to arrest the disorder. But, if the inflammatory swelling is well developed, the best remedy will be *Belladonna*, especially if there is erysipelatous redness; or *Bryonia* if Belladonna is not sufficient, and if the tumor is very red, with lancinating or tensive pains. If an ABSCESS should threaten, the best remedy is *Mercurius*, especially if it can be used as soon as the first signs of suppuration are perceived; but if the pus is already formed, and the suppurative process has become quite evident, *Phosphorus* will be found the best remedy. If FISTULOUS ulcers develop themselves, *Silicea* is the best remedy. All these remedies should be administered as follows: 6 globules in half a tumblerful of water, a dessertspoonful of which solution is to be given every three hours. If the suppuration should have become chronic, or should have been going on for months before the physician is called, the same medicines may be administered, except that the above-mentioned dose should be given every morning only, or even 3 globules dry on the tongue every three or four days at most. With my late friend Croserio, I repudiate with all my might the use of poultices in these tumors. Poultices promote the suppuration and the formation of chronic engorgements which occur so frequently under old school treatment.

PHTHISIS of nurses, when induced either by a too profuse flow of milk, or by excessively prolonged nursing, is generally ushered in by great weakness, depression of spirits, constant desire to weep; after a while the patient experiences acute drawing pains in the forepart of the chest and in the back, between the shoulder-blades, with loss of appetite or else canine hunger, burning at the stomach, in the fauces, chest, or sense of emptiness at the pit of the stomach, violent thirst and exacerbation of all the pains during and after nursing; afterwards a hectic fever sets in, which is sometimes accompanied by paroxysms of hypochondria or hysteria, and, if the disease is not arrested, the emaciation and prostration may rapidly lead to death. The first thing to be done, as soon as the first symptoms of consumption make their appearance, is to wean the child. In most cases the secretion of milk ceases shortly after weaning, and the health of the patient is restored again shortly after, especially if a substantial and easily digested nourishment is resorted to. Exercise in the open air should not be neglected. If this change of regimen is not sufficient, a few small doses of *China*, 6 globules of the 15th attenuation in half a tumblerful of water, a dessertspoonful morning and evening, will soon bring about a favorable change, so much so that the patient is sometimes enabled to resume her nursing. If the disease is too far advanced to yield to the action of China, *Calcarea*, *Sulphur*, or *Lycopodium* will render good service. In CRAMPS OF THE STOMACH which sometimes set in after exhausting nursing, *China* may be given, and, if this does not help, *Carbo vegetabilis*.

SECTION 152.

WEANING.—If nothing occurs to force the mother to wean her infant, the best period for weaning is the time when the child has cut its first teeth, and is able to digest the new nourishment for the use of which the organs of the child have gradually been prepared. Few women, however, can await this period: the reappearance of the menses, the diminution of milk, a new pregnancy, marked debility and other accidents of this kind, may compel her, and often do compel her, to wean her child sooner than she would wish. The nearer to the period when the first dentition is accomplished, the better for the child to be weaned. In any case, as soon as the milk commences to give out, or if the breast remains empty even after the child makes an effort to draw milk, it is time to wean the child, both on the mother's account as well as for the sake of the child's own health. The child should not be weaned suddenly, but gradually by lengthening the intervals between the hours when the child is put to the breast. It is likewise proper to gradually diminish the period during which the child is kept at the breast. If the period for weaning the child altogether, has finally arrived, it may be well for the mother to keep her bed for a day or two, and to use nothing but gruels or light broths for her nourishment. By this means the secretion of milk will soon cease; a dose of *Pulsatilla* or *Calcarea* may sometimes be necessary to facilitate this result. As regards the engorgements of the breasts which sometimes take place after weaning, they have to be treated like the engorgements of which mention was made in the preceding paragraph.

Section 153.

Milk-affections. — We cannot conclude this chapter without alluding to those pretended metastases or displacements of the milk to which a good many affections of mothers who have weaned their children are attributed by ignorant persons. Nevertheless, like the sudden suppression of the menses or lochia, so may the sudden suppression of the milky secretion give rise to many troublesome and even dangerous symptoms. If the sudden suppression of the milk in consequence of a fright or of some other emotion, should be followed by acute inflammation of some viscus or some acute eruption, we may safely infer that the suppression is the cause of this acute disorder. Whether such a suppression may likewise be followed by chronic disorders, remains yet to be decided. Nor do we exactly know what these disorders are. But inasmuch as the other suppressions may lead to functional derangements in almost any organ, it is fair to suppose that the suppression of milk may be followed by similar affections, and that these affections may, by improper management or neglect, become more or less chronic. As far as homœopathic treatment is concerned, this pathological distinction is of very little consequence. By selecting a remedy in accordance with the existing symptoms, we not only pursue the right treatment, but likewise cure the disease. If it should be certain, however, that an existing affection was caused by sudden suppression of the milk, the following remedies may deserve a preference over any other: *Belladonna*, *Pulsatilla*, *Agnus*, *Rhus*, *Bryonia*, *Calcarea*, *Sulphur*, *Dulcamara*, *Mercurius*, *Lachesis*, *Lycopodium*, *Sepia*, *Cina*, *Zincum*.

And in particular:

In metastasis to the abdominal viscera: *Pulsatilla*, *Rhus*, *Belladonna*, *Bryonia*, *Sulphur*.

In metastasis to the chest: *Bryonia*, *Calcarea*, *Belladonna*, *Sulphur*, *Lycopodium*, *Lachesis*, *Rhus*, *Pulsatilla*.

In metastasis TO THE BRAIN: *Belladonna, Rhus, Bryonia, Zincum, Lachesis, Mercurius, Sulphur, Pulsatilla, Cina.*

In metastasis TO THE SKIN: *Sulphur, Calcarea, Dulcamara, Causticum, Rhus.*

Of these remedies dissolve 6 globules of the 12th attenuation in about half a tumblerful of water, and give the patient a dessertspoonful of this solution every 3 hours.

ARTICLE X.

ATTENTIONS TO NEW-BORN INFANTS AND TO CHILDREN AT THE BREAST.

SECTION 154.

GENERAL OBSERVATIONS.—The object and narrow limits of this work do not permit us to enter upon long details concerning the diseases to which little children are subject, and still less concerning the diseases of children generally. In order to do justice to this subject, a separate volume would have to be written, perfectly distinct from the present work which is exclusively devoted to diseases of women. However, inasmuch as the life of new-born children is intimately connected with that of their mother, we will offer a few remarks about the attentions to be bestowed upon infants at the breast until the first dentition is accomplished. This period comprises four distinct intervals, namely: 1st, *the moment of birth;* 2d, *the first few days of their existence;* 3d, *the period of nursing;* 4th, *the period of dentition.* Each of these periods is liable to peculiar ailments and derangements, which we shall describe as they occur according to the order of these periods corresponding as they do to similar periods in the life of the mother, namely: 1, *labor;* 2, *confinement;* 3, *nursing;* 4, *weaning.* If the same ailments should occur in more than one of these periods, we shall allot them to the period when they occur most frequently.

Section 155.

First attentions to the infant.—The first thing to be done after the child is born, is to place it so as to enable it to breathe freely, and not to deliver the placenta until the pulsations in the cord have either ceased or become considerably weaker. If the cord is twisted round the neck or round any other part of the child's body, the parts are disembarrassed, after which the child is placed on one side with its face turned away from the vulva, by this means the mucus which may be in the mouth, will flow out without causing any trouble, and the blood discharged from the vulva will be prevented from obstructing the nostrils of the infant. After tying the cord a few inches from its attachment to the infant, previous to which operation we have to ascertain whether a portion of bowel has not slipped into the cord, we sever the cord between the ligature and the placenta. The cord having been tied, all the impurities which may be found in the child's mouth and nostrils, are removed by means of a soft piece of linen, the child's body is carefully washed with tepid water, the navel is dressed, a bandage is applied round the abdomen, and the child is comfortably and warmly dressed, so as neither to interfere with the breathing nor the circulation, nor with the free motion of its limbs. We do not approve of washing the child's body with brandy or alcohol, which some accouchers recommend for the purpose of dissolving the fatty matter with which the newborn infant is often covered; alcohol does not act upon this substance, and, moreover, irritates the delicate skin of the child. It is much better to use sweet oil or cream for this purpose.

After dressing the child, it may be laid close to the mother who may commence nursing it after ten or twelve hours. The first milk which is drawn from the mother's breast, called *colostrum*, is not very nutritive, and will help to expel the *meconium* if this substance should have remained in the bowels. No mother should deprive her infant of the nourishment which nature seems to have destined for it, except in case of absolute necessity. No animal refuses to nurse its young; it is only among the human species that we find mothers cruel enough to deprive a newborn infant of its natural food. If this is done from wilful neglect or indifference, mothers often pay dearly for such violations of nature's laws. If compelled by weakness to renounce the pleasure of nursing their infants, a nurse should be obtained whose milk is as nearly as possible like that of the mother; if the milk is too old, it becomes so strong and fat that the child cannot assimilate it, in consequence of which the tender being languishes, and gradually perishes. If no nurse that has suitable milk for the baby, can be had, it should be fed on fresh cow's milk mixed with one-third tepid water, and sweetened with a little loaf sugar; a few teaspoonfuls of this milk may be fed every now and then, increasing the quantity and the consistence of this nourishment in proportion as the infant grows stronger. Nursing bottles should never be used for this purpose. Whatever care we may bestow upon them, it is impossible to keep them clean. Nor can the instrument with which they are stopped, and which is in imitation of a nipple, be washed with sufficient care to prevent some particles of the milk from penetrating the pores in the ivory. This milk turns sour, of which we may convince ourselves by the smell; and it is this sour milk which frequently causes aphthæ. The silver nursing spoons which are used in Germany, are much better than our nursing bottles. They are shaped like bottles with long necks, and can be opened and closed at pleasure. Being accessible in every part, they can be kept perfectly clean and polished, and the infant can drink out of them with the most perfect ease.

In order to keep the infant clean, it should be washed every day in tepid or cold water, according to the season. After the first teething, cold water may be used altogether.

It is a bad habit to put the infant into a tepid bath every day. Such a proceeding is highly favorable to the development of a lymphatic constitution, and, moreover, weakens the child, and renders it unnecessarily sensitive to changes in the weather or temperature. It is not to be wondered that in England where the use of tepid baths is quite prevalent, a number of individuals should be affected with tubercular diseases.

Section 156.

Diseases of new-born children.—The arrival of a new being in this world of misery and strife is not always exempt from difficulties and pains. Tears and cries mark its first entry into life. The first cries of a child which are caused by the irritating effect of the air upon the lungs, need not alarm any one; on the contrary, they show that the child is born with a healthy and strong constitution, and it is right and proper that young mothers should be delighted to hear these first cries of their little ones. Sometimes, however, these joyful scenes are closed by sorrow. Respiration, which is an indispensable condition of life, is sometimes wanting, and all the other functions remain suspended; the child seems asphyxiated. In other cases the child is alive, but its head is ecchymosed or swollen, or its skin is blue, yellow or indurated, and sometimes the child is born with malformations. All these conditions may require the immediate attention of the practitioner. We will describe the treatment which sometimes has to be instituted in the case of children, under the following heads: *apoplexy*, *asphyxia*, *cyanosis*, *jaundice*, *ecchymoses and swelling of the head*, *cellular indurations*, *swelling of the breasts*, *congenital malformations*, *and hernia.*

The apoplectic condition in which children sometimes are born, is caused by long and painful labor; the surface of the body seems swollen; the face and the whole body are of a violet, or rather blackish-blue color; the muscles do not move; the limbs preserve their flexibility and the body its heat; the pulsations of the cord, pulse and even those of the heart are either imperceptible or at any rate very feeble, and the breathing does not take place. In such cases allœopathic accouchers are in the habit of promptly severing the cord and letting a few teaspoonfuls of blood flow from it. Instead of resorting to such a proceeding and depriving these little beings of the blood which constitutes the principal support of their feeble existence, we have it in our power to remove the difficulty by the exhibition of *Aconitum*, *Tartar emetic*, or *Opium*. A single pellet of *Aconitum*, 18th attenuation, dry on the tongue, sometimes changes this unfavorable condition visibly; if no improvement should take place after ten or fifteen minutes, we may have recourse to *Tartar emetic*, which will generally help. If the body of the child is violet-colored, *Opium* will sometimes prove efficient. This apoplectic condition must not be confounded with asphyxia; for this last named condition requires a treatment different from the one required by apoplexy.

ASPHYXIA of new-born infants generally occurs among feeble children, or among such as have been weakened by tedious labor, or by flooding during pregnancy, or by other affections with which the mother had been attacked during the period of utero-gestation. In these children the circulation is neither arrested nor impeded, but the breathing and the muscular movements are wanting, the skin is extremely pale, the flesh is flabby and soft, and the child almost looks like a corpse. In such a case the umbilical cord should be left undivided as long as we discover pulsations in the cord, and the mucus which is in the nostrils should be removed by means of a little linen rag; afterwards we place three pellets of *China* 18th, on the child's tongue, wrap it in warm flannel, and rub the chest and hands with a similar material. If the child does not commence to breathe soon, or if the pulsations cease entirely, the cord may be severed after tying it; this being done, we place the child in a warm bath in order to preserve the temperature of the body, and we endeavor to excite muscular action by gentle strokes on the limbs and chest. If *China* does not bring on any change within ten or fifteen minutes, a similar dose of *Tartarus emeticus* may be given, which may be alternated with *China* every fifteen minutes; if no change takes place in two hours, we may give *Lachesis.* At the same time a young person in good health may place her mouth close over the mouth of the infant, and endeavor to blow air into the child's lungs, during which operation the nostrils of the child have to be closed with the fingers. Insufflation of the lungs is best accomplished by means of the laryngeal tube which, passing as it does into the larynx, prevents the air from being blown into the œsophagus and distending the stomach, which would increase the compression of the lungs. These insufflations, however, do not always respond to the object we seek to attain; sometimes the best means to excite action in the muscles of the thorax, is to sprinkle the chest with cold water, especially the left side; or to blow a little brandy and water out of one's own mouth against the anterior wall of the child's thorax. It often happens that respiration commences immediately after resorting to the sprinkling. We should not give up too soon in our efforts to restore animation. Sometimes it takes several hours to accomplish this result; but even, if all our endeavors should prove fruitless, the child ought nevertheless to be kept warm for some time, for in more cases than one, animation set in spontaneously after all the efforts of art seemed to have proved fruitless. As soon as we perceive the first signs of life, our efforts to restore animation should be discontinued; nor should the child be left in the warm bath after it has commenced to cry and to breathe freely.

CYANOSIS of new-born infants results from a mixture of the arterial and venous blood caused by an imperfect closure of the foramen ovale, on which account the blood of the right ventricle, instead of passing into the lungs and there being arterialised, passes directly into the left ventricle whence it is propelled into the general circulation. We may try *Sulphur*, *Calcarea* or *Digitalis* for the purpose of removing this malformation, small doses should be given at long intervals.

ICTERUS of new-born children is often caused by exposure

to cold at the time of birth, resulting from the carelessness of nurses; sometimes it is owing to the retention of the meconium in the bowels. This trouble is not serious; in most cases it gets well of itself without any treatment; if, however, this should not be the case, and the skin should at the same time be dry and hot, we may give three globules of *Aconitum*, 12th attenuation, in half a tumblerful of water, of which solution a dessertspoonful should be given twice a day.

The INDURATION OF THE CELLULAR TISSUE is almost always a very serious difficulty, which attacks children during the first ten days after their birth. It generally commences at the lower extremities or cheeks, when it soon extends to the abdomen and chest. The skin which covers the diseased parts is slightly rose-colored or purple, violet, livid. If the disease runs a rapid course, the temperature of the body decreases rapidly, the pulse is scarcely perceptible, the breathing becomes more and more labored, the child's cries diminish and gradually cease altogether, the face becomes livid, and the little ones die as of suffocation, generally on the third day. Sometimes the disease is more chronic, and passes off again from the fourth to the eighth day; but these cases are exceedingly rare, and under the old treatment most children die in a few days. Under homœopathic treatment this disease is readily cured by *Aconitum*, 18th attenuation, six globules in half a tumblerful of water, a dessertspoonful of which solution may be given every three or four hours. If there should be no improvement after a few doses of *Aconitum*, we may give *Bryonia* in a similar manner. If the disease grows obstinate, three globules of *Sulphur*, dry on the tongue, may be administered once only as an intercurrent remedy.

The ECCHYMOSES and SWELLING of the head with which children are sometimes born, are caused by the instruments which had been applied during delivery, or by the contusions which the head receives in passing through the straits. They generally disappear after bathing the head with a mixture of ten drops of tincture of Arnica in half a tumblerful of water; if any swelling should remain after applying the Arnica, we may give *Rhus*, three globules dry on the tongue. This will remove the difficulty; but if ulcers should form, give *Silicea* the same as Rhus.

SWELLING OF THE BREASTS in new-born children often results from pressing the breasts after birth, which is a habit with a great many nurses. If the swelling is not inflamed, a single dose of *Arnica* will remove it; if it is red, give *Belladonna*, three globules dry on the tongue; if suppuration is to be feared, we may give *Mercurius* or *Hepar*, or even *Silicea* if suppuration should have set it. For scirrhous induration of the breasts *Chamomilla* is the specific remedy.

UMBILICAL OR INGUINAL HERNIA of new-born infants often yields to *Nux vomica* and *Sulphur*, three globules alternately every week, dry on the tongue. If no better in six weeks, give *Cocculus*, or *Aurum*, or *Veratrum*, *Lachesis*, *Sulphuris acidum*.

MALFORMATIONS, CONGENITAL EXCRESCENCES, TUMORS, etc., sometimes disappear of themselves as the child grows older; hence operations should not be performed too soon. In many cases three globules of *Sulphur*, dry on the tongue, will prove useful; in five or six weeks we may give a similar dose of *Calcarea*. These two remedies are likewise excellent for NÆVI MATERNI, unless we should have to give *Carbo vegetabilis*, *Platina*, *Sepia*, *Thuja*, *Zincum*. If the skull-bones should slip one over the other, as is often the case after instrumental labor, and should remain in this situation, making the child look old, emaciated, with flabby muscles, *Opium* will sometimes remove these symptoms.

SECTION 157.

DISEASES OF INFANTS AT THE BREAST.—After children have passed through the first moments of their existence, and draw their sustenance regularly from the breast of their mother, they are still exposed to many derangements incidental to their condition. These are: *hiccough*, *stoppage of the nose*, *asthma, cardiospasm, sleeplessness, cries, colic, diarrhœa, constipation, falling of the rectum, retention of urine, erythema, aphthæ, ophthalmia, erysipelas* and *rash.* In this paragraph we will treat successively of each of these affections, reserving for the last paragraph all that has to be said concerning dentition and the disorders inherent in this period.

Hiccough is sometimes very troublesome to little children, without however being a serious complaint. It generally passes off shortly after the infant gets warm again in its mother's bosom, and takes a few teaspoonfuls of fresh water. If the attack should take place frequently, a few globules of *Aconitum,* or *Nux vomica,* or *Pulsatilla,* dry on the tongue, will soon stop it.

STOPPAGE OF THE NOSE often renders it impossible for infants to nurse. Sometimes rubbing a little goose-grease on the nose will cure the trouble; if not, we may give *Nux vomica,* or *Sambucus* if Nux is insufficient. If mucus should flow from the nose, we may give *Chamomilla;* or *Carbo vegetabilis,* if the trouble gets worse toward evening; or *Dulcamara* if the aggravation takes place in the open air.

CARDIOSPASM or liver-grown, is a sudden bloating and hardness of the pit of the stomach and hypochondria, with sense of suffocation; the children are restless, cry, toss about, draw their thighs up, and are out of breath. *Chamomilla* is specific for this trouble.

ASTHMA of infants, which is sometimes mistaken by the uninformed for croup, consists in a sort of spasm of the chest which arrests the breathing, and imparts a violent color to the face; the children wake suddenly, with anxiety, hollow and dry cough, and plaintive cries. A few magnetic passes quiet the child; if not, two globules of *Ipecacuanha* may be given dry on the tongue, or *Sambucus,* both of which are specific remedies for this condition.

SLEEPLESSNESS of infants is generally owing to a vicious regimen on the part of the mother, the use of coffee, chamomile or other teas, heating food, etc., or the child does not lie well, is bandaged too tightly, etc. If, after the removal of these causes, the sleeplessness still continue, a pellet of *Coffea* may be given dry on the tongue, or, if insufficient, a dose of *Chamomilla*, especially if the child is troubled with flatulence; or *Opium* may be given if the blood goes to the head and the face is very red. For simple wakefulness without nervousness, we try *Ranunculus, bulbosus.*

CRYING WITHOUT A CAUSE probably never occurs. If a child cries, it feels uncomfortable, a pin pricks it, or the skin itches, etc. We should make every effort to discover the true cause of the trouble; but if, after removing it as well as we know, the crying still continues, we may give for crying from ANGER:—*Aconitum*, *Chamomilla* or *Arnica;* from FRIGHT: *Opium*, *Belladonna*, *Ignatia;* for crying followed by CONVULSIONS, with rigidity of the body, raising of the abdomen, and throwing the head back: *Chamomilla;* if the children are restless with a burning skin: *Coffea* or *Aconitum;* if the FACE IS RED: *Aconitum* or *Belladonna;* if they cry and CANNOT BE QUIETED: *Belladonna*, *Aconitum*, or *Coffea;* if they become *furious*, and kick and demean themselves: *Tartar emetic;* if the crying is caused by ear-ache, colic, etc., give the remedies indicated for these affections.

COLIC is easily recognized by the twisting of the child, emission of flatulence, drawing up of the legs, crying, etc., *Chamomilla* is a specific remedy for this trouble, especially if there is greenish and watery diarrhœa, with constant crying, distension of the abdomen, starting of the limbs and cold feet; or *China* may be given, if the colic occurs towards evening, with hardness of the abdomen, absence of stool or whitish stool, or resembling stirred eggs. *Pulsatilla* for flatulence, rumbling, frequent shuddering, pale face and no thirst. *Ipecacuanha*, for fermented diarrhœa having a foul smell, and the children uttering violent and piercing cries.

DIARRHŒA of infants generally yields to a few doses of *Ipecacuanha*, eighteenth attenuation, three globules in half a tumblerful of water, a dessert-spoonful of which solution should be given every three hours. If this should not help, we may give *Rhabarbarum*, if the evacuations and the child's whole body smell sour; *Chamomilla*, if the child cries a good deal, draws up its legs, with distension of the bowels and frequent emission of flatulence; *Antimonium*, if the tongue is coated white or yellow; *Dulcamara*, if the diarrhœa arises from a cold or from exposure to cold air; *Bryonia*, if caused by summer-heat; *Belladonna*, if the evacuations are greenish, the child sleeps a good deal, but the sleep is restless, with pale face; *Arsenicum* or *Secale*, if the child is very feeble; *Sulphur*, *Calcarea* or *Nux moschata*, in obstinate cases where nothing else will help.

CONSTIPATION of little children is often caused by heating food, and yields to a change of diet. If medicine is required, *Bryonia*, *Nux vomica*, *Opium*, will be found sufficient. Give one or two pellets dry on the tongue, and again in twenty-four hours, changing the medicine, if no improvement takes place after the second dose. For chronic constipation we may give three pellets of *Sulphur* or *Alumina*, every three or four days, dry on the tongue; if no evacuation should take place within twenty-four hours, we may resort to injections of tepid milk and water.

FALLING OF THE RECTUM in the case of little children, occurs quite frequently, generally after long lasting diarrhœa or violent straining at stool when the fæces are hard and large. The best medicines are *Ignatia* or *Nux vomica*. These medicines may be given at the time when the trouble takes place; sometimes they act on the spot, and the rectum returns to its normal position without any manual assistance.

RETENTION OF URINE, generally yields to *Pulsatilla*, or *Nux vomica;* if these medicines are not sufficient, we may give *Aconitum*, or the child may smell of the tincture of *Camphor*.

EXCORIATIONS, SORENESS, INTERTRIGO, are very troublesome to little children; generally they are seated in the groin between the genital organs and the thighs, but often they invade the parts between the nates, the genital organs and the axilla. The best remedy is *Sulphur*, two globules dry on the tongue, which generally effect an improvement in a few days; if not sufficient, we may give *Chamomilla*, especially if the children cry a good deal and seem ill-natured; or *Carbo vegetabilis*, if Chamomilla renders the symptoms worse; or *Mercurius*, if the child looks yellow, the excoriation extends behind the ears, with redness of the sore places. Semetimes *Graphites* renders good service; *Lycopodium* is seldom indicated. The SORENESS behind the ears requires *Sulphur*, *Calcarea* or *Graphites*.

ERYSIPELAS of infants generally proves fatal unless checked. It is always seated on the abdomen, spreading from the navel over the abdomen to the genital parts, and the inner surface of the thighs. The affected parts are warm, hard and painful to the touch, the urine stains the linen yellow and reddish; the fever is generally high, with frequent pulse, dry and hot skin; and coated tongue. This erysipelas generally yields to *Belladonna*, 18th attenuation, three pellets in half a tumblerful of water, a dessertspoonful every three hours; if *Belladonna* does not help, we may give *Rhus*.

RASH of infants is generally caused by excessive covering, and passes off again after the cause is removed; if not, we may give *Aconitum* if there is fever, with dry skin and frequent pulse; or *Ipecacuanha*, if diarrhœa is present; or *Bryonia*, if there is constipation and distension of the bowels.

FEVER of little children, unless caused by teething, is generally a sign that some other acute affection is approaching, such as inflammation of some organ, or an eruptive disease. But in many cases these diseases may be prevented by attending to the precursory symptoms. If the child is hot, restless, with quick and strong pulse, dissolve three pellets of *Aconitum*, 18th attenuation, in half a tumblerful of water, and give a dessertspoonful of this solution every few hours until the fever ceases, or until other symptoms develop themselves, pointing to some other remedy. In most cases, the fever will cease in about twenty-four hours, or, at any rate, the disease will run a much milder course, provided it was impossible to arrest it.

APHTHÆ are small white specks in the mucous lining of the mouth, which spread, and form irregular and thin patches that either remain distinct or run into each other. If remaining distinct, the disease is not very serious, and the inflammation runs its course in one or two weeks; but if these patches unite, the whole mouth becomes lined with a creamy crust that thickens from day to day; this crust soon turns yellow; the inflammation spreads to the digestive organs, and the little patient becomes weaker and weaker, and finally dies. The most frequent causes of this affection are: sucking when the breast is empty; too substantial food; old milk; want of cleanliness; the use of ordinary sugar-tits, or nursing-bottles that are not kept clean. The best remedy for this affection is *Sulphuris acidum*, six pellets of third attenuation in half a tumblerful of water, in dessertspoonful doses every three hours; if this remedy is not sufficient, we may give *Mercurius;* or *Sulphur*, if Mercurius does not help. *Borax* may be given, if the urine smells like cat's urine, or if no other medicine helps.

OPHTHALMIA of infants is characterized by an enormous swelling of the lids with accumulation of a purulent matter between the eyeball and the lower lids; it principally occurs among children of a bad constitution and who are not kept clean. The best remedy for this affection is *Aconitum*, 6th attenution, 6 globules in half a tumblerful of water, in dessertspoonful doses every three hours; if the affection is more chronic, we may give *Sulphur*. In some cases the favorable action of *Aconitum* is very appropriately succeeded by *Dulcamara*, *Mercurius*, *Chamomilla*, *Belladonna*, or by *Pulsatilla*, and after Sulphur we may give *Calcarea*, *Lycopodium*, *Silicea*, *Arsenicum*.

OTALGIA and OTITIS of infants, (earache and inflammation of the ears) generally announce themselves by cries, restlessness, starting during sleep, fever; the child continually grasps at the ear, and is very uneasy. The best remedies are: 1. *Chamomilla*. 2. *Pulsatilla*, *Belladonna*, *Mercurius* or *Sul-*

phur. And if there is discharge, we give *Pulsatilla*, *Mercurius* or *Sulphur.*

CONVULSIONS of children are generally frightful to those who are unacquainted with medicine, but they scarcely ever fail to yield to homœopathic treatment. In many cases these convulsions cease by rubbing the upper lip of the child, under the nose, with a finger moistened with the tincture of *Camphor.* If this is not sufficient, and the paroxysms return, we may give *Ignatia*, *Belladonna*, *Chamomilla*, *Coffea*, *Ipecacuanha*, *Mercurius*, *Opium*, *Sulphur.*

IGNATIA is indicated, if the attack comes on without any apparent cause, especially every other day at the same hour, or if worms or teething seem to be the cause of it; BELLADONNA, if the convulsions are accompanied by cerebral symptoms, such as vertigo, sparks before the eyes, loss of consciousness, etc.; CHAMOMILLA, if the convulsions affect the arms, legs, and head, the eyes are half closed; one cheek is red, the other pale; COFFEA, suitable to feeble children, when the convulsions are not accompanied by other symptoms; IPECACUANHA, if the children are oppressed on the chest, with eructations, vomiting or diarrhœa, tetanic rigidity of the whole body; MERCURIUS, if the abdomen is hard and distended, with eructations, water in the mouth, fever, prostration after every attack; OPIUM, if, after a fright, the body trembles, the arms and legs are thrown about, the child cries without consciousness, with stupor, distension of the abdomen, retention of stool and urine; SULPHUR, if the convulsions recur constantly in spite of treatment.

The presence of WORMS is often suspected where other causes induce derangements. If worms are really present, we may give alternately *Sulphur* and *Cina*, two pellets dry on the tongue, every week. In case of fever, *Aconitum* or *Mercurius* will soon dispel it.

SECTION 158.

AILMENTS DURING DENTITION.—The process of dentition, which generally commences a few months after birth, develops various ailments which generally disappear again after this period, but which may become so violent as to require the interference of a physician. These are, *affections of the gums, nervous excitement, fever, convulsions, diarrhœa, cough, and general derangements.* We shall treat of each of these affections in particular.

The AFFECTIONS OF THE GUMS are generally the first visible signs of dentition. The gums become swollen, hot, painful and whitish at the borders; they itch; the child's mouth is hot, and there is a constant flow of saliva from the mouth; the child has difficulty in nursing, and crowds everything into its mouth in order to bite. If this condition does not last too long, it does not require any treatment; otherwise, if the gums remain swollen and the teeth do not break through, or if the teething takes place in an irregular manner, three pellets of *Sulphur*, 30th attenuation, may be given dry on the tongue, and in about a week a dose of *Calcarea;* if necessary, another dose of *Calcarea* may be given in a week. By this mode of treatment the necessity of lancing the gums will always be avoided.

THE NERVOUS IRRITATION caused by the teething is sometimes exceedingly troublesome. The child does not sleep, is restless, capricious, laughs or weeps about trifles. The best remedies for these symptoms are *Aconitum* or *Coffea*, especially if the child's cheeks are alternately red and pale; or *Chamomilla* if one cheek is red, the other pale, with starting in the limbs; or *Nux vomica*, if there is constipation and nervous hacking cough, and if *Aconitum* and *Coffea* remain without effect, sometimes *Belladonna* or *Borax* are indicated.

THE FEVER OF DENTITION generally yields to *Aconitum*, six pellets in half a tumblerful of water, in dessertspoonful doses every three hours; we may also give *Chamomilla*, *Belladonna*, *Coffea*, *Nux vomica* or *Silicea*. CHAMOMILLA, if the child is restless at night, with continual tossing, marked thirst, short breathing with anxiety and moanining, oppression on the chest, warm head with sweat of the hair and scalp, redness of one cheek and paleness of the other, starting of the limbs; *Belladonna*, if *Chamomilla* is not sufficient, eyes and skin are red, a good deal of thirst, disposition to start, anguish, dry cough like whooping-cough; *Coffea*, if the fever is accompanied by nervousness, with cries, weeping, disconsolate restlessness, *Aconitum* having been given without effect; *Nux vomica*, for constipation, nervous, hacking cough, aggravation towards morning; *Silicea*, suitable to scrofulous children, if the fever will not yield to any medicine, the child's body is burning hot, face red and bloated, distension of the abdomen, swelling and hardness of the cervical glands, which feel like dry peas.

CONVULSIONS caused by teething are sometimes prevented by a small dose of *Chamomilla*, 18th attenuation, three pellets dry on the tongue, if the medicine can be administered in time, as soon as diarrhœa, paleness of the face, dulness of the eyes, loss of appetite, prostration which induces the child to lay its head upon the shoulder of the nurse, are perceived. If *Chamomilla* is not sufficient, we may give *Ignatia*, *Belladonna*, *Cina*, *Tartarus*, *Calcarea*, *Stramonium* or *Sulphur*.—*Ignatia* is suitable if Chamomilla proves insufficient during the precursory stage, especially if the convulsions resemble epilepsy, or break out at once without any precursory symptoms; *Belladonna*, if Ignatia is insufficient, and if the child is drowsy between the attacks, with involuntary emission of urine during sleep, waking as if in affright, with restless looks, dilated pupils, immovable eyes, burning hands and head; *Cina*, suitable for children who wet their beds, have worms, or who have a cough like whooping-cough, or if the convulsions resemble epilepsy; *Tartarus*, if the children cough and gape a good deal between the attacks, with drowsiness, convulsive movements of the facial muscles, continual crying, anxiety in the features, greenish diarrhœa; *Calcarea*, especially suitable for fat and lymphathic children, if no other medicine helps; *Stannum*, for epileptiform convulsions, for which Ignatia or Cina remains powerless; *Sulphur*, as an intercurrent remedy, if the convulsions recur in spite of temporary palliation produced by other remedies; if the brain should be affected between the attacks, as may be inferred from such symptoms as these: glazed and dull eyes, drowsiness, sleeplessness, desire to bury the head into the pillow or to roll it about constantly, pale or animated face, or if the children bite the glass when drinking, we may give *Belladonna* and *Cina*, or sometimes *Hyoscyamus*, *Cuprum*, *Sulphur*, *Calcarea*.

CONSTIPATION may aggravate the condition of the child, it should be wet by *Bryonia*, *Nux vomica*, *Magnesia muriatica*.

DIARRHŒA during dentition should never be stopped suddenly, for it frequently acts as a natural outlet for the cerebral irritation which sometimes takes place during this period; but if the diarrhœa lasts too long, we may treat it with *Mercurius*, *Sulphur*, *Ipecacuanha*.

The cough which frequently affects children during dentition, is very much like whooping-cough. It is hollow, dry and more or less spasmodic. The best medicines for this cough are *Cina*, *Chamomilla*, *Nux vomica*, *Belladonna*, *Ipecacuanha*.

There are various derangements which attack children during dentition, and which may be arranged as follows: 1st, STROPHULUS, consisting of red, prominent, more or less inflamed patches, scattered over the forearms, the back of the hand, but especially over the cheeks, and sometimes intermingled with erythematous patches. 2d, IMPETIGINOUS ECZEMA, or scald-head, consisting of inflamed vesicles which sometimes resemble impetigo-pustules and form yellowish and soft crusts that sometimes discharge a profuse quantity of purulent mucus; 3d, MILK-CRUSTS, (impetigo larvalis,) resembling the former eruption, except that it is seated in the face, these two eruptions are often accompanied with swelling of the glands of the neck and back of the neck. Strophulus generally disappears without medicine; but if the blotches become troublesome, we may give *Sulphur* or *Mercurius*, or sometimes *Chamomilla*, *Cina*, *Rhus*, *Graphites* or *Causticum*. The best remedy for milk-crust or scald-head, is *Rhus*, 18th attenuation, six globules in half a tumblerful of water, a dessertspoonful morning and evening. If there should be no improvement within six or eight days, three pellets of *Sulphur* may be given dry on the tongue, and if no change takes place within a week, *Rhus* may again be given for a week, to be followed by a second dose of *Sulphur;* and, if things remain unchanged, we may give *Calcarea*, three pellets dry on the tongue, which may be allowed to act one, two or more weeks. In some cases *Mercurius*, *Staphysagria*, *Arsenicum*, may be given. Other medicines, such as *Viola tricolor*, *Aconitum*, *Chamomilla*, *Dulcamara*, *etc.*, scarcely ever do any good, unless they are indicated very particularly by the symptoms. *Cicuta*, *Baryta*, *Lycopodium*, *Graphites*, *Sarsaparilla*, are likewise rarely indicated. If the cervical glands are swollen and the crusts itch a good deal, *Ammonium carbonicum*, will be found very useful.

Section 159.

Chronic derangements of little children.—Little children are subject to various chronic derangements, which sometimes affect them immediately after birth. The principal are: *large head*, *retarded closing of the fontanelles*, *deviations of the spinal column*, *muscular weakness*, which prevents children from learning to walk, *large abdomen*, *spontaneous limping*, *stammering and wetting the bed.*

A large head often arises from an excessive development of the brain. This may facilitate in one respect the growth of the mind, but, on the other hand, predisposes children to acute hydrocephalent. Hence it is of importance that this excessive development of the brain should be arrested as soon as possible. We accomplish this result by means of *Sulphur*, *Calcarea*, *Silicea*, *Mercurius*, of which three pellets may be taken dry on the tongue, allowing each dose of the selected remedy to act three or more weeks, as long as the good effect continues.

Retarded closing of the fontanelles, arises from the fact that the process of ossification from the centre to the circumference of the skull-bones takes place too slowly. This same defect affects also other bones of the body, so that children in whom the fontanelles remain open, often labor under deviations of the spinal column, curvatures, etc., arising to excessive softness of the osseous substance. The best remedies for this difficulty are: *Sulphur*, *Calcarea*, *Silicea*, *Mercurius*, to be administered as before, under *large heads*.

DEVIATIONS OF THE SPINE arises, as was stated above, from deficient ossification, owing to which the bones do not offer sufficient resistance to the muscle, and hence, deviate from their true direction. These deviations of the bones are likewise successfully treated by the same remedies which we have proposed for retarted closing of the fontanelles, namely: *Sulphur*, *Calcarea*, *Pulsatilla*, *Silicea*. And sometimes we may use with success: *Mercurius*, *Lycopodium*, *Rhus*, *Staphysagria*, *Ammoniacum*, *Hepar*, *Phosphorus*, *Plumbum*.

MUSCULAR DEBILITY which incapacitates children from learning to walk, generally depends upon the presence of some scrofulous taint which likewises causes the slow development of the osseous system. Hence *Sulphur*, *Calcarea*, *Silicea*, are likewise eminently serviceable in the difficulty. Sometimes *Belladonna*, *Causticum* or *Pinus silvestris* may be given with advantage.

ABDOMINAL ENLARGEMENT is likewise a sign of scrofulous diathesis. It is a tuberculous affection of the mercuteric ganglia, with swelling and hardness of the abdomen, emaciation and general derangement of the functions of nutrition, with or without diarrhœa. This serious malady often yields to a dose of *Sulphur*, 18th attenuation, three pellets dry on the tongue, to be permitted to act three, four or more weeks, and to be followed by a similar dose of *Calcarea*, if Sulphur should be insufficient. If there should be diarrhœa and debility, *Arsenicum*, 30th attenuation may be given, six pellets in half a tumblerful of water, a dessertspoonful of this solution, morning and evening for a week. After *Arsenicum* we give *Nux vomica*, 30th attenuation, three pellets dry on the tongue, and in about a week after we give *Sulphur*, as above.

In SPONTANEOUS LUXATION of the femur, one limb is shorter than the other, and the children limp. This defect is likewise owing to a scrofulous taint which induces an inflammation and subsequent ulceration of the articular surfaces. This disease which, if it lasts any length of time, causes incurable disorganizations in the joints, is a most obstinate malady; sometimes however we succeed in arresting and removing the inflammation. The best remedies are *Sulphur* and *Calcarea*, to be administered as for abdominal enlargement. If the inflammatory symptoms are not yet fully developed, and the child simply limps without complaining of pains in the thigh, it is best to use *Mercurius* and *Belladonna* alternately, first three pellets of *Mercurius* dry on the tongue, and in two or three days a similar dose of *Belladonna*, continuing this alternate use for a fortnight, unless the improvement produced by one of these remedies, should indicate its exclusive use without the other. If these two remedies cease to do any good, *Rhus*, 18th attenuation, three pellets every four days, may be given, until an improvement is perceived, after which we may discontinue the use of medicine until the improvement ceases to progress, after which *Sulphur* may be given as above; this medicine should likewise be prescribed, if Rhus effects no improvement within a week.

STAMMERING should be attended to as soon as the first signs of it are perceived. Sometimes we cure it by making the child draw a long breath and hold it as long as possible; during the expiration they should be made to pronounce a few words. This exercise should be continued for several months with great patience and kindness. A dose of *Belladonna*, three pellets dry on the tongue, every few days, or a dose of *Mercurius* may be given from the commencement. *Platina*, *Sulphur*, *Euphrasia*, *Bovista*, are likewise useful.

WETTING THE BED, is a very troublesome and distressing weakness with which many children are afflicted. The best remedies for this weakness are: *Belladonna* or *Cina*, three pellets dry on the tongue every three or four days; first we give *Belladonna*, and if this remedy affects no improvement within a week, two doses of *Cina.* If this does not help, three pellets of *Sulphur* dry on the tongue: or *Sepia*, three globules every eight days, for four weeks, if *Sulphur* is insufficient. If none of these remedies help, we may resort to *Silice*a, 30th attenuation, three pellets dry on the tongue, every week, until the patient is better.

ALPHABETICAL INDEX

OF THE

SUBJECTS TREATED OF IN THIS VOLUME.

A.

B.

D.

E.

F.

G.

H.

I.

J.

L.

M.

N.

O.

P.

U.

V.

W.

www.ingramcontent.com/pod-product-compliance
Lightning Source LLC
LaVergne TN
LVHW021132110826
845150LV00005B/1002

* 9 7 8 1 4 2 5 5 5 0 1 5 8 *